Bayesian Brain

Computational Neuroscience

Terrence J. Sejnowski and Tomaso A. Poggio, editors

Bayesian Brain

Probabilistic Approaches to Neural Coding

Kenji Doya, Shin Ishii, Alexandre Pouget, and Rajesh P. N. Rao

The MIT Press
Cambridge, Massachusetts
London, England

First MIT Press paperback edition, 2011

MIT Press books may be purchased at special quantity discounts for business
or sales promotional use. For information, please email special_sales@mitpress.mit.edu
or write to Special Sales Department, The MIT Press, 55 Hayward Street, Cambridge, MA 02142.

This book was typeset by the authors using LaTeX 2_ε and *fbook* style file by Christo-
pher Manning. Printed and bound in the United States of America.

Library of Congress Cataloging-in-Publication Data
Bayesian brain : probabilistic approaches to neural coding / Kenji Doya ... [et
al.].
p. cm. — (Computational neuroscience)
Includes bibliographical references.
ISBN-13: 978-0-262-04238-3 (alk. paper) – 978-0-262-51601-3 (pb. : alk. paper)

1. Brain. 2. Neurons. 3. Bayesian statistical decision theory. I. Doya, Kenji.

QP376.B39 2007   612.8′2—dc22   2006049827

10 9 8 7 6 5 4

Contents

Series Foreword

Computational neuroscience is an approach to understanding the information content of neural signals by modeling the nervous system at many different structural scales, including the biophysical, the circuit, and the systems levels. Computer simulations of neurons and neural networks are complementary to traditional techniques in neuroscience. This book series welcomes contributions that link theoretical studies with experimental approaches to understanding information processing in the nervous system. Areas and topics of particular interest include biophysical mechanisms for computation in neurons, computer simulations of neural circuits, models of learning, representation of sensory information in neural networks, systems models of sensory-motor integration, and computational analysis of problems in biological sensing, motor control, and perception.

Terrence J. Sejnowski
Tomaso Poggio

Preface

When we perceive the physical world, make a decision, and take an action, a critical issue that our brains must deal with is uncertainty: there is uncertainty associated with the sensory system, the motor apparatus, one's own knowledge, and the world itself. The Bayesian framework of statistical estimation provides a coherent way of dealing with these uncertainties. Bayesian methods are becoming increasingly popular not only in building artificial systems that can handle uncertainty but also in efforts to develop a theory of how the brain works in the face of uncertainty.

At the core of the Bayesian way of thinking is the Bayes theorem, which maintains, in its simplest interpretation, that one's belief about the world should be updated according to the product of what one believed in before and what evidence has come to light since. The strength of the Bayesian approach comes from the fact that it offers a mathematically rigorous computational mechanism for combining prior knowledge with incoming evidence.

A classical example of Bayesian inference is the Kalman filter, which has been extensively used in engineering, communication, and control over the past few decades. The Kalman filter utilizes knowledge about the noise in sensory observations and the dynamics of the observed system to keep track of the best estimate of the system's current state and its variance. Although Kalman filters assume linear dynamics and Gaussian noise, recent Bayesian filters such as particle filters have extended the basic idea to nonlinear, non-Gaussian systems. However, despite much progress in signal processing and pattern recognition, no artificial system can yet match the brain's capabilities in tasks such as speech and natural scene recognition. Understanding how the brain solves such tasks could offer considerable insights into engineering artificial systems for similar tasks.

A Bayesian approach can contribute to an understanding of the brain at multiple levels. First, it can make normative predictions about how an ideal perceptual system combines prior knowledge with sensory observations, enabling principled interpretations of data from behavioral and psychophysical experiments. Second, algorithms for Bayesian estimation can provide mechanistic interpretations of neural circuits in the brain. Third, Bayesian methods can be used to optimally decode neural data such as spike trains. Lastly, a better understanding the brain's computational mechanisms should have a synergistic impact on the development of new algorithms for Bayesian computation, leading to new applications and technologies.

About This Book

This book is based on lectures given at the First Okinawa Computational Neuroscience Course, held in November 2004 at Bankoku Shinryokan, Okinawa, Japan. The intention of the course was to bring together both experimental and theoretical neuroscientists employing the principles of Bayesian estimation to understand the brain mechanisms of perception, decision, and control.

The organization of the book is as follows. In the Introduction, Doya and Ishii give the mathematical preliminaries, including the Bayes theorem, that are essential for understanding the remaining chapters of the book. The second part of the book, Reading Neural Codes, introduces readers to Bayesian concepts that can be used for interpretation of neurobiological data. The chapters by Fairhall, Pillow, and Richmond and Wiener explore methods for characterizing what a neuron encodes based on its spike trains. The chapter by Penny and Friston describes how Bayesian theory can be used for processing and modeling functional brain imaging data. The third part, entitled Making Sense of the World, assembles chapters on models of sensory processing. Pouget and Zemel review ideas about how information about the external world can be coded within populations of neurons. Latham and Pouget explore the use of such codes for neural computation. Lee and Yuille consider how top-down and bottom-up information can be combined in visual processing, while Knill uses Bayesian models to investigate optimal integration of multiple sensory cues. The final part, Making Decisions and Movements, explores models of the dynamic processes governing actions and behaviors. The chapter by Shadlen, Hanks, Churchland, Kiani, and Yang focuses on neurons in higher visual cortex that accumulate evidence for perceptual decisions over time. Rao discusses a model of how cortical circuits can implement "belief propagation," a general method for Bayesian estimation. Todorov reviews optimal control theory from the viewpoint of Bayesian estimation. Finally, Körding and Wolpert utilize Bayesian decision theory to understand how humans make decisions about movements.

It is our hope that this book will stimulate further research into Bayesian models of brain function, leading to a deeper, mathematically rigorous understanding of the neural processes underlying perception, decision, and action.

Acknowledgments

We wish to thank The Cabinet Office, Japanese Neural Network Society, Tamagawa University, and Kyushu Institute of Technology for sponsoring Okinawa Computational Neuroscience Course 2004, and Sydney Brenner, President of Okinawa Institute of Science and Technology, for advocating the course.

The course and the subsequent book publication would have been impossible without all the secretarial work by Izumi Nagano. Emiko Asato and Yasuhiro Inamine also helped us in manuscript preparation. Our thanks go to MIT Press editors Barbara Murphy and Kate Blakinger and to Terry Sejnowski for supporting our book proposal.

AP would like to thank the National Science Foundation (NSF) for their support. RPNR would like to acknowledge the support of the National Science Foundation (NSF), the ONR Adaptive Neural Systems program, the Sloan Foundation, and the Packard Foundation.

PART I

Introduction

1 A Probability Primer

Kenji Doya and Shin Ishii

1.1 What Is Probability?

The subtitle of this book is "Probabilistic Approaches to Neural Coding," so, to start with, we have to be clear about what is probability [1].

A classical notion of probability is the so-called frequentist view. If you toss a coin or roll a die infinitely many times, the ratio of having a particular outcome among all possible outcomes would converge to a certain number between zero and one, and that is the probability. An alternative idea of probability is the "Bayesian" view [2], which regards probability as a measure of belief about the predicted outcome of an event.

There has been a long debate between the two camps; the frequentists refuse to include a subjective notion like "belief" into mathematical theory. Bayesians say it is OK, as long as the way a belief should be updated is given objectively [3]. The Bayesian notion of probability fits well with applied scientists' and engineers' needs of mathematical underpinnings for measurements and decisions. As we will see in this book, the Bayesian notion turns out to be quite useful also in understanding how the brain processes sensory inputs and takes actions.

Despite the differences in the interpretation of probability, most of the mathematical derivation goes without any disputes. For example, the Bayes theorem, at the core of the Bayesian theory of inference, is just a straightforward fact derived from the relationship between joint probability and conditional probability, as you will see below.

1.1.1 Probability Distribution and Density

We consider a random variable X, which can take either one of discrete values $x_1, ..., x_N$ or continuous values, for example, $x \in R^n$. We denote by $P(X = x)$, or just $P(x)$ for short, the probability of the random variable X taking a particular value x.

For discrete random variables, $P(X)$ is called *the probability distribution* function. The basic constraint for probability distribution function is non-negativity and unity, i.e.,

$$P(x_i) \geq 0, \qquad \sum_{i=1}^{N} P(x_i) = 1. \tag{1.1}$$

If X takes a continuous value, its probability of taking a particular value is usually zero, so we should consider a probability of X falling in a finite interval $P(X \in [x1, x2])$. Here $P(X)$ gives a *probability density* function, whose constraint is given by

$$P(x) \geq 0, \qquad \int_X P(x)dx = 1. \tag{1.2}$$

Here the integral is taken over the whole range of the random variable X.

Despite these differences, we often use the same notation $P(X)$ for both probability distribution and density functions, and call them just *probability* for convenience. This is because many of the mathematical formulas and derivations are valid for both discrete and continuous cases.

1.1.2   Expectation and Statistics

There are a number of useful quantities, called *statistics*, that characterize a random variable. The most basic operation is to take an *expectation* of a function $f(X)$ of a random variable X following a distribution $P(X)$

$$E_{P(X)}[f(X)] = \sum_{i=1}^{N} P(x_i)f(x_i), \tag{1.3}$$

or a density $P(X)$ as

$$E_{P(X)}[f(X)] = \int_X P(x)f(x)dx. \tag{1.4}$$

We often use shorthand notations $E_X[\ ]$ or even $E[\ ]$ when the distribution or density that we are considering is apparent. Table 1.1 is a list of the most popular statistics.

1.1.3   Joint and Conditional Probability

If there are two or more random variables, say X and Y, we can consider their *joint probability* of taking a particular pair of values, $P(X = x, Y = y)$. We can also consider a *conditional probability* of X under the condition that Y takes a particular value y, $P(X = x|Y = y)$.

Table 1.1 Most popular statistics

name	notation	definition
mean	$<X>, \mu_X$	$E[X]$
variance	$Var[X], \sigma_X^2$	$E[(X - E[X])^2] = E[X^2] - E[X]^2$
covariance	$Cov[X,Y]$	$E[(X - E[X])(Y - E[Y])] = E[XY] - E[X]E[Y]$
correlation	$Cor[X,Y]$	$\frac{Cov[X,Y]}{E[X]E[Y]}$

The joint and conditional probabilities have a natural relationship

$$P(X,Y) = P(X|Y)P(Y) = P(Y|X)P(X). \tag{1.5}$$

When we start from the joint probability $P(X,Y)$, $P(X)$ and $P(Y)$ are derived by summing or integrating the two-dimensional function toward the margin of the X or Y axis, i.e.

$$P(X) = \sum_{i=1}^{N} P(X, Y = y_i), \tag{1.6}$$

or

$$P(X) = \int_Y P(X, Y = y)dy, \tag{1.7}$$

so they are often called *marginal probablity*.

1.1.4 Independence and Correlation

When the joint probability is just a product of two probabilities, i.e.,

$$P(X,Y) = P(X)P(Y), \tag{1.8}$$

the variables X and Y are said to be *independent*. In this case we have

$$P(X|Y) = P(X), \qquad P(Y|X) = P(Y).$$

Otherwise we say X and Y are dependent.

A related but different concept is *correlation*. We say two variables are uncorrelated if

$$E[XY] = E[X]E[Y]. \tag{1.9}$$

In this case the covariance and correlation are zero.

If two variables are independent, they are uncorrelated, but the reverse is not true. Why? Let's imagine a uniform probability $P(X,Y)$ over a rhombus around the origin of $X - Y$ space. From symmetry, X and Y are obviously uncorrelated, but the marginal probabilities $P(X)$ and $P(Y)$ are triangular, so their product will make a pyramid rather than a flat rhombus, so X and Y are dependent.

1.2   Bayes Theorem

From the two ways of representing the joint probability (1.5), we can relate the two conditional probabilities by the following equation:

$$P(X|Y) = \frac{P(Y|X)P(X)}{P(Y)},$$ (1.10)

as long as $P(Y)$ never becomes exactly zero. This simple formula is famous as *the Bayes theorem* [2]. The Bayes theorem is just a way of converting one conditional probability to the other, by reweighting it with the relative probability of the two variables. How can we be so excited about this?

This is quite insightful when we use this theorem for interpretation of sensory data, for example,

$$P(hypothesis|data) = \frac{P(data|hypothesis)P(hypothesis)}{P(data)}.$$

Here, the Bayes theorem dictates how we should update our belief of a certain hypothesis, $P(hypothesis)$ based on how well the acquired data were predicted from the hypothesis, $P(data|hypothesis)$. In this context, the terms in the Bayes theorem (1.10) have conventional names: $P(X)$ is called the *prior probability* and $P(X|Y)$ is called the *posterior probability* of X given Y. $P(Y|X)$ is a *generative model* of observing Y under hypothesis X, but after a particular observation is made it is called the *likelihood* of hypothesis X given data y.

The marginal probability $P(Y)$ serves as a normalizing denominator so that the sum of $P(X|Y)$ for all possible hypotheses becomes unity. It appears as if the marginal distribution is there just for the sake of bookkeeping, but as we will see later, it sometimes give us insightful information about the quality of our inference.

1.3   Measuring Information

Neuroscience is about how the brain processes information. But how can we define "information" in a quantitative manner [4]? Let us consider how informative is an observation of a particular value x for a random variable X with probability $P(X)$. If $P(X = x)$ is high, it is not so surprising, but if $P(X = x)$ is close to zero, it is quite informative. The best way to quantify the *information* or "surprise" of an event $X = x$ is to take the logarithm of the inverse of the probability

$$\log \frac{1}{P(X = x)} = -\log P(X = x).$$ (1.11)

Information is zero for a fully predicted outcome x with $P(X = x) = 1$, and increases as $P(X = x)$ becomes smaller. The reason we take the logarithm is that we can measure the information of two independent events x and y, with joint probability $P(x, y) = P(y)P(y)$, by the sum of each event, i.e.

$$\log \frac{1}{P(x,y)} = \log \frac{1}{P(x)P(y)} = \log \frac{1}{P(x)} + \log \frac{1}{P(y)}.$$

It is often convenient to use a binary logarithm, and in this case the unit of information is called a *bit*.

1.3.1 Entropy

By observing repeatedly, x should follow $P(X)$, so the average information we have from observing this variable is

$$H(X) = E[-\log P(X)] = \sum_X -P(X) \log P(X), \tag{1.12}$$

which is called *the entropy* of X. Entropy is a measure of randomness or uncertainty of the distribution $P(X)$, since the more random the distribution, the more information we gather by observing its value. For instance, entropy takes zero for a deterministic variable (as $H(X) = 0$ for $P(X = x) = 1$ and $P(X \neq x) = 0$), and takes the largest positive value $\log N$ for a uniform distribution over N values.

1.3.2 Mutual Information

In sensory processing, it is important to quantify how much information the sensory input Y has about the world state X. A reasonable way is to ask how much uncertainty about the world X decreases by observing Y, so we take the difference in the entropy of $P(X)$ and $P(X|Y)$,

$$I(X;Y) = H(X) - H(X|Y), \tag{1.13}$$

where $H(X|Y)$ is the *conditional entropy*, given by the entropy of conditional distribution $P(X|Y = y)$ averaged over the probability of observation $P(Y = y)$,

$$H(X|Y) = E_{P(Y)}[E_{P(X|Y)}[-\log P(X|Y)]] = \sum_Y P(Y) \sum_X -P(X|Y) \log P(X|Y).$$
$$\tag{1.14}$$

$I(X;Y)$ is called the *mutual information* of X and Y. It is symmetric with respect to X and Y. This can be confirmed by checking that the entropy of the joint probability $P(X, Y) = P(Y|X)P(X) = P(X|Y)P(Y)$ is given by

$$H(X, Y) = H(X) + H(Y|X) = H(Y) + H(X|Y), \tag{1.15}$$

and hence the mutual information can be presented in three ways:

$$I(X;Y) = H(X) - H(X|Y) = H(Y) - H(Y|X) = H(X) + H(Y) - H(X,Y).$$
$$\tag{1.16}$$

1.3.3   Kullback-Leibler Divergence

We often would like to measure the difference in two probability distributions, and the right way to do it is by information. When we observe an event x, its information depends on what probability distribution we assume for the variable. The difference in information with distributions $P(X)$ and $Q(X)$ is

$$\log \frac{1}{Q(x)} - \log \frac{1}{P(x)} = \log \frac{P(x)}{Q(x)}.$$

If x turns out to follow distribution $P(X)$, then the average difference is

$$D(P;Q) = E_{P(X)} \left[\log \frac{P(x)}{Q(x)} \right] = \sum_X P(x) \log \frac{P(x)}{Q(x)}, \tag{1.17}$$

which is called *the Kullback-Leibler (KL) divergence*. This is a good measure of the difference of two distributions, but we cannot call it "distance" because it does not usually satisfy the symmetry condition, i.e., $D(P,Q) \neq D(Q,P)$.

1.4   Making an Inference

Let us now consider the process of perception in a Bayesian way. The brain observes sensory input Y and makes an estimate of the state of the world X.

1.4.1   Maximum Likelihood Estimate

The mechanics of the sensory apparatus determines the conditional probability $P(Y|X)$. One way of making an inference about the world is to find the state X that maximizes the likelihood $P(Y = y|X)$ of the sensory input y. This is called the *maximum likelihood (ML)* estimate. Although the ML estimate is quite reasonable and convenient, there are two possible drawbacks. First, in the world, there are more probable and less probable states, so inference just by the present sensory input may not be the best thing we can do. Second, using just a single point estimate of X can be dangerous because it neglects many other states that are nearly likely.

1.4.2   Maximum a Posteriori Estimate

This is why the Bayes theorem can be useful in perceptual inference. If we express the probability of different world states as a prior probability $P(X)$, we can combine the sensory information and this prior information according to the Bayes therorem:

$$P(X|Y) = \frac{P(Y|X)P(X)}{P(Y)}. \tag{1.18}$$

If we put aside the normalizing denominator $P(Y)$, the posterior probability $P(X|Y)$ of the world state X given sensory input Y is proportional to the product of the likelihood $P(Y|X)$ and the prior probability $P(X)$. The state X that maximizes the posterior probability is called *the maximum a posterioir (MAP) estimate*.

1.4.3   Bayesian Estimate

The MAP estimate can incorporate our prior knowledge about the world, but it still is a point estimate. We can instead use the full probability distribution or density of the posterior $P(X|Y)$ as our estimate. For example, if we make a decision or motor action based on the estimated world state X, how sharp or flat is the posterior distribution gives us the confidence of our estimate. When the distribution is wide or even has multiple peaks, we can average the corresponding outputs to make a more conservative decision rather than just using a single point estimate.

1.4.4   Bayes Filtering

A practically important way of using the posterior probability is to use it as the prior probability in the next step. For example, if we make multiple independent sensory observations

$$y = (y_1, y_2, ..., y_t),$$

the likelihood of a state given the sequence of observations is the product

$$P(y|X) = P(y_1|X)P(y_2|X)...P(y_t|X).$$

The posterior is given by

$$P(X|y) = \frac{P(y_1|X)P(y_2|X)...P(y_t|X)P(X)}{P(y)}, \tag{1.19}$$

but this can be recursively computed by

$$P(X|y_1, ..., y_t) \propto P(y_t|X)P(X|y_1, ..., y_{t-1}). \tag{1.20}$$

Here, $P(X|y_1, ..., y_{t-1})$ is the posterior of X given the sensory inputs till time $t - 1$ and serves as the prior for further estimation at time t.

So far we assumed that the world state X stays the same, but what occurs if the state changes while we make sequential observations? If we have the knowledge about how the world state would change, for example, by a state transition probability $P(X_t|X_{t-1})$, then we can use the posterior at time $t - 1$ multiplied by this transition probability as the new prior at t:

$$P(X_t|y_1, ..., y_{t-1}) \propto P(X_t|X_{t-1})P(X_{t-1}|y_1, ..., y_{t-1}). \tag{1.21}$$

Table 1.2 Popular probability distribution and density functions

name	definition	range	mean	variance
Binomial	$\binom{N}{x}\alpha^x(1-\alpha)^{N-x}$ $\binom{N}{x}=\frac{N!}{(N-x)!x!}$	$x=0,1,...,N$	$N\alpha$	$N\alpha(1-\alpha)$
Poisson	$\frac{1}{x!}\alpha^x e^{-\alpha}$	$x=0,1,2,...$	α	α
Gaussian or normal	$\frac{1}{\sqrt{2\pi}\sigma}e^{-\frac{(x-\mu)^2}{2\sigma^2}}$	$x\in R$	μ	σ^2
Gamma	$\frac{1}{\Gamma(a)}b^a x^{a-1}e^{-bx}$ $\Gamma(a)=\int_0^\infty x^{a-1}e^{-x}dx$ ($\Gamma(a)=a!$ if a is an integer)	$x\geq 0$	$\frac{a}{b}$	$\frac{a}{b^2}$

Thus the sequence of the Bayesian estimation of the state is given by the following iteration:

$$P(X_t|y_1,...,y_t) \propto P(y_t|X_t)P(X_t|X_{t-1})P(X_{t-1}|y_1,...,y_{t-1}). \qquad (1.22)$$

This iterative estimation is practically very useful and is in general called *the Bayes filter*. The best known classical example of the Bayes filter is the *Kalman filter*, which assumes linear dynamics and Gaussian noise. More recently, a method called *particle filter* has been commonly used for tasks like visual tracking and mobile robot localization [5].

1.5   Learning from Data

So far we talked about how to use our knowledge about the sensory transformation $P(Y|X)$ or state transition $P(X_t|X_{t-1})$ for estimation of the state from observation. But how can we know these transformation and transition probabilities? The brain should *learn* these probabilistic models from experience.

In estimating a probablistic model, it is convenient to use a *parameterized family* of distributions or densities. In this case, the process of learning, or system identification, is regarded as the process of *parameter estimation*. Table 1.2 is a list of popular parameterized distribution and density functions.

When we make an estimate of the parameter, we can use the same principle as we did in the world state estimation above. For example, when the observation Y is a linear function of the state X with Gaussian noise, we have a parameterized model

$$P(y|x,w,\sigma) = \frac{1}{\sqrt{2\pi}\sigma}e^{-\frac{(y-wx)^2}{2\sigma^2}},$$

where $\theta=(w,\sigma)$ is a parameter vector. From the set of input-output observations $\{(x_1,y_1),...,(x_T,y_T)\}$, we can derive a maximum likelihood estimation by searching for the parameter that maximizes

$$P(y_1, ..., y_T | x_1, ..., x_T, \theta) = \prod_{t=1}^{T} P(y_t | x_t, \theta).$$

A convenient way of doing ML estimation is to maximize the log-likelihood:

$$\log P(y_1, ..., y_T | x_1, ..., x_T, \theta) = \sum_{t=1}^{T} \log P(y_t | x_t, \theta) = \sum_{t=1}^{T} -\frac{(y_t - wx_t)^2}{2\sigma^2} - T \log \sqrt{2\pi}\sigma.$$

From this, we can see that finding the ML estimate of the linear weight w is the same as finding the *least mean-squared error (LMSE)* estimate that minimizes the mean-squared error

$$E = \frac{1}{T} \sum_{t=1}^{T} (y_t - wx_t)^2.$$

1.5.1   Fisher Information

After doing estimation, how can we be certain about an estimated parameter $\hat{\theta}$? If the likelihood $P(Y|\theta)$ is flat with respect to the parameter θ, it would be difficult to make a precise estimate. The *Fisher information* is a measure of the steepness or curvature of the likelihood:

$$I_F(\theta) = E_Y \left[\left(\frac{\partial \log P(Y|\theta)}{\partial \theta} \right)^2 \right] = E_Y \left[-\frac{\partial^2 \log P(Y|\theta)}{\partial \theta^2} \right]. \qquad (1.23)$$

A theorem called *Cramér-Rao inequality* gives a limit of how small the variance of an *unbiased* estimate $\hat{\theta}$ can be, namely,

$$Var(\hat{\theta}) \geq I_F(\hat{\theta})^{-1}. \qquad (1.24)$$

For example, after some calculation we can see that the Fisher information matrix for a Gaussian distribution with parameters $\theta = (\mu, \sigma^2)$ is

$$I_F(\theta) = \begin{pmatrix} \frac{1}{\sigma^2} & 0 \\ 0 & \frac{1}{2\sigma^4} \end{pmatrix}.$$

If data $Y = (y_1, ..., y_T)$ are given by repeated measures of the same distribution, from $\log P(Y|\theta) = \sum_{t=1}^{T} \log P(y_t|\theta)$, the Fisher information is T times that of a single observation. Thus Cramér-Rao inequality tells us how good estimate of the mean μ we can get from the observed data Y depends on the variance and number of observations, $\frac{\sigma^2}{T}$.

1.5.2 Bayesian Learning

We can of course use not only ML, but MAP or Bayesian estimation for learning parameter θ, for example, for the sensory mapping model $P(Y|X, \theta)$ by

$$P(\theta|X, Y) = \frac{P(Y|X, \theta)P(\theta)}{P(Y|X)}. \tag{1.25}$$

In the above linear example, if we have a prior knowledge that the slope is not so steep, we can assume a Gaussian prior of w,

$$P(w) = \frac{1}{\sqrt{2\pi}\sigma_w} e^{-\frac{||w||^2}{2\sigma_w^2}}.$$

Then the log posterior probability is

$$\log P(w|Y, X) = \sum_{t=1}^{T} -\frac{(y_t - wx_t)^2}{2\sigma^2} - \frac{||w||^2}{2\sigma_w^2} - T\log\sqrt{2\pi}\sigma - \log\sqrt{2\pi}\sigma_w - \log P(Y|X),$$

so maximizing it with respect to w is the same as minimizing the least mean-squared error with a penalty term

$$E = \frac{1}{T}\sum_{t=1}^{T}\frac{(y_t - wx_t)^2}{2\sigma^2} + \frac{||w||^2}{2T\sigma_w^2}.$$

Such estimation with additional regularization terms is used to avoid extreme solutions, often in an adhoc manner, but the Bayesian framework provides a principled way of how to design them [6].

1.5.3 Marginal Likelihood

The normalizing denominator $P(Y|X)$ of the posterior distribution (1.25) is given by integrating the numerator over the entire range of the paremeter

$$P(Y|X) = \int P(Y|X, \theta)P(\theta)d\theta, \tag{1.26}$$

which is often called *marginalization*. This is a hard job in a high-dimensional parameter space, so if we are just interested in finding a MAP estimate, it is neglected.

However, this marginal probability of observation Y given X, or *marginal likelihood*, conveys an important message about the choice of our prior $P(\theta)$. If the prior distribution is narrowly peaked, it would have little overlap with the likelihood $P(Y|X, \theta)$, so the expectation of the product will be small. On the other hand, if the prior distribution is very flat and wide, its value is inversely proportional to the width, so the marginal will again be small. Thus the marginal probability $P(Y|X)$ is a good criterion to see whether the prior is consistent with the observed data, so it is also called *evidence*. A parameter like σ_w of the prior probability for a parameter w is called a *hyperparameter*, and the evidence is used for selection of prior probability, or hyperparameter tuning.

The same mechanism can also be used for selecting one of discrete candidates of probabilistic models $M_1, M_2, \dots$. In this case the marginal probability for a model $P(M_i)$ can be used for *model selection*, then called *Bayesian criterion* for model selection.

1.6 Graphical Models and Other Bayesian Algorithms

So far we dealt with just two or three random variables, but in real life there are many states, observations, and parameters, some of which are directly or indirectly related. To make such dependency clear, graphical representations of random variables are useful. They are called *graphical models*, and the Bayes rule is used for estimation of the latent variables and parameters. Especially when a graphical model is represented by a *directed acyclic graph* (DAG), or equivalently, for an n-dim. variable vector X,

$$P(X) = \prod_{i=1}^{n} P(X_i | Pa_i), \tag{1.27}$$

where Pa_i denotes the parent variables of the variable X_i in the DAG, such a model is called a *Bayesian network*. For estimation of any missing variable in a Bayesian network, various *belief propagation* algorithms, the most famous one being the *message passing algorithm*, have been devised in recent years, and there are excellent textbooks to refer to when it becomes necessary for us to use one.

References

[1] Papoulis A (1991) *Random Variables, and Stochastic Process*. New York: McGraw-Hill.

[2] Bayes T (1763) An essay towards solving a problem in the doctrine of chances. *Philosophical Transactions of Royal Society*, **53**, 370-418.

[3] Cox RT (1946) Probability, frequency and reasonable expectation. *American Journal of Physics*, **14**, 1-13.

[4] Shanon CE (1948) A mathematical theory of communication. *Bell System Technical Journal*, **27**, 379-423, 623-656.

[5] Doucet A, de Freitas ND, Gordon N, eds. (2001) *Sequential Monte Carlo Methods in Practice*. New York: Springer-Verlag.

[6] MacKay DJC (2003) *Information Theory, Inference, and Learning Algorithms*. Cambridge, UK: Cambridge University Press.

PART II

Reading Neural Codes

2 *Spike Coding*

Adrienne Fairhall

2.1 Spikes: What Kind of Code?

Most neurons in the brain convey information using action potentials, or spikes. This chapter will examine the coding properties of the spike train outputs recorded from individual neurons. What kind of code do these spike trains represent? How do spikes encode complex inputs; how can they be decoded?

Spike trains are the primary means of communication in the nervous system. All current approaches to neural coding assume that the arrival times of spikes comprise all that needs to be known about them. While variations in spike height and width occur as a result of stimulus and prior spiking history [19], it is generally assumed that these variations disappear in transmission through the axon and downstream synapses and thus are incapable of conveying differentiated information about the stimulus. This picture is a great simplification, allowing us to think about the spike code in terms of a time series of all-or-none events. However, there are still many possible ways in which these events might communicate information through the nervous system. Does the exact timing of spikes matter, and if so, at what accuracy? Perhaps precise timing is irrelevant, and all that matters is the total number of spikes produced over some time window, or in aggregate by a population of neurons. If spike timing is important, what are the elementary symbols of the code: single spikes or patterns of spikes such as bursts? What do these symbols represent in the stimulus? How do groups of neurons work together to transmit information: independently or through intricate correlations capable of representing complex stimulus patterns?

In figure 2.1, we show rasters of spike trains recorded from retinal ganglion cells during the repeated viewing of a natural movie. Responses occur reliably at fixed times, with a precision on the order of one to several milliseconds. Different neurons in the ganglion cell array respond at different times during the stimulus presentation, signaling distinct features of the visual input. This is the form in which visual information is transmitted from our eye to the rest of the brain. In this chapter, we will concentrate on spike trains from single neu-

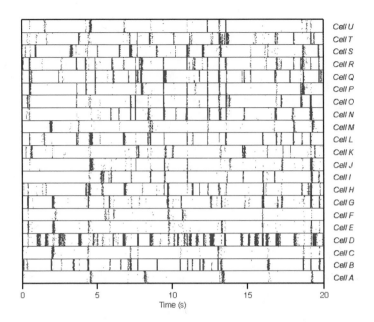

Figure 2.1 Simultaneously recorded spike trains from twenty retinal ganglion cells firing in response to a repeated natural movie. Figure courtesy of J. Puchalla and M. Berry.

rons to show how stimuli are encoded in the arrival times of single spikes, and conversely, how one may go about decoding the meaning of single spikes as a representation of stimulus features. We will show how information theory has been applied to address questions of precision and reliability in spike trains, and to evaluate the role of multiple-spike symbols.

2.1.1   From Rate to Spikes

The measurement of a *tuning curve* is a classic method for establishing and quantifying the correlation of neural activity with an external signal or a behavior generated by the animal. As an external parameter varies systematically, the response of the neuron is measured in terms of the mean number of spikes per second, counted in a time bin often of hundreds of milliseconds in length. Stimuli are typically well separated in time so that responses unambiguously belong to a single stimulus category. While such characterizations are valuable, information relevant for behavior must often be conveyed over shorter time scales [58], bringing into question whether the integration of spike count over long time scales is an appropriate representation. Researchers have therefore been motivated to study responses to dynamically varying stimuli [14, 40, 18, 20], both in order to take contextual effects into account and to characterize coding under more naturalistic conditions.

Despite internal noise sources, many neuron types are capable of firing in response to a repeated direct current input with reproducible responses of high temporal precision [38]. Even when stimuli are transmitted through a neural circuit, the firing of single neurons can still be remarkably precise. While temporal precision has been documented most extensively in invertebrate identified neurons [21] and in the sensory periphery [43, 10], time-locked spiking to dynamic stimuli has been observed under anesthesia in the lateral geniculate nucleus (LGN) [16, 57, 76], and in somatosensory [50], auditory [24, 23] and visual cortex [81, 60]. Recent evidence suggests that temporal locking is also observed in cortex in awake, behaving animals [29].

2.1.2 Timing and Information

The ability of a code to transmit information is limited by the fidelity with which a given symbol of the code represents a given input. The quality of a code can be quantified using information theory [66, 67, 15]. When considering neural firing as a code, information theory allows us to evaluate the power of different representations for encoding a stimulus. For example, imagine that one is given a series of spikes recorded in response to a variety of stimuli. What is the appropriate time bin at which to measure the response? We can answer this question by computing how much information the response contains about the stimulus when represented using different time bins. Very coarse time bins may lose information by averaging away temporal structure in the spike train; yet using overly fine time bins will simply proliferate the number of interchangeable output symbols corresponding to a given input, due to spike timing jitter. Computing information can reveal the appropriate time bin for representing the response. Later we will show an example of the application of this procedure to neural responses in the LGN.

The Shannon information [66, 67] of a random variable X, distributed according to $P(X)$, is defined as $-\log_2 P(X)$. This quantity is the number of bits, or the number of yes/no questions, required to establish the value of the random variable: for example, if something is located somewhere in a 4 x 4 grid with equal probability $P(X) = 1/16$, it would take $-\log_2(1/16) = 4$ yes/no questions to locate it (think of performing a binary search!). This definition is clear for a discrete variable. For a continuous variable, characterized by a probability density function $p(X)$, the probability of any particular value $X = x$ is zero, hence the information is infinite: no number of yes/no questions will establish the value to infinite precision. A sensible answer is obtained only by integrating the probability density over an interval of x. In real systems, the presence of noise imposes a precision limit, or an effective natural discretization scale.

The overall variability or uncertainty of X is measured by its *entropy*,

$$H[P(X)] = - \sum_{x \in X} P(x) \log_2 P(x). \tag{2.1}$$

This is simply an average over the Shannon information, or the average number of bits required to specify the variable. Here we will mostly be concerned with the *mutual information*, the amount by which knowing about one random variable reduces uncertainty about another. For our purposes, one of these variables will be the stimulus, S, and the other, the response, R. The response R must clearly be variable (that is, have nonzero entropy) in order to encode a variable stimulus. However, the variability observed in the response might reflect variability in the input, or it might be due to noise. Mutual information quantifies the amount of *useful* variability, the amount of entropy that is associated with changes in the stimulus rather than changes that are not correlated with the stimulus— i.e. noise.

The mutual information is defined as

$$I(S; R) = \sum_{s \in S, r \in R} P(s, r) \log_2 \frac{P(s, r)}{P(s)P(r)}. \tag{2.2}$$

This representation shows that the mutual information is simply the Kullback-Leibler divergence between the joint distribution of S and R and their marginal distributions, and therefore measures how far S and R are from independence. Another way to write the mutual information is

$$I(S; R) = H[P(R)] - \sum_{s \in S} P(s)H[P(R|s)] = H[P(S)] - \sum_{r \in R} P(r)H[P(S|r)]. \tag{2.3}$$

In this form, it is clear that the mutual information is the difference between the **total entropy** of the response and the entropy of the response *to a fixed input*, averaged over all inputs. This averaged entropy is called the **noise entropy**, and quantifies the "blurring" of the responses due to noise. We emphasize that "noise" here is not necessarily noise in the physical sense; it is simply any nonreproducibility in the mapping from S to R. This "noise" may in fact be informative about some other variable not included in our definition of S or R. Mutual information is symmetric with respect to S and R. It represents the amount of information about S encoded in R, or equivalently, the amount of information about R that can be predicted from a known S.

2.1.3   Information in Single Spikes

To compute the information in a spike train, we will first discuss a method [13] to compute the information conveyed about the stimulus by the arrival of a single spike. This method has the advantage that it makes no assumptions about the nature of the encoding or decoding process. By symmetry, the information gained about the stimulus given that one observes a single spike is the same as the information gained about the arrival time of a spike, given that one knows the stimulus. The key idea is that this mutual information is the reduction in entropy between the prior distribution, the spike time distribution when the stimulus is unknown, and the spike time distribution when the stimulus is known. Let us consider a single time bin of size Δt, where Δt is small enough to contain a maximum of one spike only. Knowing nothing about the stimulus, the probability to observe either a spike, $r = 1$, or no spike, $r = 0$, in this time bin is

$$P(r = 1) \quad = \quad \bar{r}\Delta t, \tag{2.4}$$
$$P(r = 0) \quad = \quad 1 - \bar{r}\Delta t, \tag{2.5}$$

where $\bar{r}$ is the mean firing rate.

When the neuron is given a particular random, dynamic stimulus sequence, $s(t)$, the result is a particular pattern of output. Averaged across many repetitions, one obtains a temporally modulated firing pattern, $r(t)$, such as would be obtained by averaging the rasters in figure 2.1. Depending on the system, the modulations in $r(t)$ may be very sharp and well-isolated, as in figure 2.1, or there may be relatively small modulations around some mean firing rate. Intuitively, in the former case the stimulus and spikes are highly correlated; in the latter, less so. Now we can compute the noise entropy from the conditional distributions:

$$P(r = 1|s(t)) \quad = \quad r(t)\Delta t, \tag{2.6}$$
$$P(r = 0|s(t)) \quad = \quad 1 - r(t)\Delta t. \tag{2.7}$$

Denoting $p = \bar{r}\Delta t$ and $p(t) = r(t)\Delta t$, the information is given by

$$I(r;s) = [-p\log_2 p - (1-p)\log_2(1-p)] + \frac{1}{T}\int_0^T dt[p(t)\log_2 p(t) + (1-p(t))\log_2(1-p(t))]. \tag{2.8}$$

Here a time average, $\frac{1}{T}\int_0^T dt$, has been substituted for the average over the ensemble of stimuli, $\int ds P(s)$, or its discrete equivalent appearing in equation (2.3). This is valid if the random sequence $s(t)$ is sufficiently long. Assuming that $p \ll 1$, we may expand $\log(1 - p) \sim p$ and use $\frac{1}{T}\int_0^T dt\, p(t) \to p$ for $T \to \infty$ to obtain

$$I(r;s) = \frac{1}{T}\int_0^T dt\, r(t)\Delta t \log_2 \frac{r(t)}{\bar{r}} + \text{Var}(p(t))/2\log 2 + O(p^3). \tag{2.9}$$

To obtain information per spike rather than information per second, we divide by the mean number of spikes per second, $\bar{r}\Delta t$, and truncate to first order:

$$I(r;s) = \frac{1}{T}\int_0^T dt\, \frac{r(t)}{\bar{r}} \log_2 \frac{r(t)}{\bar{r}}. \tag{2.10}$$

While $p \ll 1$, $p(t)$ may be large, and one might worry that one is discarding an important component of the information, this truncation amounts to computing only information in spikes, and neglecting the information contributed by the lack of spikes, or silences. For salamander retinal ganglion cells, this contribution turns out to be very small: we found it to be less than 1% of the total information (A. L. Fairhall and M. J. Berry II, unpublished observations). This result may break down for neurons with higher firing rates.

2.1.4   Information in Spike Sequences

While this formulation is simple and elegant, it is limited to the computation
of information in single spikes. A more general method was introduced by
Strong et al. [75]. Here, the neural response is represented by discretizing the
spike train into bins of size Δt. For simplicity, let us again take Δt to be shorter
than the refractory period of the neuron, so that bins will contain either a single spike and be given the value 1, or no spikes, given the value 0. Sequences
of N bins are then N-letter binary words, w (figure 2.2). (One could of course
use larger bins and generalize to ternary or quaternary words, to dubious advantage.) We need now to compute the **total entropy** and the **noise entropy**.
The total entropy will be given by the entropy $H[P(w)]$ of all words observed
in response to a long random stimulus. The noise entropy can be found by
repeating a segment of a random stimulus sequence, $s(t)$, many times. In this
case, at every time t, the same stimulus was presented, and the word distribu-
tion at time t provides a conditional distribution $P(w|s(t))$. Taken from LGN
data, figure 2.3a shows an example of the full distribution $P(w)$ generated from
the long random stimulus. Figure 2.3b shows one of the conditional distribu-
tions $P(w|s(t))$ sampled at a particular time in the repeated sequence. We now
need, according to equation (2.3), to average the entropy of $P(w|s(t))$ over the
conditioning variable, the stimulus s. As above, if the repeated segment is
long enough, a time average samples the ensemble of s so is equivalent to an
average over $P(s)$.

There are two parameters in this choice of representation of the spike train:
the temporal precision, or the bin width Δt, and the total duration of the word,
$L = N\Delta t$. To ensure that all correlations in the spiking output have been taken
into account, one would like to examine the limit where $N \to \infty$. In practice
this is not possible as the number of possibilities for w increases as 2^N, so that
$P(w)$ and $P(w|s)$ rapidly become impossible to sample. In general, the issue
of finite sampling poses something of a problem for information-theoretic approaches and has accordingly been an active area of study. This topic deserves
a chapter on its own and so we will simply point the reader in the direction
of a few recent papers addressing finite size biases in information estimates,
with particular application to neuroscience [75, 49, 77, 45, 44, 34, 80]. Within
sampling limits, Reinagel and Reid [57] examined the information content of
spike words from responses of LGN neurons. Figure 2.4 shows the information rate (bits per second) about the stimulus conveyed by the spike train as
a function of the temporal precision of the spike binning Δt and the inverse
word duration $1/L$. For this neuron, the information rate is maximal at higher
precisions, up to around 1 ms, for all word lengths. The drop in information for
decreasing $1/L$ is a result of sampling. For a fixed Δt, the information varies
approximately linearly with $1/L$. The information value plotted in the narrow
bar $1/l \to 0$ is the value obtained by extrapolating the total and noise entropies
as a function of $1/L$ from their approximately linear regimes to the origin at
infinite word length [75].

Information has also used to assess the importance of particular complex

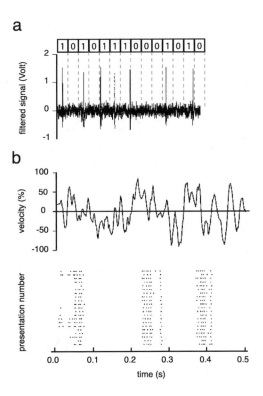

Figure 2.2   (a). A spike train and its representation in terms of binary "letters." A word consists of some number of sequential binary letters. (b). A randomly varying Gaussian stimulus (here, a velocity stimulus) and the spike-train responses from fly visual neuron H1 for many repetitions. Adapted from Strong et al.[73]

symbols. Let us consider the symbol defined by the joint occurrence of some pair of output events, E_1 and E_2. The *synergy* [13] is defined as the difference between the mutual information between output and stimulus obtained from the joint event compared with that obtained if the two events were observed independently,

$$Syn(E_1, E_2; s) = I(E_1, E_2; s) - [I(E_1; s) + I(E_2; s)] . \qquad (2.11)$$

A positive value for $Syn(E_1, E_2; s)$ indicates that E_1 and E_2 encode the stimulus synergistically; a negative value implies that the two events are redundant. This and related quantities [27, 48, 57] have been applied to multiple-spike outputs to assess the contribution to stimulus encoding of timing relationships among spikes in the fly visual neuron H1 [13] and the LGN [57]. Petersen et al. [47, 52] found that, for responses in rat barrel cortical neurons, the first spike of a burst conveyed most of the information about the stimulus.

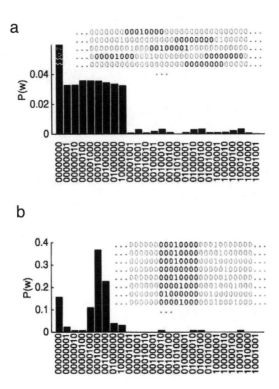

Figure 2.3 (a). The probability distribution $P(w)$ of all words w generated by a long random stimulus. (b). The word distribution $P(w|s(t))$ generated at a particular time t by a given repeated stimulus sequence $s(t)$.

Another type of complex symbol is that produced by simultaneous firing responses of multiple cells. The retina provides a perfect system for the study of population coding, since it is easy to stimulate with dynamical stimuli and its output, the planar layer of retinal ganglion cells, is accessible to multielectrode array recording (figure 2.1). These neurons form a mosaic with overlapping receptive fields [41, 55, 64]. It has been shown that pairs of neurons convey largely redundant information [55]. Recently, information-theoretic tools have been developed to assess the information gain resulting from simultaneous observation of groups of N neurons due to successive higher-order correlations [63]. Application of these tools to retinal ganglion cell recordings demonstrates that pairwise correlations dominate the additional information encoded in the population [62]. Similar questions have also been addressed in cortex, e.g. [42, 51].

The question "what kind of code?" has different answers in different sys-

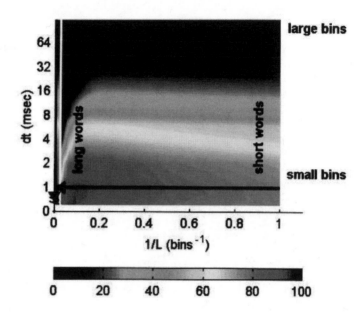

Figure 2.4 Information rate in spikes per second as a function of parameters of the spike-train representation, the bin width Δt, and the inverse total word length $1/L$. Reproduced with permission from Reinagel and Reid,[55] (see color insert).

tems, and for neural populations, we are only beginning to have the available experimental and theoretical methods to address it. Here we have seen that information-theoretic tools allow us to address the question in a quantitative way.

2.2   Encoding and Decoding

How is the stimulus encoded by the spike train? In other words, given the stimulus, can one predict the timing of a spike? For a single neuron, the conversion from current or conductance stimulus to spiking response is a function of the detailed biophysics of the neuron. For an external stimulus, the entire network between the environment and the recorded neuron contributes to the transformation. One might also "take the organism's point of view" [58], or the inference problem that downstream neurons are in some sense solving: what is the stimulus given observation of the spike train?

2.2.1 Linear Decoding

The first-pass approach to the decoding problem is to assume a linear relationship between input and output [17, 58]. Since the input is time-varying, we seek a linear relationship between the instantaneous firing rate, $r(t)$, and the recent stimulus history, i.e. a linear kernel $K(\tau)$. Given a rate response, $r(t)$, we therefore seek the optimal linear estimator $K(\tau)$ such that a linear estimate of the rate, $r_{\text{est}}(t)$, is as close as possible to $r(t)$:

$$r_{\text{est}}(t) = \bar{r} + \int d\tau\, s(t - \tau)K(\tau). \tag{2.12}$$

Setting $r_{\text{est}}(t) = r(t)$ gives us an equation for the unknown linear kernel $K(t)$. Let's multiply both sides with $s(t - \tau')$ and integrate over t:

$$\int dt\, s(t - \tau')r(t) = \int dt \int d\tau s(t - \tau')s(t - \tau)K(\tau). \tag{2.13}$$

Now on both sides, we have correlation functions, on the left C_{rs}, the correlation between r and s, and on the right, the stimulus autocorrelation C_{ss}:

$$C_{rs}(-\tau') = \int d\tau\, C_{ss}(\tau' - \tau)K(\tau). \tag{2.14}$$

Fourier-transforming this expression,

$$\int d\tau'\, e^{i\omega\tau'} C_{rs}(-\tau') = \int d\tau' e^{i\omega\tau'} \int d\tau\, C_{ss}(\tau' - \tau)K(\tau), \tag{2.15}$$

we obtain an algebraic equation for $K(\omega)$:

$$\tilde{C}_{rs}(-\omega) = \tilde{C}_{ss}(\omega)K(\omega). \tag{2.16}$$

Solving by inverse transform for the kernel in the time domain, one arrives at:

$$K(t) = \frac{1}{2\pi} \int d\omega\, e^{-i\omega t} \frac{\tilde{C}_{rs}(-\omega)}{\tilde{C}_{ss}(\omega)}. \tag{2.17}$$

For white noise stimuli, the stimulus autocorrelation function $C_{ss}(\omega)$ is uniform in ω or a delta function in time, a considerable simplification. In the limit that $r(t)$ is defined as a sequence of spike times, $r(t) = \sum_i \delta(t - t_i)$ where t_i are the times of spikes, the correlation C_{rs} between the stimulus and the response becomes the *spike-triggered average* or STA. The correlation function corresponds to the average of all stimulus histories preceding every spike. This linear approximation is equivalent to a first-order Wiener [82] or Volterra [40] kernel.

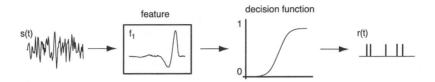

Figure 2.5 A simple cascade or linear/nonlinear model. The incoming stimulus $s(t)$ is filtered by the linear filter or feature f. The filtered stimulus is then passed through a static nonlinearity, or a decision function $P(\text{spike}|s)$, to produce a spiking probability $r(t)$. This can be turned into a discrete spike train by treating $r(t)$ as a Poisson rate in every time bin.

2.2.2 Cascade Models

While the linear model can be a reasonable approximation in some cases, it fails to account for the basic nonlinearities of spike generation, such as saturation and rectification. A much better approximation to the stimulus-to-rate mapping can be found by retaining the linear filter, and adding an additional nonlinear stage. Models of this type are known as linear-nonlinear (LN) models, or cascade models, (figure 2.5). The computation that the system performs can be thought of as first, feature selection, whereby the complex stimulus is reduced to its similarity (linear projection) to a single stimulus *feature*, then second, a nonlinear decision or threshold function on the outcome of the filter which determines the probability to fire. This formulation is an elegant generalization of the tuning curve concept: the "relevant stimulus parameter" is replaced by a complex feature, which may have arbitrary— e.g., spatial, temporal, or spectral— characteristics depending on the experimental design. As we saw above, the spike-triggered average is the optimal estimator of the stimulus given a spike and is a natural choice for the relevant feature.

The nonlinear threshold function, $P(\text{spike}|\text{stimulus})$, may also be computed directly from data for a given feature. From Bayes' rule,

$$P(\text{spike}|\text{stimulus}) = P(\text{spike})\frac{P(\text{stimulus}|\text{spike})}{P(\text{stimulus})}. \tag{2.18}$$

All of the quantities on the right-hand side can be found empirically. $P(\text{spike})$ is a scaling factor proportional to the overall mean firing rate; the prior stimulus distribution, $P(\text{stimulus})$, is determined by the experimental design. The conditional distribution, $P(\text{stimulus}|\text{spike})$, is sampled from data by forming a histogram of the stimulus values at the times of spikes. Recall that, for the model of figure 2.5, the stimulus at any time is represented by a single number, the projection of the time-varying, complex stimulus onto the relevant feature. If the feature is truly relevant for the system, $P(\text{stimulus}|\text{spike})$ will be distinct from the prior distribution, $P(\text{stimulus})$, and their ratio will be a nontrivial function over the projected stimulus.

LN models have provided a quite successful description of a variety of neural systems [40], including retinal ganglion cells [68, 35, 10] and the LGN [16, 74]. However, the model has two principal weaknesses. The first is that it is limited to only one linear feature. The assumption of feature selectivity means that the system is sensitive not to the entire stimulus history but only to certain aspects of it. Another way to put this is that the neural system is only sensitive to certain *dimensions* of the high-dimensional input. There is no *a priori* reason to expect only a single dimension to be relevant. Indeed, it is easy to design a case in which a single linear dimension will fail to capture the relevant sensitivity of the system. Take, for instance, a model for a high-frequency auditory neuron. This neuron is sensitive to power at a particular frequency, ω, in the auditory spectrum, but is insensitive to the phase. As spikes occur at random phases with respect to the sound wave, the spike-triggered average is zero. The appropriate stimulus space is spanned by the two unit vectors, $\sin(\omega)$ and $\cos(\omega)$, which can be linearly combined to produce a wave at frequency ω with arbitrary phase. We will later see experimental data from a system showing exactly this property. In the next section we will discuss methods for discovering feature selectivity for multiple dimensions.

The second weakness of the model as a predictor for neural output is that it generates only a time-varying probability, or rate. A purely rate-based description of neural response does not account for individual spike times. Typically one might use such a rate model to generate spiking responses by assuming that single neurons fire with Poisson statistics: the probability of a spike in a time bin of length Δt is determined solely by the instantaneous rate at time t, $r(t)$: in other words, $P(\text{spike at } t) = r(t)\Delta t$. Under this scheme, every spike is independent. A Poisson model on its own makes no assumption about the cause of the modulations of $r(t)$. The simplest case is as above, where $r(t)$ is purely a function of the stimulus s: $r(t) \propto P(\text{spike at } t|s)$. However, the biophysics of neurons and neural circuits– e.g. ion channel dynamics and short-term synaptic plasticity– can prevent spikes from being truly independent of one another and introduce a dependence on the history of activity. These properties can endow multiple-spike symbols with meanings that are distinct from those inferred from spikes treated independently. One could, as discussed in the previous section, take the output to consist of symbols that are sufficiently long to include any correlations between spikes. Alternatively, from a mechanistic viewpoint, one could consider $r(t)$ to depend jointly on stimulus *and* spike history. In figure 2.6, we refer to three possible ways to include the effects of previous spikes: a change in the threshold or decision function, a change in the effective input to the decision function, or a change in the relevant features [54]. In the spike response model [28], previous spikes add an effective input to the external stimulus, and the stimulus filter is also taken to depend on the time to the last spike.

Recent work has shown that integrate-and-fire (IF) models, which provide a semirealistic yet simple description of neural spiking dynamics, can exhibit some of the important statistical characteristics of real neurons, and may be tractably used (like the cascade-type models described above) to provide a de-

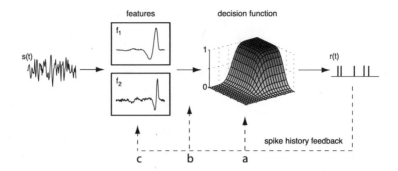

Figure 2.6 Modified cascade model: in general one would like to allow for multiple spike-triggering features, which combine in a general multidimensional nonlinearity. One would also like to include the effects of spike history. There are at least three possible ways to do so: a. a modification of the decision function, for example, an effective increase in threshold following a spike; b. an afterhyperpolarization or other current waveform is added to the filtered stimulus prior to input into the decision function; or c. the features themselves are altered by the previous occurrence of a spike.

scription of neural encoding [56, 32, 53].

Figure 2.7 shows a schematic diagram of a "generalized" IF model [46, 53]. It consists of a standard leaky IF component driven by three time-varying input currents: a stimulus-dependent current, a spike-history dependent current, and a noise current. The stimulus-dependent current is the linear convolution of the stimulus with input filter k, which represents the neuron's spatiotemporal receptive field. The history-dependent current results from a current waveform h injected following each spike, and captures the influence of spike train history. This is equivalent to convolving h with the spike train; h can also be thought of as a linear filter operating on the spike train. The noise current accounts for intrinsic variability in the neural response, and introduces a probability measure on the set of observable spike trains.

Recent work has shown that this model can be efficiently fit using maximum likelihood: the parameters describing the receptive field f, the spike history filter h, and the statistics of the noise a are determined as those under which the observed spike responses are most likely given the stimulus. A related approach uses a similar set of stimulus and spike-history filters to predict intracellular voltage, but uses an instantaneous nonlinearity (followed by Poisson spike generation) instead of an IF compartment to convert voltage to spikes. This model can also be estimated using the maximum-likelihood framework [46, 78].

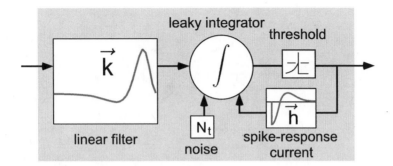

Figure 2.7 The generalized integrate-and-fire model. The stimulus is filtered by f, then integrated to threshold. A Gaussian time-varying noise is added to the filtered stimulus, as is a post-spike current waveform h. Figure courtesy of Jonathan Pillow.

2.2.3   Finding Multiple Features

Let us backtrack and take a more formal and more geometric perspective on the ground we have covered so far. Let us consider a stimulus s— spatial, temporal, spatiotemporal, spectrotemporal, or otherwise– as a vector of discrete values, where the discretization scale may be set by the correlation length. The length of the vector will be determined by the number of components of the stimulus and its extent in time, space, etc., that is relevant to the firing of the neuron, i.e. the outer boundary of the receptive field. Even for a stimulus with a single time-varying component, such as a current input into a neuron, the number of dimensions D required to specify the stimulus may be as many as 500. If the stimulus has multiple components (e.g. spatial dimensions), we consider it to be flattened or "unfolded" into a vector. Every sample of the stimulus history is then a point in a D-dimensional space. If we use a Gaussian stimulus with zero mean, the prior distribution of stimuli will fill a D-dimensional Gaussian ball in this space. (Note that it is not necessary that the true stimulus has zero mean, but the analysis is simplified by expressing the true stimulus as a difference from its mean.) The marginal distribution of the prior along any arbitrary direction in this space is then also Gaussian, with the same mean (zero) and variance. Linear filtering with unit norm is precisely such a stimulus projection, with direction vector given by the filter components.

The spike-triggered ensemble is a limited subset of the prior distribution, not necessarily Gaussian. Looking along a direction to which the neuron is sensitive, the distribution of spike-triggered samples will differ from the prior; along irrelevant dimensions, the spike-triggered ensemble will be indistinguishable from the prior.

Our goal is to capture a compact description of this spike-triggering stimulus distribution given a cloud of points in D-dimensional space, each a measured spike-inducing stimulus history. The obvious first approximation is the one we have already discussed: the centroid of the cloud of points. This is simply the STA (figure 2.8a). This geometrical picture makes it easy to imagine cases where the STA is an incomplete or even useless description. Let's assume the system is sensitive to a particular feature, but insensitive to the sign: an example is an ON/OFF retinal ganglion cell [25]. Then the spike-triggered ensemble will form two symmetric clouds in this space, and the STA will be zero (figure 2.8b). In the case of our auditory neuron, the spike-triggered ensemble will lie on a ring around the origin due to the phase invariance, and again the centroid will be at or close to zero, (figure 2.8c). Even without these exotic structures, the cloud that describes the spike-triggered ensemble may have interesting geometry that extends through multiple dimensions. Thus it is appropriate to proceed to the next order statistic, the covariance [20, 12].

The covariance matrix $\mathbf{C}$ is given by an average over all spike histories, indexed by i:

$$C_{jk} = \left\langle \left(s^{(i)}(\tau_j) - \bar{s}(\tau_j) \right) \left(s^{(i)}(\tau_k) - \bar{s}(\tau_j) \right) \right\rangle_i, \tag{2.19}$$

where for an s consisting of an ordinary (scalar) time series, the index τ runs over time prior to the spike, and otherwise over time and all components of the stimulus; and $\bar{s}$ is the STA. The average $\langle \cdot \rangle_i$ is over all spikes. In some applications, one further computes the difference between the spike-triggered covariance matrix and that of the prior,

$$\hat{\mathbf{C}} = \mathbf{C} - \mathbf{C}^{\text{prior}}. \tag{2.20}$$

One then finds the eigenvalue decomposition of $\hat{\mathbf{C}}$. This procedure identifies the dimensions $\mathbf{e}_1, \mathbf{e}_2, \cdots, \mathbf{e}_N$ in stimulus space that are most relevant to the neuron: those eigenvectors corresponding to the largest (in absolute value) eigenvalues. Due to the subtraction of the prior, the eigenvalues can have either positive or negative sign. The sign of the eigenvalue indicates how the variance along a particular dimension differs from that of the prior. Irrelevant dimensions will have eigenvalues close to zero. Relevant dimensions may have variance either less than the prior— for example, a thresholding neuron— or greater, as will be the case for the auditory example, as stimuli are distributed to either side of the origin. Computing the eigensystem of $\mathbf{C}$ directly is known as principal components analysis (PCA); in this case the eigenvalues will be strictly positive. Significant directions will appear associated with eigenvalues significantly differing from the prior variance. In what follows we will consider the eigensystem of $\hat{\mathbf{C}}$ only.

Due to finite size effects, many eigenvalues may differ from zero. To determine which eigenvalues are *significantly* nonzero, one could track the eigenvalues as a function of the number of spikes, to determine the noise floor [4, 3]. We will see an example of this in figure 2.11b. Another method for determining the noise floor is the bootstrap method, where the same number of stimuli as there are spikes is chosen randomly from the prior and the covariance matrix computed. Repeating this many times determines a threshold for the size of eigenvalues arising randomly [71, 60].

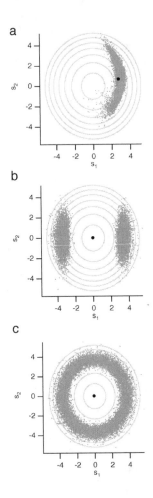

Figure 2.8 Spike-triggered stimuli projected onto two stimulus dimensions when spikes have been generated in response to zero-mean white noise current (a) by a slowly firing (1 Hz) Hodgkin-Huxley model neuron, (b) by thresholding the absolute value of the stimulus, and (c) by thresholding the sum of two independent squared stimulus projections. Each point represents one spike-inducing stimulus history. The dark black circle denotes the spike-triggered average stimulus. Concentric circles exclude $10^{-1}\%$, $10^{-2}\%$, $10^{-3}\%$, and so on of the Gaussian prior stimulus.

Once one has found the N relevant eigenvectors, one can then compute a multidimensional cascade model (see figure 2.6). This requires determining the nonlinear threshold function over the space of relevant dimensions, $P(\text{spike}|s_1, s_2, \cdots, s_N)$, where s_j is the stimulus component along the direction $\mathbf{e}_j$. In principle one can compute this function by direct sampling, as for the one-dimensional case (equation (2.18)). However, given the number of spikes typically obtainable from an experiment (of order several thousand), it is unlikely that one can sample a function over more than two or perhaps three dimensions. Significant improvements in the performance of a 2D model over a 1D, STA model have been shown in several cases [4, 25, 60, 72]. Rust et al. [60] found a large number of relevant eigenvalues— up to 14— for neurons in visual cortex. They reduced this large number by combining pairs in quadrature and fitted a parametric nonlinear function over the resulting variables.

One of the limitations in applying this approach is the restriction to Gaussian stimuli. One would like to be able to study neural coding in the context of natural stimuli, which have highly non-Gaussian statistics, in particular long-range correlations [59, 70]. Sharpee et al. [69] directly maximized mutual information between the stimulus and the spiking response to determine the maximally informative stimulus dimensions for arbitrary stimulus ensembles.

2.2.4 Examples of the Application of Covariance Methods

Neural Models

To develop an intuition for this procedure, it is useful to apply it to some simple model neurons. The first is a variant of a spike response model: a cascade model, as in figure 2.5, augmented by the addition of an afterhyperpolarization (AHP) [33], similar to figure 2.7. The stimulus is filtered by a linear filter f, (figure 2.9). When the filtered stimulus reaches a threshold θ, the neuron fires a spike. Following the spike, a negative current waveform is added to the filtered stimulus, moving the system away from threshold temporarily until the sum of filtered stimulus and AHP is again sufficient to cross threshold. A Gaussian noise current $a(t)$ is added to the filtered stimulus. This model implements some of the interspike dependencies that real neurons show.

This system depends explicitly on a single feature, f, so one might expect that there will be a single significant eigenvalue. The spike-triggering stimuli will show a reduced variance along this direction as generally [25],

$$\int d\tau f(\tau)s(t - \tau) \geq \theta. \tag{2.21}$$

If not for the AHP, the threshold condition in equation (2.21) would be an equality. For spikes that follow other spikes within the time scale of the AHP, the sum of the filtered stimulus and the (negative) AHP must exceed θ. Upon reflection, a second filter should appear: the time derivative $f' \equiv df/dt$. When

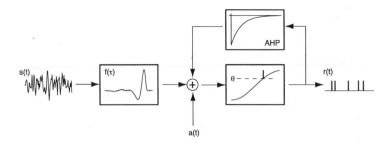

Figure 2.9 Threshold-crossing model with interspike interaction through an afterhyperpolarization. a. The incoming current stimulus is filtered by filter f. The input to the threshold function is the sum of the filtered stimulus and the afterhyperpolarization. When threshold θ is crossed, a spike is fired. Following the spike, the afterhyperpolarization current waveform is added to the input.

the filtered stimulus crosses threshold, it generally does so from below,

$$\frac{d}{dt} \int d\tau f(\tau) s(t - \tau) > 0 \implies \int d\tau f'(\tau) s(t - \tau) > 0, \tag{2.22}$$

and again one expects the variance in the direction of f' to be reduced relative to the prior. For threshold crossings that occur during the influence of the AHP, equation (2.22) is not necessarily satisfied.

The covariance analysis, as expected, shows two significant modes (or eigenvectors), with negative eigenvalues; the spectrum of eigenvalues is plotted in figure 2.10a. The significant modes are plotted in figure 2.10b, along with the STA. As expected, the leading mode is f; the second eigenvalue is f'. Note that the STA is not the filter f; in fact it is a linear combination of f and f'. It is interesting to look at the spike-triggering stimuli in the space of the two modes, (figure 2.10c). The points all lie approximately to the left of the threshold value, shown as a dotted line, and approximately in the positive half-plane with respect to f'. The blur around the threshold value is due to added noise. The spread of points below zero in the f' direction and throughout the quadrant in the f direction is an example of how spike interdependence can affect the covariance analysis, but the presence of the AHP does not lead to any additional filters.

This simplicity does not hold for a more common model neuron, the leaky integrate-and-fire (LIF) neuron. The LIF model is described by

$$C\frac{dV}{dt} = I(t) - \frac{V}{R} - CV_c \sum_i \delta(t - t_i), \tag{2.23}$$

where C is a capacitance, R is a resistance, and V_c is the voltage threshold for spiking. The first two terms on the right-hand side model an RC circuit; the

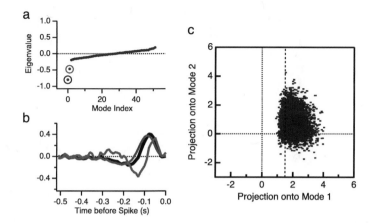

Figure 2.10 Covariance analysis of the threshold crossing model. (a). Spectrum of eigenvalues from $\hat{\mathbf{C}}$, showing two significant modes. (b). Labeled with the same colors as indicated in a., the two significant eigenvectors $\mathbf{e}_1$ and $\mathbf{e}_2$ and the spike-triggered average (black). The true filter f coincides with $\mathbf{e}_1$. (c). Spike-triggering stimuli projected into the space of $\mathbf{e}_1$ and $\mathbf{e}_2$. The threshold value is plotted as a dotted line.

capacitor integrates the input current as a potential V while the resistor dissipates the stored charge (hence "leaky"). The third term implements spiking and reset: spikes are defined as the set of times $\{t_i\}$ such that $V(t_i) = V_c$. When the potential reaches V_c, a restoring current is instantaneously injected to bring the stored charge back to zero, resetting the system.

Integrating equation (2.23) away from spikes, we obtain

$$CV(t) = \int_{-\infty}^{t} d\tau \exp\left(\frac{\tau - t}{RC}\right) I(\tau), \tag{2.24}$$

assuming initialization of the system in the distant past at zero potential. The right-hand side can be rewritten as the convolution of $I(t)$ with the causal exponential kernel

$$f_\infty(\tau) = \begin{cases} 0 & \text{if } \tau \leq 0 \\ \exp(-\tau/RC) & \text{if } 0 < \tau, \end{cases} \tag{2.25}$$

so the condition for a spike at time t_1 is that this convolution reach threshold:

$$CV_c = \int_{-\infty}^{\infty} d\tau f_\infty(\tau) I(t_1 - \tau). \tag{2.26}$$

In this case, the interaction between spikes has a severe impact. If the system spiked last at time $t_0 < t_1$, we must replace the lower limit of integration in equation (2.24) with t_0, as no current injected before t_0 can contribute to the accumulated potential. Equivalently, we can replace f_∞ with a family of kernels,

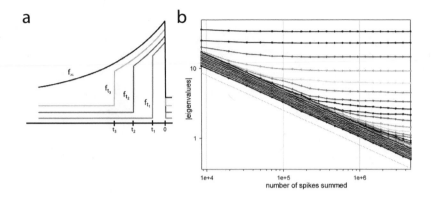

Figure 2.11   Apparent high dimensionality in the integrate-and-fire model due to spike interaction. (a). Family of filters labeled by the time to the last spike. (b). Spectrum of eigenvalues, plotted as a function of the number of spikes N. The noise floor goes down as $1/N$. Many modes emerge as significant with large enough N (see color insert).

(figure 2.11a), dependent on the time to the previous spike, $\Delta t = t_1 - t_0$:

$$f_{\Delta t}(\tau) = \begin{cases} 0 & \text{if } \tau \le 0 \\ \exp(-\tau/RC) & \text{if } 0 < \tau < \Delta t \\ 0 & \text{if } \Delta t \le \tau. \end{cases} \tag{2.27}$$

Let's look at the consequences of this for the covariance analysis. The spectrum, instead of showing one or two large eigenvalues, shows a broad range of eigenvalues. The eigenvalues are certainly significant, as one can demonstrate by plotting them over a wide range of N, the number of spikes used in the covariance calculation (figure 2.11b). The STA and the leading mode do *not* correspond to the exponential filter, f_∞, but are considerably steeper (figure 2.12a).

We found [3] that the correct exponential filter, (figure 2.12b), could be found by limiting the analysis to isolated spikes only, i.e. spikes that are separated from the previous spike by a sufficient time. The isolation requirement was determined from data by examining the interspike interval distribution: at large Δt the distribution becomes exponential, as for a Poisson process, indicating that the spikes become statistically independent.

Single Neurons

One can use the covariance method to characterize the computation performed by single neurons on their current inputs. In particular, one would like to know how changes in the neuron's biophysics lead to changes in its computation.

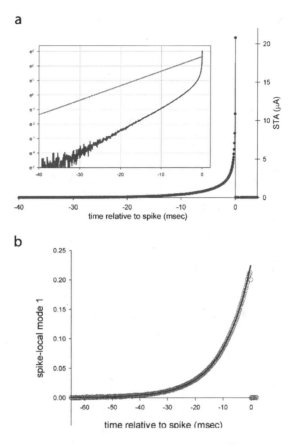

Figure 2.12   (a). The spike-triggered average (STA) is very different from exponential. The inset shows on a linear-log scale the STA in red and for comparison, the true exponential filter of the system. (b). The leading eigenmode when using isolated spikes only matches the true exponential kernel f_∞, shown in red. Reproduced with permission from Agüera y Arcas et al., [4].

Such an analysis was applied by Slee et al. [72] to neurons of nucleus magnocellularis (NM) in the avian brainstem. These neurons are a stage for the transmission of timing information about auditory signals, allowing the animal to perform sound localization. They show a strong DC filtering, responding only to the initial deflection of a DC current step.

Using injection of white noise currents, the STA and the covariance matrix were computed to derive 1D and 2D cascade models of the stimulus/response mapping. The STA had a unimodal form, and can be interpreted as a pure integrating filter. A model based on this feature alone fails to reproduce the basic DC filtering property of NM neurons. However, covariance analysis re-

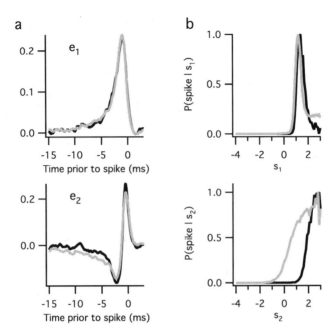

Figure 2.13 Covariance analysis results for neurons in avian nucleus magnocellularis before and after the addition of DTX, which blocks certain potassium channels. (a). The leading two eigenmodes, e_1 and e_2, before (black) and after (gray) treatment with DTX. (b). The decision functions computed for each eigenmode independently, before (black) and after (grey) DTX. While the dependence on the first mode hardly changes, the threshold with respect to e_2 shifts to a dramatically lower point.

vealed two leading features: a unimodal, integrating feature, and a bimodal, differentiating feature (figure 2.13). A third mode was also obtained but was considerably less reproducible. The combination of the two leading modes recovered the DC filtering property.

The DC filtering property is destroyed by pharmacological block of potassium channels (Kv 1.1, 1.2, and 1.6) by dendrotoxin (DTX). By probing the system with white noise during block by DTX, covariance analysis revealed that while the form of the two modes was almost unchanged, the contribution of the differentiating feature was significantly weakened. A new 2D model built from the new decision function reproduced the experimental results.

Systems Analysis: Cortical Neurons

A final very interesting example of the application of covariance analysis comes from the work of Rasmus Petersen and colleagues [50] on the responses of neurons in rat barrel cortex to externally driven vibration of the rat's whiskers. The whisker array was attached to a grid which was moved through a vertical white noise trajectory. Reverse correlation was then applied to discover the features to which the system was sensitive. The authors found an STA with a very small amplitude. However, covariance analysis revealed a number of similarities with complex cells in visual cortex [76, 60]. Several pairs of significant eigenmodes were observed. The leading two modes are a bimodal fluctuation and its derivative. These modes equivalently form a conjugate pair, with one mode phase-shifted by 90 degrees with respect to the other (analogous to a sine/cosine pair). The input/output relations, $P(\text{spike}|s_1)$ and $P(\text{spike}|s_2)$, derived with respect to these two modes independently increase symmetrically away from the origin: the firing rate increases with increasing projection, but with sign invariance. In the 2D space of this pair of modes, this turns out to be an example such as in figure 2.8c: a ringlike structure. Thus the system is sensitive to the *power*, or sum in quadrature, of the two leading features. One can therefore reduce these two modes to one dimension by forming the (nonlinear) quadratic sum of the two filter outputs, similar to the pooling procedures applied in visual cortex by Rust et al. [60]. With respect to this new variable, the input/output relation is a simple threshold.

Two more conjugate pairs of modes with significant eigenvalues were found; one with negative eigenvalues, (e_3, e_4), and one with positive, (e_{100}, e_{101}); eigenvalues are ordered by size and $\mathbf{C}$ was 101-dimensional. The positive eigenmodes have an oscillation at a frequency quite similar to the leading mode, but displaced back in time by ~ 50 ms. The input/output relation, $P(\text{spike}|s_{100}, s_{101})$, was again invariant with respect to phase, as one might by now expect. However, the structure of $P(\text{spike}|s_{100}, s_{101})$ is dramatically different from the leading modes; it shows a *maximal* predicted firing rate for zero projections, and decreases with increasing value of the projection. These modes can be thought of as *suppressive* modes; their presence induces a *decrease* in the firing rate [65, 60]. In figure 2.14 we show an example of the same phenomenon of pairs of excitatory and suppressive conjugate modes from complex cells in V1 [60].

Along with the examples already cited, covariance analysis has been applied to computation in the retina [65, 25] and color-opponency neurons in V1 [30], revealing unexpected structure. All of these examples show how such multi-dimensional cascade models allow us to put the notion of computation in different systems on a common footing. It is particularly fascinating that similar computational structures emerge analogously in different sensory systems.

2.2.5 Using Information to Assess Decoding

How does one evaluate the success of a reduced dimensional model in capturing the behavior of the system? One reasonable approach is to construct the predictive model and compare the output of the model to experimental data [60, 53]: this evaluates the features in terms of their success in building the encoding model and reproducing the spike train. An alternative is to concentrate on *decoding*: to what extent has one captured what is relevant about the stimulus? This can be done by making use of the information-theoretic methods

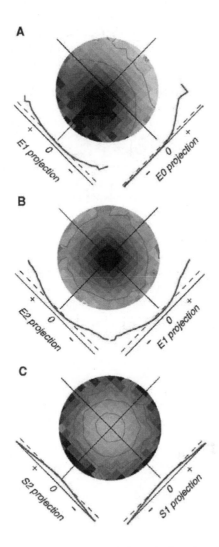

Figure 2.14 Examples of two-dimensional decision functions from a complex cell in V1; lighter color means higher predicted firing rate. Many of the neurons recorded showed a large number of relevant eigenmodes, generally occurring in conjugate pairs. The decision functions shown are constructed from (A). The projections onto the STA ($E0$) and the first excitatory mode, $E1$, (B). The projections onto the first pair of excitatory modes $E1$ and $E2$, showing an increase in firing (lighter colors) with increasing radius in the 2D plane, (C). The leading two suppressive modes, $S1$ and $S2$, showing a decrease in firing with increasing radius. Reproduced with permission from Rust et al., [58].

introduced previously. The method of Brenner et al. [13] described in §2.1.3 allows one to compute the amount of information that the arrival of a single spike conveys about the stimulus, without any assumptions about the encoding or the decoding process. One can then compare this information with the information extracted by the reduced model [4, 1].

Starting with equation (2.9),

$$I_{\text{one spike}} = \frac{1}{T} \int_0^T dt \, \frac{r(t)}{\bar{r}} \log_2 \frac{r(t)}{\bar{r}}.$$

note that by definition,

$$\frac{r(t)}{\bar{r}} = \frac{P(\text{spike at } t | \mathbf{s})}{P(\text{spike at } t)}. \tag{2.28}$$

Previously we used Bayes rule, (equation (2.18)), to invert the relationship between stimulus and spikes:

$$\frac{P(\text{spike at } t | \mathbf{s})}{P(\text{spike})} = \frac{P(\mathbf{s} | \text{spike at } t)}{P(\mathbf{s})},$$

where $\mathbf{s}$ as before represents the complete stimulus description. In forming our reduced N-dimensional model, we have replaced $\mathbf{s}$ with some limited number of dimensions, $s_1, s_2, \cdots, s_N$. That is,

$$\frac{P(\mathbf{s} | \text{spike at } t)}{P(\mathbf{s})} \rightarrow \frac{P(s_1, s_2, \cdots, s_N | \text{spike at } t)}{P(s_1, s_2, \cdots, s_N)} \tag{2.29}$$

So the single-spike information in the N-dimensional model is evaluated using the distribution of projections:

$$I^N_{\text{one spike}} = \int d^N s \, P(s_1, s_2, \cdots, s_N | \text{spike at } t) \log_2 \left[\frac{P(s_1, s_2, \cdots, s_N | \text{spike at } t)}{P(s_1, s_2, \cdots, s_N)} \right]. \tag{2.30}$$

The information in the reduced model is bounded from above by the directly computed information,

$$I^N_{\text{one spike}} \leq I_{\text{one spike}}, \tag{2.31}$$

so that one has an objective measure of the improvement in quality gained by adding additional dimensions. This was applied to the analysis of the NM neurons described previously; it was found that the 1D STA-based model recovers $\sim 63\%$ of the direct information, while a 2D model recovers $\sim 75\%$ [72]. Very similar results were found for the Hodgkin-Huxley model [4].

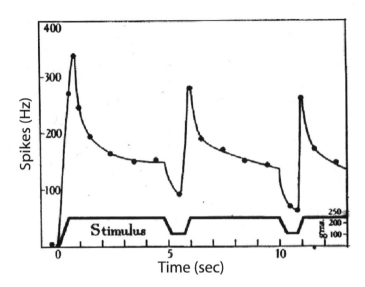

Figure 2.15   Spike rate recorded from cutaneous nerve fibers in a cat's toepad produced in response to pressure applied to the toe. Reproduced with permission from Adrian, [2].

2.3   Adaptive Spike Coding

In all of our discussions so far, we have regarded a neuron's mapping from input to output as a fixed relationship. However, from the earliest measurements of neural spiking by Adrian [2], it has been observed that neural systems show *adaptation*. In the simplest case, in response to a sustained, constant stimulus, the firing rate may decay in time, (figure 2.15). This is sometimes known as spike frequency adaptation. The ubiquity of adaptation suggests that it serves some useful function. At a basic level, this role might be to save the brain from using energetically expensive spikes to transmit stimuli that contain no new information. In the 1950s, Barlow [9] and Attneave [7] hypothesized that efficient representation and *redundancy reduction* is a design principle of neural coding. For a code to be efficient, it should take advantage of statistical regularities in the input. As we have discussed already, one may make a model

for neural response in terms of feature selectivity and an input/output relation. The efficient coding hypothesis suggests that either or both of these parts
of the neural encoding process should be determined by the statistical properties of the stimulus. In particular, output symbols should convey maximum
information. Recall that the mutual information is the difference between the
total entropy of the output and the noise entropy, (equation (2.3)). The entropy
of the output distribution will depend on the mapping from input to output,
$r = g(s)$, where g is some nonlinear function. Hence the output entropy must
depend on the input distribution. With the reasonable assumption that the
noise entropy is constant across stimuli and does not depend on the stimulus
distribution, information transmission can be maximized by maximizing the
total entropy of the output, given the statistics of the input and subject to any
physical constraints on the output.

In 1981, Laughlin [37] made a direct test of the idea that the input/output
relation of fly large monopolar cells (LMCs) might depend on the statistical
properties of natural contrasts. He took images of natural scenes to derive a
histogram of natural contrasts, $P(c)$, (figure 2.16a). LMCs do not spike but
rather show analog dependence of the output voltage on the inputs, so the response r here represents instantaneous voltage. To solve for the optimal mapping $r = g(s)$, Laughlin postulated that the output distribution r has maximum entropy, subject to a bound on the firing rate, $r \leq \alpha$. The solution for the
maximum entropy distribution for r given this constraint is simply a uniform
distribution over the interval $r \in [0, \alpha]$. To determine $g(s)$, we integrate

$$P(r)dr = P(s)ds \tag{2.32}$$

to obtain

$$r = g(s) = \frac{1}{\alpha} \int_{-1}^{s} ds' \, P(s'), \tag{2.33}$$

showing that the mapping to output $g(s)$ is simply given by a scaling of the
cumulative distribution of the contrast inputs (figure 2.16b). The prediction
compares well with experimental data (figure 2.16c).

While Laughlin's work implies that evolution or development has sculpted
the neural response to match the natural environment, it is possible that adaptive processes occur on much faster time scales. For the motion-sensitive neuron H1 in the blowfly, in response to a Gaussian stimulus with a variance σ^2,
the input/output relation adapts such that the stimulus appears to be scaled
in units of its standard deviation [12]. Furthermore, it was shown that this
rescaling, analogous to Laughlin's results, optimizes information transmission
through the system [12]. These experiments were done in the steady state,
with measurements made minutes after the adapting stimuli began. However,
adaptive processes occur in real time in response to changes in stimulus statistics. In retinal ganglion cells, adaptation of the firing rate was observed as the
stimulus variance was switched between two values with switches occurring
every 30 seconds [73]. This switching method has been used to probe the time

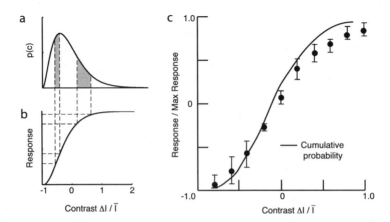

Figure 2.16 Fly large monopolar cells show response properties that match the contrast distribution in natural scenes. (a). The distribution of contrasts, $p(c)$, sampled from natural scenes. To obtain a uniform distribution of responses, r, the mapping from input to output should follow the cumulative distribution, (b), derived from $p(c)$. Equal areas under the curve $p(c)$ map to equal segments along the response axis. (c). Measured data match this prediction well. Adapted from Laughlin, [35].

scales and mechanisms of adaptation in the visual, auditory and somatosensory systems [73, 26, 35, 8, 36, 39].

In the fly neuron H1, it was shown that adaptation of the firing rate and adaptation of the input/output relation are two separate processes that occur on very different time scales [26]. The rescaling of the input/output relation with local variance occurs continuously, with a time scale that is difficult to measure through direct reverse correlation. This is illustrated in figure 2.17, where we plot the input/output relations derived during the presentation of Gaussian white noise that is modulated by a variance envelope, $\sigma(t)$, that varies over orders of magnitude. The input/output relations change continuously, but rescale when plotted with the stimulus normalized by the local standard deviation.

Although the firing rate is changing, we can use a variant of the information methods outlined above to compute the information transmission through the neuron as a function of time during a variance switch [26]. A limited number N of white noise sequences, $\{s_i\}$, of 2 seconds duration were presented. Each sequence was modulated by a multiplicative amplitude envelope that switches between two values, σ_1 and σ_2, every 4 seconds. The sequences s_i straddle the switches in σ. The spike trains are then divided into words, of total length 20 ms, with bin size $\Delta t = 2$ms. Taking time t to be measured relative to the time of the switch (either from σ_1 to σ_2 or vice versa), the word distribution $P(w(t))$ was collected for every time slice $t \in [-1, 1]$ s. Now we can sort the words produced at time t into conditional distributions, $P(w(t)|s_i)$ and $P(w(t)|\sigma_i)$, to

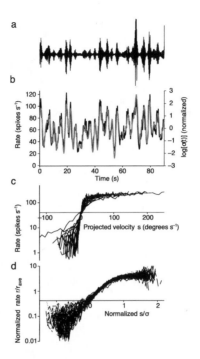

Figure 2.17 The input/output relation of the fly motion-sensitive neuron H1 adapts continuously to the local variance. (a). A white noise Gaussian motion stimulus, modulated by a Gaussian envelope $\sigma(t)$. (b). The rate measured in response follows $\log \sigma(t)$. (c). Input/output relations measured at time bins throughout the response differ considerably in their horizontal scale. (d). However, when the projected stimulus s is normalized by the local standard deviation, the input/output relations overlay. Reprinted with permission from Fairhall et al., [24].

compute either the information in the words about the white noise stimulus $s \in \{s_i\}$,

$$I(w; s) = H[P(w(t))] - \sum_{i=1}^{N} P(s_i)H[P(w(t)|s_i)], \qquad P(s_i) = \frac{1}{N}, \qquad (2.34)$$

or the information about the standard deviation σ_i:

$$I(w; \sigma) = H[P(w(t))] - \sum_{i=1}^{2} P(\sigma_i)H[P(w(t)|\sigma_i)], \qquad P(\sigma_i) = \frac{1}{2}. \qquad (2.35)$$

Using an inappropriately scaled input/output relation should result in less than optimal information transmission. Thus we expect that the adaptation of the input/output relation following a switch will lead to a recovery of information transmission. The results are shown in figure 2.18 in terms of information/spike. Information about the variance remains at a constant ~ 0.5

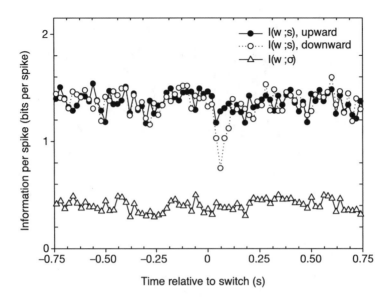

Figure 2.18 Information/spike conveyed about the rapidly varying normalized stimulus (circles), both during an upward and a downward transition in variance. Reproduced with permission from Fairhall et al., [24].

bits, while the information about the rapidly varying component of the signal indeed declines during the downward transition. However, recovery to the same information rate occurs within less than 100 ms. For an upward switch, there is no resolvable loss in information transmission. Thus, we have been able to use an information measure to estimate a time scale for the functional consequences of adaptation.

Although we have concentrated so far on the adaptation of the input/output relation, the first stage of neural computation as we framed it earlier is feature selectivity. Adaptation may also alter the relevant features, or receptive fields of the system. Atick proposed and demonstrated [5, 6] that the structure of receptive fields in the retina reduces redundancy in natural visual scenes. Receptive fields in the fly visual system were also successfully predicted analytically from an information-theoretic principle [79]. If the optimization of information transmission is indeed a "design principle," one would expect, as for the input/output relation, that changing the statistical structure of the inputs might change the receptive field properties [22, 11, 61]. A variety of spatial, temporal, and spatiotemporal correlations have been shown to affect retinal receptive field structure in a predictable way [31].

Returning to the results from Adrian with which we began, we used these to demonstrate that the relationship between input and output is not fixed, but may change with stimulus history. Another valid interpretation is that there is a fixed relationship, but one that depends, as with all of the examples we have previously considered, on the stimulus history over some range of time. A simple cascade model could produce the rate dynamics of figure 2.15 if, as for the NM neurons discussed in §2.2.4, the system showed sensitivity both to an integrating component and a differentiating component. Closer examination of figure 2.15 shows that there is another level of "adaptation": while exactly the same recent stimulus history occurs at 5 seconds and 10 seconds, the amplitude of the spiking response has decreased. Thus, as we discussed for the fly neuron H1, there appear to be adaptation-like effects happening on several time scales. An open question is whether one might be able to incorporate all "adaptive" effects in a single, unified, static model by considering the input/output relation to depend on longer stimulus histories.

2.4 Summary

In this chapter we have reviewed a number of methods that can be applied to a characterization of the neural code. We have distinguished between encoding and decoding. In decoding, we are trying to infer as much about the stimulus as possible given knowledge of the spike train. To do this, we need to know which of the details of the spike train are important, and information theory provides a means of evaluating this. The encoding problem touches more on mechanisms: how, given a stimulus, is a particular spike train generated? To solve this problem, we need to capture something of the nuts and bolts of the system by taking internal noise and spike dynamics explicitly into account. The dimensionality reduction tools that were so useful for decoding help us to build predictive models of the encoding process. Maximum-likelihood methods also provide an efficient way of fitting accurate parametric models.

As we have seen, adaptation has great benefits for the system in terms of information processing. The elegant predictive models we have reviewed are enriched and confused by the issue of adaptation and the dependence of these characterizations on stimulus statistics. We still seek a more general approach to decoding that integrates stimulus ensemble, and encoding models that capture the essence of the wide variety of cellular and network mechanisms that underlie adaptive phenomena.

2.5 Recommended Reading

We have taken a rather idiosyncratic path through a selection of topics on neural coding. We recommend the more extended treatment given to some aspects of this chapter in the excellent monographs *Spikes*, by Rieke et al. [58] and *Spiking Neuron Models*, by Gerstner and Kistler [28], and the textbook *Theoretical Neuroscience*, by Dayan and Abbott [17]. For a recent review of the concepts of synergy and redundancy, and the relationships between several of the theoretical approaches to multineuronal coding in the literature, see Schneidman et al. [62]. An overview of white noise analysis, including covariance analysis, is given in Simoncelli et al. [71].

References

[1] Adelman T, Bialek W, Olberg R (2003) The information content of receptive fields. *Neuron*, 40(4):823–33.

[2] Adrian E (1928) *The Basis of Sensation: The Action of the Sense Organs*. London: Christophers.

[3] Agüera y Arcas B, Fairhall AL (2003) What causes a neuron to spike? *Neural Computattion*, 15(8):1789–807.

[4] Agüera y Arcas B, Fairhall AL, Bialek W (2003) Computation in a single neuron: Hodgkin and Huxley revisited. *Neural Computation*, 15(8):1715–49.

[5] Atick J (1992) Could information theory provide an ecological theory of sensory processing? *Network: Computation in Neural Systems*, 3:213–51.

[6] Atick J, Redlich A (1992) What does the retina know about natural scenes? *Neural Computation*, 4:196–210.

[7] Attneave F (1954) Possible principles underlying the transformation of sensory messages. *Psychol. Rev.*, 61:183–193.

[8] Baccus S, Meister M (2002) Fast and slow contrast adaptation in retinal circuitry. *Neuron*, 36(5):909–19.

[9] Barlow H (1961) Possible principles underlying the transformation of sensory messages. In Rosenbluth WA eds., *Sensory Communication*, pages 217–234, Cambridge, MA: MIT Press.

[10] Berry MJ II., Meister M (1999) The neural code of the retina. *Neuron*, 22:435–450.

[11] Borst A, Egelhaaf M (1986) Temporal modulation of luminance adapts time constant of fly movement detectors. *Biological Cybernetics*, 54:223–236.

[12] Brenner N, Bialek W, de Ruyter van Steveninck R (2000) Adaptive rescaling maximizes information transmission. *Neuron*, 26:695–702.

[13] Brenner N, Strong S, Koberle R, Bialek W, de Ruyter van Steveninck RR (2000) Synergy in a neural code. *Neural Computation*, 12:1531–1552.

[14] Bryant H, Segundo JP (1978) Spike initiation by transmembrane current: a white-noise analysis. *Journal of Physiology*, 260:279–314.

[15] Cover T, Thomas J (1991) *Elements of Information Theory*. New York: Wiley.

[16] Dan Y, Alonso J, Usrey W, Reid R (1998) Coding of visual information by precisely correlated spikes in the lateral geniculate nucleus. *Nat. Neuroscience*, 1(6):501–7.

[17] Dayan P, Abbott LF (2001) *Theoretical Neuroscience: Computational and Mathematical Modeling of Neural Systems*. Cambridge, MA: MIT Press.

[18] de Boer E, Kuyper P (1968) Triggered correlation. *IEEE Transactions in Biomedical Engineering*, 15:169–179.

[19] de Polavieja GG, Harsh A, Kleppe I, Robinson H, Juusola M (2005) Stimulus history reliably shapes the action potential waveform of cortical neurons. *Journal of Neuroscience*, 25:5657–5665.

[20] de Ruyter van Steveninck RR, Bialek W (1988) Real-time performance of a movement sensitive in the blowfly visual system: information transfer in short spike sequences. *Proceedings of Royal Society of London, B*, 234:379–414.

[21] de Ruyter van Steveninck R, Lewen G, Strong S, Koberle R, Bialek W (1997) Reproducibility and variability in neural spike trains. *Science*, 275(5307):1805–8.

[22] de Ruyter van Steveninck R, Zaagman WH, Mastebroek H (1986) Adaptation of transient responses of a movement-sensitive neuron in the visual system of the blowfly *Calliphora erythrocephala*. *Biological Cybernetics*, 54:223–226.

[23] deWeese M, Hromadka T, Zador A (2005) Reliability and representational bandwidth in the auditory cortex. *Neuron*, 48(3):479–488.

[24] deWeese M, Zador A (2005) Shared and private variability in the auditory cortex. *Journal of Neurophysiology*, 92(3):1840–1855.

[25] Fairhall A, Burlingame C, Narasimhan R, Harris R, Puchalla J, Berry MJ II. (2006) Selectivity for multiple stimulus features in retinal ganglion cells. *Journal of Neurophysiology*, in press.

[26] Fairhall A, Lewen G, Bialek W, de Ruyter van Steveninck, RR (2001) Efficiency and ambiguity in an adaptive neural code. *Nature*, 412:787–792.

[27] Gawne T, Richmond B (1993) How independent are the messages carried by adjacent inferior temporal cortical neurons? *Journal of Neuroscience*, 13(7):2758–71.

[28] Gerstner W, Kistler WM (2002) *Spiking Neuron Models: Single Neurons, Populations, Plasticity*. Cambridge, UK: Cambridge University Press.

[29] Gur M, Snodderly D (2005) High response reliability of neurons in primary visual cortex (V1) of alert, trained monkeys. *Cerebral Cortex*. 16(6):888–895.

[30] Horwitz G, Chichilnisky E, Albright T (2005) Blue-yellow signals are enhanced by spatiotemporal luminance contrast in macaque v1. *Journal of Neurophysiology*, 93(4):2263–78.

[31] Hosoya T, Baccus S, Meister M (2005) Dynamic predictive coding by the retina. *Nature*, 436(7047):71–7.

[32] Jolivet R, Lewis T, Gerstner W (2004) Generalized integrate-and-fire models of neuronal activity approximate spike trains of a detailed model to a high degree of accuracy. *Journal of Neurophysiol.*, 92(2):959–76.

[33] Keat J, Reinagel P, Reid RC, Meister M (2001) Predicting every spike: a model for the responses of visual neurons. *Neuron*, 30(3):803–817.

[34] Kennel M, Shlens J, Abarbanel H, Chichilnisky E (2005) Estimating entropy rates with bayesian confidence intervals. *Neural Computation*, 17(7):1531–76.

[35] Kim K, Rieke F (2001) Temporal contrast adaptation in the input and output signals of salamander retinal ganglion cells. *Journal of Neuroscience*, 21:287–299.

[36] Kvale M, Schreiner C (2004) Short-term adaptation of auditory receptive fields to dynamic stimuli. *Journal of Neurophysiology*, 91(2):604–12.

[37] Laughlin SB (1981) A simple coding procedure enhances a neuron's information capacity. *Z. Naturforsch.*, 36c:910–912.

[38] Mainen Z, Sejnowski T (1995) Reliability of spike timing in neocortical neurons. *Science*, 268(5216):1503–6.

[39] Maravall M, Petersen R, Fairhall A, Arabzadeh E, Diamond M (2005) Adaptive encoding of whisker motion in rat barrel cortex. *submitted*.

[40] Marmarelis P, Naka K (1972) White-noise analysis of a neuron chain: an application of the Wiener theory. *Science*, 175:1276–8.

[41] Masland R (2001) The fundamental plan of the retina. *Nature Neuroscience*, 4(9):877–86.

[42] Narayanan N, Kimchi E, Laubach M (2005) Redundancy and synergy of neuronal ensembles in motor cortex. *Journal of Neuroscience*, 25(17):4207–16.

[43] Nelken I, Rotman Y, Yosef O (1999) Response of auditory-cortex neurons to structural features of natural sounds. *Nature*, 397:154–156.

[44] Nemenman I, Bialek W (2002) Occam factors and model independent bayesian learning of continuous distributions. *Physical Review E*, 65(2):026137.

[45] Nemenman I, Bialek W, de Ruyter van Steveninck R (2004) Entropy and information in neural spike trains: progress on the sampling problem. *Physical Review E*, 69(5):056111.

[46] Paninski L, Pillow J, Simoncelli E (2004) Maximum likelihood estimation of a stochastic integrate-and-fire neural encoding model. *Neural Computation*, 16(12):2533–61.

[47] Panzeri S, Petersen R, Schultz S, Lebedev M, Diamond M (2001) The role of spike timing in the coding of stimulus location in rat somatosensory cortex. *Neuron*, 29:769–77.

[48] Panzeri S, Schultz S, Treves A, Rolls E (1999) Correlations and the encoding of information in the nervous system. *Proc. Biological Sciences*, 266(1423):1001–12.

[49] Panzeri S, Treves A (1996) Analytical estimates of limited sampling biases in different information measures. *Network: Computation in Neural Systems*, 7:87–107.

[50] Petersen R, Diamond M (2003) Coding of dynamic whisker stimulation by neurons in the rat somatosensory cortex. *Society for Neuroscience Abstract*, 29:51.1.

[51] Petersen R, Panzeri S, Diamond M (2001) Population coding of stimulus location in rat somatosensory cortex. *Neuron*, 32(3):503–14.

[52] Petersen R, Panzeri S, Diamond M (2002) The role of individual spikes and spike patterns in population coding of stimulus location in rat somatosensory cortex. *Biosystems*, 67(1-3):187–93.

[53] Pillow J, Paninski L, Uzzell V, Simoncelli E, Chichilnisky E (2005) Prediction and decoding of retinal ganglion cell responses with a probabilistic spiking model. *Journal of Neuroscience*, 25(47):11003–13.

[54] Powers R, Dai Y, Bell B, Percival D, Binder M (2005) Contributions of the input signal and prior activation history to the discharge behaviour of rat motoneurones. *Journal of Physiology*, 562(3):707–24.

[55] Puchalla J, Schneidman E, Harris R, Berry M (2005) Redundancy in the population code of the retina. *Neuron*, 46(3):493–504.

[56] Reich D, Victor J, Knight B (1998) The power ratio and the interval map: spiking models and extracellular recordings. *Journal of Neuroscience*, 18(23):10090–104.

[57] Reinagel P, Reid C (2000) Temporal coding of visual information in the thalamus. *Journal of Neuroscience*, 20:5392.

[58] Rieke F, Warland D, Bialek W, de Ruyter van Steveninck RR (1997) *Spikes: Exploring the Neural Code*. Cambridge, MA: MIT Press.

[59] Ruderman D, Bialek W (1994) Statistics of natural images: scaling in the woods. *Physical Review Letters*, 73(6):814–817.

[60] Rust N, Schwartz O, Movshon J, Simoncelli E (2005) Spatiotemporal elements of macaque v1 receptive fields. *Neuron*, pages 945–56.

[61] Sceniak MP, Ringach DL, Hawken MJ, Shapley R (1999) Contrast's effect on spatial summation by macaque v1 neurons. *Nature Neuroscience*, 2:733–739.

[62] Schneidman E, Bialek W, Berry MJ II. (2003) Synergy, redundancy, and independence in population codes. *Journal of Neuroscience*, 23(37):11539–53.

[63] Schneidman E, Still S, Berry MJ II., Bialek W (2003) Network information and connected correlations. *Physical Review Letters*, 91(23):238701.

[64] Schnitzer M, Meister M (2003) Multineuronal firing patterns in the signal from eye to brain. *Neuron*, 37(3):499–511.

[65] Schwartz O, Chichilnisky E, Simoncelli E (2002) Characterizing neural gain control using spike-triggered covariance. In Dieterich TG, Becker S, Ghahramani Z, eds., *Advances in Neural Information Processing Systems*, volume 14, pages 269–276.

[66] Shannon CE (1948) A mathematical theory of communication. *Bell System Technical Journal*, 27:379–423.

[67] Shannon CE (1948) A mathematical theory of communication. *Bell System Technical Journal*, 27:623–656.

[68] Shapley R, Victor J (1979) The contrast gain control of the cat retina. *Vision Research*, 19:431–434.

[69] Sharpee T, Rust N, Bialek W (2004) Analyzing neural responses to natural signals: maximally informative dimensions. *Neural Computation*, 16(2):223–50.

[70] Simoncelli E, Olshausen B (2001) Natural image statistics and neural representation. *Annual Review of Neuroscience*, 24:1193–214.

[71] Simoncelli E, Pillow J, Paninski L, Schwartz O (2004) Characterization of neural responses with stochastic stimuli. In Gazzaniga M, eds., *The Cognitive Neurosciences*, 3rd edition, Cambridge MA: MIT Press.

[72] Slee S, Higgs M, Fairhall A, Spain W (2005) Two-dimensional time coding in the auditory brainstem. *Journal of Neuroscience*, 25(43):9978–88.

[73] Smirnakis SM, Berry MJ II., Warland DK, Bialek W, Meister M (1997) Adaptation of retinal processing to image contrast and spatial scale. *Nature*, 386:69–73.

[74] Stanley G, Li F, Dan Y (1999) Reconstruction of natural scenes from ensemble responses in the lateral geniculate nucleus. *Journal of Neuroscience*, 19(18):8036–42.

[75] Strong S, Koberle R, de Ruyter van Stevenick R, Bialek W (1998) Entropy and information in neural spiketrains. *Physical Review Letters*, 80:197–200.

[76] Touryan J, Lau B, Dan Y (2002) Isolation of relevant visual features from random stimuli for cortical complex cells. *Journal of Neuroscience*, 22(24):10811–8.

[77] Treves A, Panzeri S (1995) The upward bias in measures of information derived from limited data samples. *Neural Computation*, 7:399–407.

[78] Truccolo W, Eden U, Fellows M, Donoghue J, Brown E (2005) A point process framework for relating neural spiking activity to spiking history, neural ensemble, and extrinsic covariate effects. *Journal of Neurophysiology*, 93(2):1074–89.

[79] van Hateren JH (1992) Theoretical predictions of spatiotemporal receptive fields of fly LMCs, and experimental validation. *Journal of Comparative Physiology A*, 171:157–170.

[80] Victor J (2002) Binless strategies for estimation of information from neural data. *Physical Review E*, 66(5):051903.

[81] Vinje W, Gallant J (2000) Sparse coding and decorrelation in primary visual cortex during natural vision. *Science*, 287(5456):1273–6.

[82] Wiener N (1958) *Time Series.* Cambridge MA: MIT Press.

3 Likelihood-Based Approaches to Modeling the Neural Code

Jonathan Pillow

One of the central problems in systems neuroscience is that of characterizing the functional relationship between sensory stimuli and neural spike responses. Investigators call this the *neural coding problem*, because the spike trains of neurons can be considered a code by which the brain represents information about the state of the external world. One approach to understanding this code is to build mathematical models of the mapping between stimuli and spike responses; the code can then be interpreted by using the model to predict the neural response to a stimulus, or to decode the stimulus that gave rise to a particular response. In this chapter, we will examine *likelihood-based* approaches, which use the explicit probability of response to a given stimulus for both fitting the model and assessing its validity. We will show how the likelihood can be derived for several types of neural models, and discuss theoretical considerations underlying the formulation and estimation of such models. Finally, we will discuss several ideas for evaluating model performance, including time-rescaling of spike trains and optimal decoding using Bayesian inversion of the likelihood function.

3.1 The Neural Coding Problem

Neurons exhibit stochastic variability. Even for repeated presentations of a fixed stimulus, a neuron's spike response cannot be predicted with certainty. Rather, the relationship between stimuli and neural responses is probabilistic. Understanding the neural code can therefore be framed as the problem of determining $p(y|x)$, the probability of response y conditional on a stimulus x. For a complete solution, we need to be able compute $p(y|x)$ for any x, meaning a description of the full response distribution for any stimulus we might present to a neuron. Unfortunately, we cannot hope to get very far trying to measure this distribution directly, due to the high dimensionality of stimulus space (e.g., the space of all natural images) and the finite duration of neurophysiology experiments. Figure 3.1 shows an illustration of the general problem.

A classical approach to the neural coding problem has been to restrict attention to a small, parametric family of stimuli (e.g., flashed dots, moving

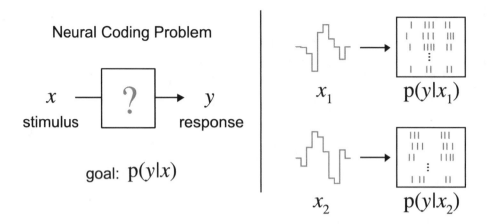

Figure 3.1 Illustration of the neural coding problem. The goal is to find a model mapping x to y that provides an accurate representation of the conditional distribution $p(y|x)$. Right: Simulated distribution of neural responses to two distinct stimuli, x_1 and x_2 illustrating (1) stochastic variability in responses to a single stimulus, and (2) that the response distribution changes as a function of x. A complete solution involves predicting $p(y|x)$ for any x.

bars, or drifting gratings). The motivation underlying this approach is the idea that neurons are sensitive only to a restricted set of *stimulus features*, and that we can predict the response to an arbitrary stimulus simply by knowing the response to these features. If $x_{\{\psi\}}$ denotes a parametric set of features to which a neuron modulates its response, then the classical approach posits that $p(y|x) \approx p(y|x_\psi)$, where x_ψ is the stimulus feature that most closely resembles x.

Although the "classical" approach to neural coding is not often explicitly framed in this way, it is not so different in principle from the "statistical modeling" approach that has gained popularity in recent years, and which we pursue here. In this framework, we assume a probabilistic model of the neural response, and attempt to fit the model parameters θ so that $p(y|x, \theta)$, the response probability under the model, provides a good approximation to $p(y|x)$. Although the statistical approach is often applied using stimuli drawn stochastically from a high-dimensional ensemble (e.g. Gaussian white noise) rather than a restricted parametric family (e.g. sine gratings), the goals are essentially similar: to find a simplified and computationally tractable description of $p(y|x)$. The statistical framework differs primarily in its emphasis on detailed quantitative prediction of spike responses, and in offering a unifying mathematical framework (likelihood) for fitting and validating models.

3.2 Model Fitting with Maximum Likelihood

Let us now turn to the problem of using likelihood for fitting a model of an individual neuron's response. Suppose we have a set of stimuli $\mathbf{x} = \{x_i\}$ and a set of spike responses $\mathbf{y} = \{y_i\}$ obtained during a neurophysiology experiment, and we would like to fit a model that captures the mapping from $\mathbf{x}$ to $\mathbf{y}$. Given a particular model, parametrized by the vector θ, we can apply a tool from classical statistics known as *maximum likelihood* to obtain an asymptotically optimal estimate of θ. For this, we need an algorithm for computing $p(\mathbf{y}|\mathbf{x}, \theta)$, which, considered as a function of θ, is called the *likelihood* of the data. The maximum likelihood (ML) estimate $\hat{\theta}$ is the set of parameters under which these data are most probable, or the maximizer of the likelihood function:

$$\hat{\theta} = \arg\max_{\theta} p(\mathbf{y}|\mathbf{x}, \theta). \tag{3.1}$$

Although this solution is easily stated, it is unfortunately the case that for many models of neural response (e.g. detailed biophysical models such as Hodgkin-Huxley) it is difficult or impossible to compute likelihood. Moreover, even when we can find simple algorithms for computing likelihood, maximizing it can be quite difficult; in most cases, θ lives in a high-dimensional space, containing tens to hundreds of parameters (e.g. describing a neuron's receptive field and spike-generation properties). Such nonlinear optimization problems are often intractable.

In the following sections, we will introduce several probabilistic neural spike models, derive the likelihood function for each model, and discuss the factors affecting ML estimation of its parameters. We will also compare ML with standard (e.g. moment-based) approaches to estimating model parameters.

3.2.1 The LNP Model

One of the best-known models of neural response is the linear-nonlinear-Poisson (LNP) model, which is alternately referred to as the linear-nonlinear "cascade" model. The model, which is schematized in the left panel of figure 3.2, consists of a linear filter (k), followed by a point nonlinearity (f), followed by Poisson spike generation. Although many interpretations are possible, a simple description of the model's components holds that:

- k represents the neuron's space-time receptive field, which describes how the stimulus is converted to intracellular voltage;

- f describes the conversion of voltage to an instantaneous spike rate, accounting for such nonlinearities as rectification and saturation;

- instantaneous rate is converted to a spike train via an inhomogeneous Poisson process.

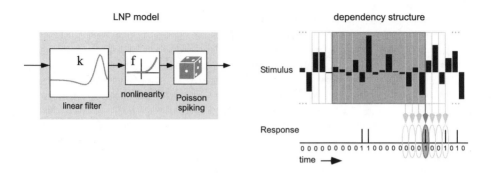

Figure 3.2 Schematic and dependency structure of the linear-nonlinear-Poisson model. Left: LNP model consists of a linear filter k, followed by a point nonlinearity f, followed by Poisson spike generation. Right: Depiction of a discretized white noise Gaussian stimulus (above) and spike response (below). Arrows indicate the causal dependency entailed by the model between portions of the stimulus and portions of the response. The highlighted gray box and gray oval show this dependence for a single time bin of the response, while gray boxes and arrows indicate the (time-shifted) dependency for neighboring bins of the response. As indicated by the diagram, all time bins of the response are conditionally independent given the stimulus (equation (3.2)).

The parameters of this model can be written as $\theta = \{k, \phi_f\}$, where ϕ_f are the parameters governing f. Although the LNP model is not biophysically realistic (especially the assumption of Poisson spiking), it provides a compact and reasonably accurate description of average responses, e.g., peri-stimulus time histogram (PSTH), in many early sensory areas.

Another reason for the popularity of the LNP model is the existence of a simple and computationally efficient fitting algorithm, which consists in using spike-triggered average (STA) as an estimate for k and a simple histogram procedure to estimate ϕ_f (see [6, 8]). It is a well-known result that the STA (or "reverse correlation") gives an unbiased estimate of the direction of k (i.e. the STA converges to αk, for some unknown α) if the raw stimulus distribution $p(x)$ is spherically symmetric, and f shifts the mean of the spike-triggered ensemble away from zero (i.e. the expected STA is not the zero vector) [7, 15]. However, the STA does *not* generally provide an optimal estimate of k, except in a special case we will examine in more detail below [16].

First, we derive the likelihood function of the LNP model. The right panel of figure 3.2 shows the dependency structure (also known as a graphical model) between stimulus and response, where arrows indicate conditional dependence. For this model, the bins of the response are conditionally independent of one another given the stimulus, an essential feature of Poisson processes, which means that the probability of the entire spike train factorizes as

$$p(\mathbf{y}|\mathbf{x}, \theta) = \prod_i p(y_i|x_i, \theta), \qquad\qquad (3.2)$$

where y_i is the spike count in the ith time bin, and x_i is the stimulus vector causally associated with this bin. Equation (3.2) asserts that the likelihood of the entire spike train is the product of the single-bin likelihoods. Under this model, single-bin likelihood is given by the Poisson distribution with rate parameter $\Delta f(k \cdot x_i)$, where $k \cdot x_i$, is the dot product of k with x_i and Δ is the width of the time bin. The probability of having y_i spikes in the ith bin is therefore

$$p(y_i|x_i, \theta) = \frac{1}{y_i!} \left[\Delta f(k \cdot x_i)\right]^{y_i} e^{-\Delta f(k \cdot x_i)}, \tag{3.3}$$

and the likelihood of the entire spike train can be rewritten as:

$$p(\mathbf{y}|\mathbf{x}, \theta) = \Delta^n \prod_i \frac{f(k \cdot x_i)^{y_i}}{y_i!} e^{-\Delta f(k \cdot x_i)}, \tag{3.4}$$

where n is the total number of spikes.

We can find the ML estimate $\hat{\theta} = \{\hat{k}, \hat{\phi}_f\}$ by maximizing the log of the likelihood function (which is monotonically related to likelihood), and given by

$$\log p(\mathbf{y}|\mathbf{x}, \theta) = \sum_i y_i \log f(k \cdot x_i) - \Delta \sum_i f(k \cdot x_i) + c, \tag{3.5}$$

where c is a constant that does not depend on k or f. Because there is an extra degree of freedom between the amplitude of k and input scaling of f, we can constrain k to be a unit vector, and consider only the angular error in estimating k. By differentiating the log-likelihood with respect to k and setting it to zero, we find that the ML estimate satisfies:

$$\lambda \hat{k} = \sum_i y_i \frac{f'(\hat{k} \cdot x_i)}{f(\hat{k} \cdot x_i)} x_i - \Delta \sum_i f'(\hat{k} \cdot x_i) x_i, \tag{3.6}$$

where λ is a Lagrange multiplier introduced to constrain k to be a unit vector. As noted in [16], the second term on the right hand converges to a vector proportional to k if the stimulus distribution $p(x)$ is spherically symmetric. (It is the expectation over $p(x)$ of a function radially symmetric around k.) If we replace this term by its expectation, we are left with just the first term, which is a weighted STA, since y_i is the spike count and x_i is the stimulus preceding the ith bin. This term is proportional to the (ordinary) STA if f'/f is constant, which occurs only when $f(z) = e^{az+b}$.

Therefore, the STA corresponds to the ML estimate for k whenever f is exponential; conversely, if f differs significantly from exponential, equation (3.6) specifies a different weighting of the spike-triggered stimuli, and the traditional STA is suboptimal. Figure 3.3 illustrates this point with a comparison between the STA and the ML estimate for k on spike trains simulated using three different nonlinearities. In the simulations, we found the ML estimate by directly maximizing log-likelihood (equation (3.5)) for both k and ϕ_f, beginning with the STA as an initial estimate for k. As expected, the ML estimate outperforms the STA except when f is exponential (rightmost column).

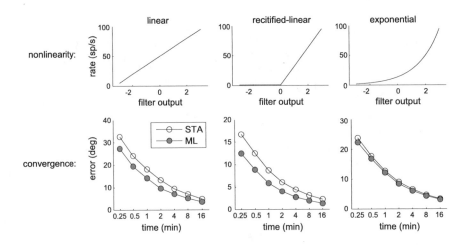

Figure 3.3 Comparison of spike-triggered average (STA) and maximum likelihood (ML) estimates of the linear filter k in an LNP model. Top row: three different types of nonlinearity f: a linear function (left), a half-wave rectified linear function (middle), and an exponential. For each model, the true k was a 20-tap temporal filter with biphasic shape similar to that found in retinal ganglion cells. The stimulus was temporal Gaussian white noise with a frame rate of 100 Hz, and k was normalized so that filter output had unit standard deviation. Bottom row: Plots show the convergence behavior for each model, as a function of the amount of data collected. Error is computed as the angle between the estimate and the true k, averaged over 100 repeats at each stimulus length.

Figure 3.4 shows a similar analysis comparing ML to an estimator derived from spike-triggered covariance (STC) analysis, which uses the principal eigenvector of the STC matrix to estimate k. Recent work has devoted much attention to fitting LNP models with STC analysis, which is relevant particularly in cases where the f is approximately symmetric [10, 22, 26, 1, 25, 3, 23]. The left column of figure 3.4 shows a simulation where f is a quadratic, shifted slightly from the origin so that both the STA and the first eigenvector of the STC provide consistent (asymptotically convergent) estimates of k. Both, however, are significantly outperformed by the ML estimator. Although it is beyond the scope of this chapter, a derivation similar to the one above shows that there is an f for which the ML estimator and the STC estimate are identical. The relevant f is a *quadratic* in the argument of an exponential, which can also be represented as a ratio of two Gaussians (see [20] for a complete discussion). The right column of figure 3.4 shows results obtained with such a nonlinearity. If we used a similar nonlinearity in which the first term of the quadratic is negative, e.g. $f(x) = \exp(-x^2)$, then f produces a reduction in variance along k, and the STC eigenvector with the *smallest* eigenvalue is comparable to the ML estimate [20].

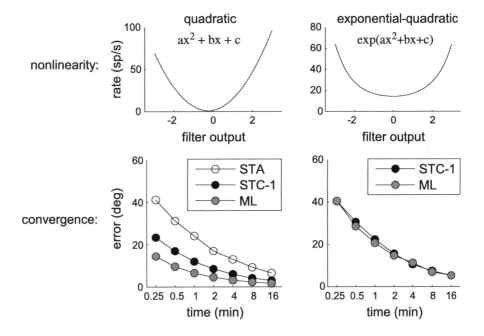

Figure 3.4   Comparison of STA, STC, and ML estimates k in an LNP model. Top row: Two types of nonlinearity functions used to generate responses; a quadratic function (left), a quadratic raised to an exponential (right). Stimulus and true k as in figure 3.3. Bottom row: Convergence behavior of the STA, first (maximum-variance) eigenvector of the STC, and ML estimate. The STA is omitted from the right plot, as it fails to converge under a symmetric nonlinearity.

Before closing this section, it is useful to review several other general characteristics of ML estimation in LNP models. Firstly, note that the LNP model can be generalized to include multiple linear filters and a multidimensional nonlinearity, all of which can be fit using ML. In this case, the likelihood function is the same as in equation (3.4), only the instantaneous spike rate is now given by:

$$\text{rate}(x_i) = f(k_1 \cdot x_i, k_2 \cdot x_i, \ldots, k_m \cdot x_i), \tag{3.7}$$

where $\{k_1, k_2, \ldots, k_m\}$ is a collection of filters and f is an m-dimensional point nonlinearity. Secondly, ML estimation of the LNP model enjoys the same statistical advantages as several information-theoretic estimators that have been derived for finding "maximally informative dimensions" or features of the stimulus space [15, 24]. Specifically, the ML estimator is unbiased even when the raw stimulus distribution lacks spherical symmetry (e.g. "naturalistic stimuli") and it is sensitive to higher-order statistics of the spike-triggered ensemble, making it somewhat more powerful and more general than STA or STC analysis. Unfortunately, ML also shares the disadvantages of these information-theoretic estimators: it is computationally intensive, difficult to use for recovering multiple (e.g. > 2) filters (in part due to the difficulty of choosing an appropriate parametrization for f), and cannot be guaranteed to converge to the true maximum using gradient ascent, due to the existence of multiple local maxima in the likelihood function.

We address this last shortcoming in the next two sections, which discuss models constructed to have likelihood functions that are free from sub-optimal local maxima. These models also introduce dependence of the response on spike-train history, eliminating a second major shortcoming of the LNP model, the assumption of Poisson spike generation.

3.2.2 Generalized Linear Model

The generalized linear model (or GLM), schematized in figure 3.5, generalizes the LNP model to incorporate feedback from the spiking process, allowing the model to account for history-dependent properties of neural spike trains such as the refractory period, adaptation, and bursting [16, 27]. As shown in the dependency diagram (right panel of figure 3.5), the responses in distinct time bins are no longer conditionally independent given the stimulus; rather, each bin of the response depends on some time window of the recent spiking activity. Luckily, this does not prevent us from factorizing the likelihood, which can now be written

$$p(\mathbf{y}|\mathbf{x}, \theta) = \prod_i p(y_i|x_i, y_{[i-k\,:\,i-1]}, \theta), \qquad (3.8)$$

where $y_{[i-k\,:\,i-1]}$ is the vector of recent spiking activity from time bin $i - k$ to $i - 1$. This factorization holds because, by Bayes' rule, we have

$$p(y_i, y_{[i-k\,:\,i-1]}|\mathbf{x}, \theta) = p(y_i|y_{[i-k\,:\,i-1]}, \mathbf{x}, \theta)p(y_{[i-k\,:\,i-1]}|\mathbf{x}, \theta), \qquad (3.9)$$

and we can apply this formula recursively to obtain equation (3.8). (Note, however, that no such factorization is possible if we allow loopy, e.g. bidirectional, causal dependence between time bins of the response.)

Except for the addition of a linear filter, h, operating on the neuron's spike-train history, the GLM is identical to the LNP model. We could therefore call it the "recurrent LNP" model, although its output is no longer a Poisson process, due to the history-dependence induced by h. The GLM likelihood function is similar to that of the LNP model. If we let

$$r_i = f(k \cdot x_i + h \cdot y_{[i-k\,:\,i-1]}) \qquad (3.10)$$

denote the instantaneous spike rate (or "conditional intensity" of the process), then the likelihood and log-likelihood, following equation (3.4) and (3.5), are

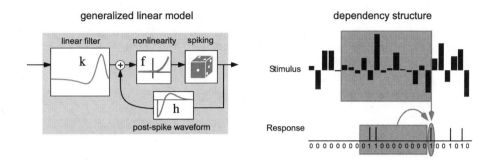

Figure 3.5   Diagram and dependency structure of a generalized linear model. Left: Model schematic, showing the introduction of history-dependence in the model via a feedback waveform from the spiking process. In order to ensure convexity of the negative log-likelihood, we now assume that the nonlinearity f is exponential. Right: Graphical model of the conditional dependencies in the GLM. The instantaneous spike rate depends on both the recent stimulus and recent history of spiking.

given by:

$$p(\mathbf{y}|\mathbf{x}, \theta) \quad = \quad \Delta^n \prod_i \frac{r_i^{y_i}}{y_i!} e^{-\Delta r_i} \tag{3.11}$$

$$\log p(\mathbf{y}|\mathbf{x}, \theta) \quad = \quad \sum_i y_i \log r_i - \Delta \sum_i r_i + c. \tag{3.12}$$

Unfortunately, we cannot use moment-based estimators (STA and STC) to estimate k and h for this model, because the consistency of those estimators relies on spherical symmetry of the input (or Gaussianity, for STC), which the spike-history input term $y_{[i-k\,:\,i-1]}$ fails to satisfy [15].

As mentioned above, a significant shortcoming of the ML approach to neural characterization is that it may be quite difficult in practice to find the maximum of the likelihood function. Gradient ascent fails if the likelihood function is rife with local maxima, and more robust optimization techniques (like simulated annealing) are computationally exorbitant and require delicate oversight to ensure convergence.

One solution to this problem is to constrain the model so that we guarantee that the likelihood function is free from (non-global) local maxima. If we can show that the likelihood function is *log-concave*, meaning that the negative log-likelihood function is convex, then we can be assured that the only maxima are global maxima. Moreover, the problem of computing the ML estimate $\hat{\theta}$ is reduced to a convex optimization problem, for which there are tractable algorithms even in very high-dimensional spaces.

As shown by [16], the GLM has a concave log-likelihood function if the nonlinearity f is itself convex and log-concave. These conditions are satisfied if the second-derivative of f is non-negative and the second-derivative of $\log f$

is non-positive. Although this may seem like a restrictive set of conditions—it rules out symmetric nonlinearities, for example—a number of suitable functions seem like reasonable choices for describing the conversion of intracellular voltage to instantaneous spike rate, for example:

- $f(z) = \max(z + b, 0)$
- $f(z) = e^{z+b}$
- $f(z) = \log(1 + e^{z+b})$,

where b is a single parameter that we also estimate with ML.

Thus, for appropriate choice of f, ML estimation of a GLM becomes computationally tractable. Moreover, the GLM framework is quite general, and can easily be expanded to include additional linear filters that capture dependence on spiking activity in nearby neurons, behavior of the organism, or additional external covariates of spiking activity. ML estimation of a GLM has been successfully applied to the analysis of neural spike trains in a variety of sensory, motor, and memory-related brain areas [9, 27, 14, 19].

3.2.3   Generalized Integrate-and-Fire Model

We now turn our attention to a dynamical-systems model of the neural response, for which the likelihood of a spike train is not so easily formulated in terms of a conditional intensity function (i.e. the instantaneous probability of spiking, conditional on stimulus and spike-train history). Recent work has shown that the leaky integrate-and-fire (IF) model, a canonical but simplified description of intracellular spiking dynamics, can reproduce the spiking statistics of real neurons [21, 13] and can mimic important dynamical behaviors of more complicated models like Hodgkin-Huxley [11, 12]. It is therefore natural to ask whether likelihood-based methods can be applied to models of this type.

Figure 3.6 shows a schematic diagram of the generalized IF model [16, 18], which is a close relative of the well-known spike response model [12]. The model generalizes the classical IF model so that injected current is a linear function of the stimulus and spike-train history, plus a Gaussian noise current that introduces a probability distribution over voltage trajectories. The model dynamics (written here in discrete time, for consistency) are given by

$$\frac{v_{i+1} - v_i}{\Delta} = -\frac{1}{\tau}(v_i - v_L) + (k \cdot x_i) + (h \cdot y_{[i-k\,:\,i-1]}) + \sigma \mathcal{N}_i \Delta^{-\frac{1}{2}}, \qquad (3.13)$$

where v_i is the voltage at the ith time bin, which obeys the boundary condition that whenever $v_i \geq 1$, a spike occurs and v_i is reset instantaneously to zero. Δ is the width of the time bin of the simulation, and $\mathcal{N}_i$ is a standard Gaussian random variable, drawn independently on each i. The model parameters k and h are the same as in the GLM: linear filters operating on the stimulus and spike-train history (respectively), and the remaining parameters are: τ, the time constant of the membrane leak; v_L, the leak current reversal potential; and σ, the amplitude of the noise.

generalized IF model

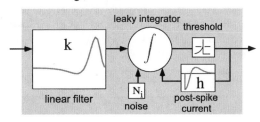

---

dependency structure

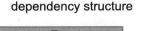

likelihood of a single ISI

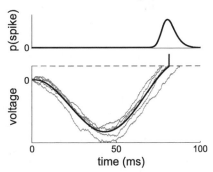

Figure 3.6   Generalized integrate-and-fire model. Top: Schematic diagram of model components, including a stimulus filter k and a post-spike current h that is injected into a leaky integrator following every spike, and independent Gaussian noise to account for response variability. Bottom left: Graphical model of dependency structure, showing that the likelihood of each interspike interval (ISI) is conditionally dependent on a portion of the stimulus and spike-train history prior to the interspike interval (ISI). Bottom right: Schematic illustrating how likelihood could be computed with Monte Carlo sampling. Black trace shows the voltage (and spike time) from simulating the model without noise, while gray traces show sample voltage paths (to the first spike time) with noise. The likelihood of the ISI is shown above, as a function of the spike time (black trace). Likelihood of an ISI is equal to the fraction of voltage paths crossing threshold at the true spike time.

The lower left panel of figure 3.6 depicts the dependency structure of the model as it pertains to computing the likelihood of a spike train. In this case, we can regard the probability of an entire interspike interval (ISI) as depending on a relevant portion of the stimulus and spike-train history. The lower right panel shows an illustration of how we might compute this likelihood for a single ISI under the generalized GIF model using Monte Carlo sampling. Computing the likelihood in this case is also known as the "first-passage time" problem. Given a setting of the model parameters, we can sample voltage trajectories from the model, drawing independent noise samples for each trajectory, and following each trajectory until it hits threshold. The gray traces show show five such sample paths, while the black trace shows the voltage path obtained in the absence of noise. The probability of a spike occurring at the ith bin is simply the fraction of voltage paths crossing threshold at this bin. The black trace (above) shows the probability distribution obtained by collecting the first passage times of a large number of paths. Evaluated at the actual spike, this density gives the likelihood of the relevant ISI. Because of voltage reset following a spike, all ISIs are conditionally independent, and we can again write the likelihood function as a product of conditionally independent terms:

$$p(\mathbf{y}|\mathbf{x}, \theta) = \prod_{t_j} p(y_{[t_{j-1}+1 \, : \, t_j]}|\mathbf{x}, y_{[0 \, : \, t_j]}, \theta), \qquad (3.14)$$

where $\{t_j\}$ is the set of spike times emitted by the neuron, $y_{[t_{j-1}+1 \, : \, t_j]}$ is the response in the set of time bins in the jth ISI, and $y_{[0 \, : \, t_j]}$ is the response during time bins previous to that interval.

The Monte Carlo approach to computing likelihood of a spike train can in principle be performed for any probabilistic dynamical-systems style model. In practice, however, such an approach would be unbearably slow and would likely prove intractable, particularly since the likelihood function must be computed many times in order find the ML estimate for θ. However, for the generalized IF model there exists a much more computationally efficient method for computing the likelihood function using the Fokker-Planck equation. Although beyond the scope of this chapter, the method works by "density propagation" of a numerical representation of the probability density over subthreshold voltage, which can be quickly computed using sparse matrix methods. More importantly, a recent result shows that the log-likelihood function for the generalized IF model, like that of the GLM, is concave. This means that the likelihood function contains a unique global maximum, and that gradient ascent can be used to find the ML estimate of the model parameters (see [17] for a more thorough discussion). Recent work has applied the generalized IF model to the responses of macaque retinal ganglion cells using ML, showing that it can be used to capture stimulus dependence, spike-history dependence, and noise statistics of neural responses recorded *in vitro* [18].

3.3   Model Validation

Once we have a used maximum likelihood to fit a particular model to a set of neural data, there remains the important task of validating the quality of the model fit. In this section, we discuss three simple methods for assessing the goodness-of-fit of a probabilistic model using the same statistical framework that motivated our approach to fitting.

3.3.1 Likelihood-Based Cross-Validation

Recall that the basic goal of our approach is to find a probabilistic model such that we can approximate the true probabilistic relationship between stimulus and response, $p(y|x)$, by the model-dependent $p(y|x, \theta)$. Once we have fit θ using a set of training data, how can we tell if the model provides a good description of $p(y|x)$? To begin with, let us suppose that we have two competing models, p_A and p_B, parametrized by θ_A and θ_B, respectively, and we wish to decide which model provides a better description of the data. Unfortunately, we cannot simply compare the likelihood of the data under the two models, $p_A(\mathbf{y}|\mathbf{x}, \theta_A)$ vs. $p_B(\mathbf{y}|\mathbf{x}, \theta_B)$, due to the problem of *overfitting*. Even though one model assigns the fitted data a higher likelihood than the other, it may not generalize as well to new data.

As a toy example of the phenomenon of overfitting, consider a data set consisting of 5 points drawn from a Gaussian distribution. Let model A be a single Gaussian, fit with the mean and standard deviation of the sample points (i.e. the ML estimate for this model). For model B, suppose that the data come from a mixture of five *very* narrow Gaussians, and fit this model by centering one of these narrow Gaussians at each of the 5 sample points. Clearly, the second model assigns higher likelihood to the data (because it concentrates all probability mass near the sample points), but it fails to generalize–it will assign very low probability to new data points drawn from the true distribution which do not happen to lie very near the five original samples.

This suggests a general solution to the problem of comparing models, which goes by the name *cross-validation*. Under this procedure, we generate a new set of "test" stimuli, $\mathbf{x}^*$ and present them to the neuron to obtain a new set of spike responses $\mathbf{y}^*$. (Alternatively, we could set aside a small portion of the data at the beginning.) By comparing the likelihood of these new data sets under the two models, $p_A(\mathbf{y}^*|\mathbf{x}^*, \theta_A)$ vs. $p_B(\mathbf{y}^*|\mathbf{x}^*, \theta_B)$, we get a fair test of the models' generalization performance. Note that, under this comparison, we do not actually care about the number of parameters in the two models: increasing the number of parameters in a model does *not* improve its ability to generalize. (In the toy example above, model B has more parameters but generalizes much more poorly. We can view techniques like regularization as methods for reducing the effective number of parameters in a model so that overfitting does not occur.) Although we may prefer a model with fewer parameters for aesthetic or computational reasons, from a statistical standpoint we care only about which model provides a better account of the novel data.

3.3.2 Time-Rescaling

Another powerful idea for testing validity of a probabilistic model is to use the model to convert spike times into a series of i.i.d. random variables. This conversion will only be successful if we have accurately modeled the probability distribution of each spike time. This idea, which goes under the name *time-rescaling* [5], is a specific application of the general result that we can convert any random variable into a uniform random variable using its cumulative density function (CDF).

First, let us derive the CDF of a spike time under the LNP and GLM models. If r_i is the conditional intensity function of the ith time bin (i.e. $f(k \cdot x_i)$ under the LNP model), then the probability that the "next" spike t_{j+1} occurs on or before bin k, given that the previous spike occurred at t_j, is simply 1 minus the probability that no spikes occur during the time bins $t_j + 1$ to k. This gives

$$p(t_{j+1} \leq k|t_j) = 1 - \left(\prod_{i \in [t_j+1,k]} e^{-\Delta r_i} \right) \tag{3.15}$$

which we can rewrite:

$$p(t_{j+1} \leq k|t_j) = 1 - \exp\left(-\Delta \sum_{t_j+1}^{k} r_i \right) \tag{3.16}$$

Note that the argument of the exponential is simply the negative integral of the intensity function since the time of the previous spike.

For the generalized IF model, computing the likelihood function involves computing the probability density function (PDF) over each interspike interval (as depicted in figure 3.6), which we can simply integrate to obtain the CDF [17].

Given the CDF for a random variable, a general result from probability theory holds that it provides a remapping of that variable to the one randomly distributed unit interval $[0, 1]$. Even though the CDF for each spike time is different, if we remap the entire spike train using $t_j \longrightarrow CDF_j(t_j)$, where CDF_j is the cumulative density of the jth spike time, then, if the model is correct, we should obtain a series of independent, uniform random variables. This suggests we test the validity of the model by testing the remapped spike times for independence; any correlation (or some other form of dependence) between successive pairs of remapped spike times (for example), indicates a failure of the model. We can also examine the marginal distribution of the remapped times (using a K-S test, for example) to detect deviations from uniformity. The structure of any deviations may be useful for understanding the model's failure modes: an excess of small-valued samples, for example, indicates that the model predicts too few short interspike intervals. If we wish to compare multiple models, we can use time-rescaling to examine which model produces the most nearly independent and most nearly uniform remapped spike times.

3.3.3   Model-Based Decoding

A third tool for assessing the validity of a probabilistic model is to perform stimulus decoding using the model-based likelihood function. Given the fitted model parameters, we can derive the *posterior* probability distribution over the stimulus given a spike train by inverting the likelihood function with Bayes' rule:

$$p(\mathbf{x}|\mathbf{y}, \theta) = \frac{p(\mathbf{y}|\mathbf{x}, \theta)p(\mathbf{x})}{p(\mathbf{y}|\theta)}, \tag{3.17}$$

where $p(x)$ is the prior probability of the stimulus (which we assume to be independent of θ), and the denominator is the probability of response y given θ. We can obtain the most likely stimulus to have generated the response y by maximizing the posterior for x, which gives the maximum a posteriori (MAP) estimate of the stimulus, which we can denote

$$\hat{\mathbf{x}}_{MAP} = \arg\max_{\mathbf{x}} p(\mathbf{y}|\mathbf{x}, \theta)p(\mathbf{x}) \tag{3.18}$$

since the denominator term $p(\mathbf{y}|\theta)$ does not vary with x.

For the GLM and generalized IF models, the concavity of the log-likelihood function with respect to the model parameters also extends to the posterior with respect to the stimulus, since the stimulus interacts linearly with model parameters k. Concavity of the log-posterior holds so long as the prior $p(\mathbf{x})$ is itself log-concave (e.g. Gaussian, or any distribution of the form $\alpha e^{-(x/\sigma)^\gamma}$, with $\gamma \geq 1$). This means that, for both of these two models, we can perform MAP decoding of the stimulus using simple gradient ascent of the posterior.

If we wish to perform decoding with a specified loss function, for example, mean-squared error, optimal decoding can be achieved with Bayesian estimation, which is given by the estimator with minimum expected loss. In the case of mean-squared error, this estimator is given by

$$\hat{\mathbf{x}}_{Bayes} = E[\mathbf{x}|\mathbf{y}, \theta], \tag{3.19}$$

which is the conditional expectation of x, or the mean of the posterior distribution over stimuli. Computing this estimate, however, requires sampling from the posterior distribution, which is difficult to perform without advanced statistical sampling techniques, and is a topic of ongoing research.

Considered more generally, decoding provides an important test of model validity, and it allows us to ask different questions about the nature of the neural code. Even though it may not be a task carried out explicitly in the brain, decoding allows us to measure how well a particular model preserves the stimulus-related information in the neural response. This is a subtle point, but one worth considering: we can imagine a model that performs worse under cross-validation or time-rescaling analyses, but performs better at decoding, and therefore gives a better account of the stimulus-related information that is conveyed to the brain. For example, consider a model that fails to account for the refractory period (e.g. an LNP model), but which gives a slightly better description of the stimulus-related probability of spiking. This model assigns non-zero probability to spike trains that violate the refractory period, thereby "wasting" probability mass on spike trains whose probability is actually zero, and performing poorly under cross-validation. The model also performs poorly under time-rescaling, due to the fact that it over-predicts spike rate during the refractory period. However, when decoding a *real* spike train, we do not encounter violations of the refractory period, and the "wasted" probability mass affects only the normalizing term $p(\mathbf{y}|\theta)$. Here, the model's improved accuracy in predicting the stimulus-related spiking activity leads to a posterior that is more reliably centered around the true stimulus. Thus, even though the model fails to reproduce certain statistical features of the response, it provides a valuable tool for assessing what information the spike train carries about the stimulus, and gives a perhaps more valuable description of the neural code. Decoding may therefore serve as an important tool for validating likelihood-based models, and a variety of exact or approximate likelihood-based techniques for neural decoding have been explored [28, 4, 2, 18].

3.4   Summary

We have shown how to compute likelihood and perform ML fitting of several types of probabilistic neural models. In simulations, we have shown that ML outperforms traditional moment-based estimators (STA and STC) when the nonlinear function of filter output does not have a particular exponential form. We have also discussed models whose log-likelihood functions are provably concave, making ML estimation possible even in high-dimensional parameter spaces and with non-Gaussian stimuli. These models can also be extended to incorporate dependence on spike-train history and external covariates of the neural response, such as spiking activity in nearby neurons. We have examined several statistical approaches to validating the performance of a neural model, which allow us to decide which models to use and to assess how well they describe the neural code.

In addition to the insight they provide into the neural code, the models we have described may be useful for simulating realistic input to downstream brain regions, and in practical applications such as neural prosthetics. The theoretical and statistical tools that we have described here, as well as the vast computational resources that make them possible, are still a quite recent development in the history of theoretical neuroscience. Understandably, their achievements are still quite modest: we are some ways from a "complete" model that predicts responses to *any* stimulus (e.g., incorporating the effects of spatial and multi-scale temporal adaptation, network interactions, and feedback). There remains much work to be done both in building more powerful and accurate models of neural responses, and in extending these models (perhaps in cascades) to the responses of neurons in brain areas more deeply removed from the periphery.

References

[1] Aguera y Arcas B, Fairhall AL (2003) What causes a neuron to spike? *Neural Computation*, 15(8):1789–1807.

[2] Barbieri R, Frank L, Nguyen D, Quirk M, Solo V, Wilson M, Brown E (2004) Dynamic Analyses of Information Encoding in Neural Ensembles. *Neural Computation*, 16:277–307.

[3] Bialek W, de Ruyter van Steveninck R (2005) Features and dimensions: motion estimation in fly vision. *Quantitative Biology, Neurons and Cognition*, arXiv:q-bio.NC/0505003.

[4] Brown E, Frank L, Tang D, Quirk M, Wilson M (1998) A statistical paradigm for neural spike train decoding applied to position prediction from ensemble firing patterns of rat hippocampal place cells. *Journal of Neuroscience*, 18:7411–7425.

[5] Brown E, Barbieri R, Ventura V, Kass R, Frank L (2002) The time-rescaling theorem and its application to neural spike train data analysis. *Neural Computation*, 14:325–346, 2002.

[6] Bryant H, Segundo J (1976) Spike initiation by transmembrane current: a white-noise analysis. *Journal of Physiology*, 260:279–314.

[7] Bussgang J (1952) Crosscorrelation functions of amplitude-distorted gaussian signals. *RLE Technical Reports*, 216.

[8] Chichilnisky EJ (2001) A simple white noise analysis of neuronal light responses. *Network: Computation in Neural Systems*, 12:199–213.

[9] Chornoboy E, Schramm L, Karr A (1988) Maximum likelihood identification of neural point process systems. *Biological Cybernetics*, 59:265–275.

[10] de Ruyter van Steveninck R, Bialek W (1988) Real-time performance of a movement-senstivive neuron in the blowfly visual system: coding and information transmission in short spike sequences. *Proceedings of Royal Society of London, B*, 234:379–414.

[11] Gerstner W, Kistler W (2002) *Spiking Neuron Models: Single Neurons, Populations, Plasticity*. Cambridge, UK: University Press.

[12] Jolivet R, Lewis T, Gerstner W (2003) The spike response model: a framework to predict neuronal spike trains. *Springer Lecture Notes in Computer Science*, 2714:846–853.

[13] Keat J, Reinagel P, Reid R, Meister M (2001) Predicting every spike: a model for the responses of visual neurons. *Neuron*, 30:803–817.

[14] Okatan M, Wilson M, Brown E (2005) Analyzing Functional Connectivity Using a Network Likelihood Model of Ensemble Neural Spiking Activity. *Neural Computation*, 17:1927–1961.

[15] Paninski L (2003) Convergence properties of some spike-triggered analysis techniques. *Network: Computation in Neural Systems*, 14:437–464.

[16] Paninski L (2004) Maximum likelihood estimation of cascade point-process neural encoding models. *Network: Computation in Neural Systems*, 15:243–262.

[17] Paninski L, Pillow J, Simoncelli E (2004) Maximum likelihood estimation of a stochastic integrate-and-fire neural model. *Neural Computation*, 16:2533–2561.

[18] Pillow JW, Paninski L, Uzzell VJ, Simoncelli EP, Chichilnisky EJ (2005) Prediction and decoding of retinal ganglion cell responses with a probabilistic spiking model. *Journal of Neuroscience*, 25:11003–11013.

[19] Pillow JW, Shlens J, Paninski L, Chichilnisky EJ, Simoncelli EP (2005) Modeling the correlated spike responses of a cluster of primate retinal ganglion cells. *SFN Abstracts*, 591.3.

[20] Pillow JW, Simoncelli EP (2006)   Dimensionality reduction in neural models: an information-theoretic generalization of spike-triggered average and covariance analysis. *Journal of Vision*, 6(4):414–428.

[21] Reich DS, Victor JD, Knight BW (1998) The power ratio and the interval map: spiking models and extracellular recordings. *Journal of Neuroscience*, 18:10090–10104.

[22] Schwartz O, Chichilnisky EJ, Simoncelli EP (2002) Characterizing neural gain control using spike-triggered covariance. In T G Dietterich, S Becker, and Z Ghahramani, editors, *Advances in Neural Information Processing Systems*, volume 14, Cambridge, MA: MIT Press.

[23] Schwartz O, Pillow JW, Rust NC, Simoncelli EP (2006) Spike-triggered neural characterization. *Journal of Vision*, 6(4):484–507.

[24] Sharpee T, Rust N, Bialek W (2004) Analyzing neural responses to natural signals: maximally informative dimensions. *Neural Computation*, 16:223–250.

[25] Simoncelli E, Paninski L, Pillow J, Schwartz O (2004) Characterization of neural responses with stochastic stimuli. In M. Gazzaniga, editor, *The Cognitive Neurosciences*, 3rd edition, Cambridge, MA: MIT Press.

[26] Touryan J, Lau B, Dan Y (2002) Isolation of relevant visual features from random stimuli for cortical complex cells. *Journal of Neuroscience*, 22:10811–10818.

[27] Truccolo W, Eden UT, Fellows MR, Donoghue JP, Brown EN (2004) A point process framework for relating neural spiking activity to spiking history, neural ensemble and extrinsic covariate effects. *Journal of Neurophysiology*, 93(2):1074–1089.

[28] Warland D, Reinagel P, Meister M (1997) Decoding visual information from a population retinal ganglion cells. *Journal of Neurophysiology*, 78:2336–2350.

4 Combining Order Statistics with Bayes Theorem for Millisecond-by-Millisecond Decoding of Spike Trains

Barry J. Richmond and Matthew C. Wiener

4.1 Introduction

Although it has been possible for many decades to measure the responses of single neurons, and more recently has become possible to record the responses of small populations of neurons, the principles through which higher brain functions arise from the activity of neuronal populations are still unknown. In some invertebrates, it is possible to record neuronal activity as it crosses synaptic layers [17], thereby providing data to assess the signal transformations taking place. This is not yet possible in vertebrates, so research has progressed using a convenient, if somewhat impoverished, metaphor regarding the brain as an information-processing machine with neurons as processing elements [5]. This metaphor makes it natural to use signal processing tools and information theory to characterize both neuronal and brain function. Frequently, candidate neural codes are evaluated by seeing how much information observed trains might carry if interpreted using the different codes, and codes that provide greater information transfer are taken to be more plausible. Other work has focused on how well a decoder could interpret the signals from either single neurons or small populations, primarily in sensory and motor areas, to recover the stimulus giving rise to a particular response.

Because neuronal responses are frequently quite variable (figures 4.1 and 4.2), statistical tools must be used for their analysis. One technique from statistical processing that has been heavily used over the past two decades is information theory. Shannon's information theory was created to analyze artificial communications systems, but shortly after its introduction information theory became a tool for analyzing brain and neuronal functions [5, 12, 13, 42]. Features that make information theory appealing to quantify neural signals are that it accounts for relations among elements in extended codes (codes with more than one element in the code word), such as correlation, and it is formulated in terms of probability distributions without assumptions about the form of the probability distributions. This latter property is helpful because the probability distributions from which neural responses are drawn have generally not been clearly known. The difficulty with information theoretical approaches is that the needed conditional probability distributions – the probability of the response given the stimulus, and the stimulus given the response – can be difficult to estimate accurately. The issues related to these estimation difficulties should not be overlooked but are beyond the scope of this presentation.

The goal of the work described here is to develop a compact description of the statistics of single neuronal spike trains, in the hope that such descriptions instantiate knowledge of basic relationships. In this vein, below we make a few simple assumptions and use them as the basis to develop an approach to decoding single (with generalization multiple) spike trains as time evolves. We make the assumptions explicit so that it can be straightforward to estimate whether any particular data set meets them.

4.2   An Approach to Decoding

Using information theory, it is possible to estimate how much less uncertainty there is about which stimulus was presented if we know the neural response elicited by that stimulus. Thus, a very important use of information theory has been to identify representations of neural responses that carry information about the stimulus, and whether the information is redundant with other representations. The usual assumption is that codes carrying more information and/or accounting for more variance or power in the signal are more likely to reflect the true neural code.

Another measure of the success, or plausibility, of a neural code is to ask how quickly and how accurately it allows a response to be decoded; that is, when in the evolution of a response can we begin to guess the identity of a stimulus, and how well can we do so as the response unfolds? In studies of sensory systems, the experimenter usually controls the stimulus, or at least the environment, and measures the responses elicited by each stimulus. After an experiment, the experimenter has a set of data that represents stimulus-response pairings. When we analyze or model the responses to each stimulus, and then seek to infer the likelihood that a particular stimulus elicited an observed response, we are trying to get from the conditional probability of a response given a stimulus to the condition probability of a stimulus given a response. This reversal suggests that a Bayesian approach is well suited to the problem of decoding neuronal responses. In Bayesian terms the procedure for identifying the stimulus from the response amounts to calculating the posterior probabilities for each of the possible stimuli and guessing the stimulus from those. This requires a rule for making a guess based on the posterior probabilities. One natural possibility, used here, is the maximum likelihood rule: pick the stimulus that was

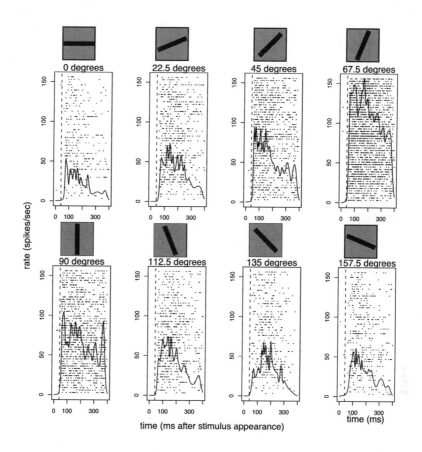

Figure 4.1 Responses of V1 supragranular complex cell in a fixating monkey to eight oriented dark bars on a gray background. The bar orientation is shown at the top of the raster. The stimuli were presented intermixed with 264 other stimuli in random order. The monkey was rewarded for fixating on a small spot, which it did for long periods. The stimuli were stepped on for 300 ms, and there was 600 ms between stimulus presentations. Each row of dots represents the spike times relative to one stimulus appearance. The stimulus presentations progress from earliest at the bottom to latest at the top of each raster. The spike densities are shown. The number of spikes elicited by one stimulus changes from trial to trial. The shapes of the spike densities depend on the stimulus. The spike density shapes are interpreted as instantaneous rates as functions of time, or if normalized, they represent the probability of spikes as a function of time.

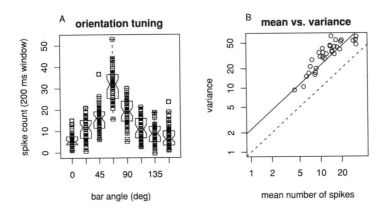

Figure 4.2 Variability of response measured by spike count. The number of spikes elicited by the trial are represented by small squares. The box plots show the median (horizontal lines in centers of boxes), 25th to 75th quantiles (the ends of the boxes), the estimated 95 % confidence interval for the median (the ends of the notch cutouts), and 1.5 times the interquartile range estimating the 95% ranges of the distributions (horizontal lines beyond the ends of the boxes). This shows that numbers of spikes vary over a large range for each stimulus. B. Variance as a function of mean for the black bars shown in figure 4.1, white bars, and gray bars. The extra responses are used here to make clearer the linear relation between the variance and mean on these log-log axes. The approximate regression line is almost parallel to the identity line but considerably higher. This illustrates the super-Poisson property often seen in cortical neuronal responses.

most likely to have elicited the response. The costs and benefits of correct and incorrect guesses could also be taken into account (for example, it might be less of a problem to mistake some food for a predator than to mistake a predator for some food), but we do not pursue that.

In parallel with the approach using information theory, we assume that decoding strategies allowing us to decode with greater speed and accuracy are more likely to reflect the true neural code. Increasing information frequently implies better decoding, but not always. For example, transmitted information will increase if small probabilities are made even smaller. However, in this case the best guess for decoding – the stimulus with the highest probability given the observed response – does not change, so the decoding accuracy does not change either.

To summarize the problem: We gather data – neuronal responses to stimuli – that might be quite variable, or noisy, and from them attempt to estimate which of the possible inputs elicited the response. A Bayesian framework nicely encapsulates the issues. We begin with a prior distribution of possible stimuli. These are chosen based on the results of previous experiments and used in the experiment, or simply assumed. We collect a set of responses, and from these we estimate the posterior probability distribution on the stimuli. We may update our posterior distribution as the response brings new information. If we are decoding, we can make decisions based on our current best estimate of what signal or input elicited the current response, or we can wait longer in the hope of enhancing the likelihood of guessing correctly. To achieve our goal of instant-by-instant decoding, we must formulate an appropriate representation of the neuronal spike trains.

If we had to have enough examples so that we had cataloged all of the possible responses, we might never finish our experiments. This extensive cataloging has been the basis for one approach to measuring information carried by motion sensitive neurons in the fly brain [35], but the general approach is impractical in vertebrates where experiments lasting 10's of hours are not generally possible, especially with some hope of system stationarity. Thus, in vertebrates, for decoding it is useful to have a model of neurons' response to stimuli when trying to decode, just as when we calculate information [44, 45, 46, 47]. One key issue for such a model is to know how stochastic or deterministic the responses are, that is, which aspects of responses are consistent and which vary from one response to another. In both the visual system and reduced systems such as tissue slice, it has been shown that neuronal spike trains can be amazingly reproducible when the driving force is fluctuating rapidly and with lots of energy [2, 9, 21]. Without such a powerful driving stimulus, for example, when a stimulus is left on a receptive field of a V1 neuron without changing for a few hundred milliseconds, responses vary substantially from one stimulus presentation to the next in both anaesthetized animals, including monkeys, and in monkeys that have been trained to fixate [15, 41].

The source of this variability is not really known. Many studies have examined the variability of the responses in some detail, and have shown that the variability is proportional to the firing rate (although not equal to it as would be the case for a pure Poisson process) [11, 15, 38, 44, 45]. It has been speculated that the variability seen during these 300 ms or longer stimulus presentations arises from small differences in eye position or eye movements. If the variability were due to the small eye movements, then in experiments with paralyzed anaesthetized animals the variability should be smaller, which it is not [11, 41]. Here we concern ourselves with responses elicited by stimuli centered on the receptive fields of V1 neurons in awake, fixating monkeys. The stimuli were stepped on for 300-400 ms (depending on the particular experiment) to mimic the time between saccadic eye movements in normal looking.

Both the firing rate and the timing of individual spikes are known to vary among individual responses to a particular stimulus. The relevance of spike count in neural coding is widely accepted, but the role of spike timing has been the focus of a great deal of debate. Which aspects of spike timing, and at what time scale, carry information, and which do not? Spike timing has been shown to carry independent information, separate from that carried by spike count. Using the spike density function [29], or, the less optimal classical peristimulus-time histogram measuring spike count in successive bins, we can ask questions about timing. We might find, for example, that spikes elicited by one stimulus are concentrated early in a response, while spikes elicited by another stimulus are spread more evenly across time (figure 4.1). Such variations in firing rate have been shown to carry information in different brain areas; that is, observing spike timing can help determine which stimulus elicited the response [22, 24, 30, 41].

To develop our approach to decoding as the response unfolds, we consider the response latency, i.e., the time at which the neuronal response to a stimulus begins. To anticipate our approach: we will develop the statistics we need to decode the responses based on the first spike, and then we will consider each subsequent spike as the "first next spike" – that is, the first spike in a response starting at the last spike considered, so, for example, the second spike is the first spike after the first spike. It is known that the time of the first spike (also called the response latency) itself carries a considerable amount of information, for example, about stimulus contrast in V1 [15].

Let us make the assumption that spikes stochastically sample an underlying rate profile over time (the spike density of figure 4.1). We make no assumption about whether the process is Poisson, that is, whether the time bins are truly independent, only that the sampling from the distribution is stochastic. To decode latency, that is, to use latency to determine which stimulus elicited a spike train, we need to have a model of the distribution of latencies elicited by each stimulus $p(L|s)$. With a sufficient number of responses from each stimulus, we could calculate the distribution of latencies directly from data, using the histogram of latencies (a strictly empirical model similar to what has been done in the fly in the reference above). Oram et al. [25] showed that spike trains from lateral geniculate nucleus (LGN) and V1 can be modeled as though the spike times for each train had been selected at random, with the probability of each spike time given by the normalized spike density function. This means that, given a spike density function (normalized to sum to 1), we can estimate the distribution of a single spike time, in a single-spike response, from the spike density function itself. In a simple (though unrealistic) special case, when each train contains only one spike, the density of latencies will be the same as the spike density function, with more trials having a spike at times of peaks than trials having a spike at times of troughs.

Oram et al. [25] used explicit simulation to derive properties of spike trains from the spike density function and count distribution. However, under the assumption of Oram et al. [25] that spike times are independently drawn from a particular density function, many properties of the trains can be calculated analytically: order statistics tell us how to estimate the distribution of first spike times no matter how many spikes occur in the responses, if the number of spikes in a train is known [1, 10, 47]. More generally, order statistics give the distribution of the kth spike out of n, for any $1 \leq k \leq n$.

Formally, order statistics describe how multiple independent draws from a probability distribution of any shape are ordered. The (k, n) order statistic describes the distribution of the kth of n draws, after those draws are sorted. In our case this will be $P(\tau_k = t_j | s, n)$, the time of the kth spike which occurs at time j, of n spikes in a train elicited by stimulus s:

$$P(\tau_k = t_j | s, n) = \frac{n!}{(k-1)!(n-k)!} F_s^{k-1}(t_j) f(t_j) [1 - F_s(t_j)]^{(n-k)} \qquad (4.1)$$

In equation (4.1), $f_s(t_j)$ is the spike density function (or normalized peristimulus time histogram), from which spike times are drawn at random in the model of Oram et al. [25], $F_s(t_j)$ is the corresponding cumulative firing rate profile, and the factor $[1 - F_s(t_j)]^{(n-k)}$ is the probability of $n - k$ spikes arriving after time t_j (figures 4.3A and B). We typically quantize time into 1-ms bins, the same precision with which spike times were recorded in our experiments. This quantization is a slight departure from the classical theory, which deals with continuous distributions, but requires only minor computational modifications. Equation (4.1) formalizes the intuition that the more spikes in a spike train, the earlier the first spike (or any other) is likely to arrive.

Order statistics give the distribution of a spike time when the total number of spikes is known. If we are trying to decode the spike train as it unfolds, we do not know in advance how many spikes a particular presentation of a particular stimulus will elicit. However, we can estimate the distribution of spike counts elicited across several (hopefully many) presentations of a stimulus, and then average the order statistics for each number of spikes n, weighted by the probability of observing each particular spike count:

$$P(\tau_1 = t_j | s) = \sum_{n=1}^{N_{\max}} \widetilde{p}(n) P(\tau_1 = t_j | s, n) \qquad (4.2)$$

The sum in equation (4.2) leaves out the term corresponding to $n = 0$, that is, to no further spikes in the train. Thus $P(\tau_1 | s)$ sums to $1 - \widetilde{p}_s(0)$. Figure 4.4 shows the count weighted first order statistics superimposed on the eight

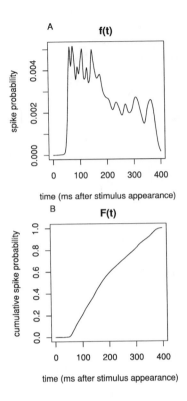

Figure 4.3   (A). Spike density normalized to unit area. The spike density functions are created using local regression fitting [20], which gives a cross-validated fitting estimate of the local density. The local neighborhood parameter was set to be 0.12, meaning the nearest 12% of available data is used to fit the regression at each point. This gives an estimate for $f(t)$, the probability of a spike at time t. (B). The cumulative spike density, $F(t)$, which is the cumulative sum from A. This gives the probability of seeing a spike up to time t.

responses shown in Figure 4.1. Figure 4.5 superimposes these count weighted order statistics (and the cumulative count weighted order statistics) so that the onset times and widths are easier to appreciate.

   As shown by equations (4.1) and (4.2), order statistics and count-weighted order statistics describe not only the distribution of the first spike in a train, but the distribution of other spike times as well. After the first spike has arrived or not arrived at a particular time (the probability of a spike not arriving is just $1 - P(\tau_1 = t_j|s)$), we have additional information. Using Bayes theorem we arrive at the desired result, the probability of the stimulus given the outcome

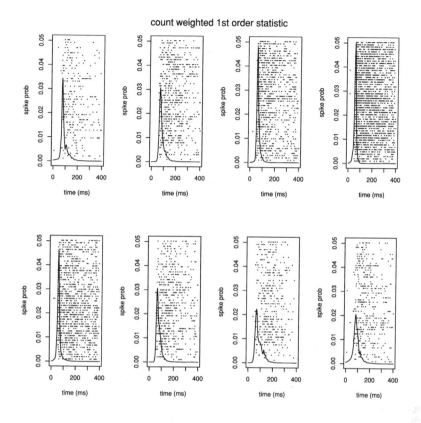

Figure 4.4   Count weighted first order statistics (equation (4.2)) for the eight stimuli in Figure 4.1. The rasters are superimposed on the order statistics. The distribution of first order statistics gives our approximation to the distribution of response latencies.

of whether or not a spike arrived:

$$p(s|\tau_1 = t_j) = \frac{p(\tau_1 = t_j|s)p(s)}{\sum\limits_{s'} p(\tau_1 = t_j|s')p(s')}. \tag{4.3}$$

This information tells us not only about what stimulus has been shown, but also about whether and when we are likely to see a next spike. Thus, after seeing a first spike at a particular time, we want to know not the distribution of second spike times across all trains, but the distribution of second spike times across trains with a first spike at the observed time. Our initial estimate of the distribution of first spike times can be regarded as a prior probability distribution, and the revised distribution after the first spike time is observed as a posterior distribution. Thus, the set of $p(s|\tau_1 = t_j)$ over the entire stimulus set

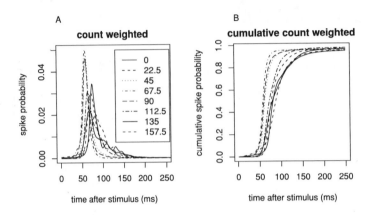

Figure 4.5 (A). Superimposed count-weighted first-order statistics from Figure 4.4. This allows the distributions to be compared more easily. (B). Cumulative count-weighted first-order statistics. These show the probability of having seen the first spike at or before time t. Following our intuition it seems likely that a spike will occur early when the firing rate for the stimulus is high. In a sense, there must be time for the rest of the spikes.

become the new priors. We have 'remembered' the firing history in our new estimated stimulus distribution. This is the only form of memory in this decoding system – we do not keep track of when previous spikes have occurred, only the stimulus-dependent estimates of when the next spike will occur.

Conditional order statistics give the distribution of the next spike times given what has already been observed; as mentioned above, we treat each spike as the "next first" spike. It can be shown [1, 10] that the $((i + j), n)$ order statistic conditioned on an observed i-th spike is simply the $(j, n - i)$ order statistic for the remaining number of spikes based on a truncated density – the portion of the density that lies to the right of the i-th spike time, re-normalized to sum or integrate to 1 (figure 4.6 A and B).

In real decoding, we do not know how many spikes remain. This requires

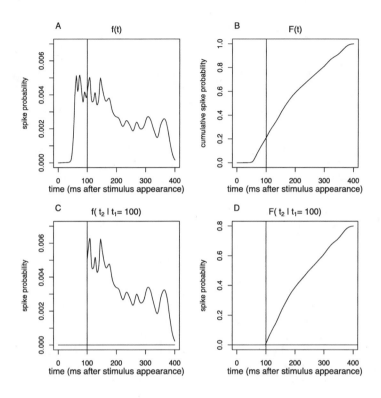

Figure 4.6   The spike density, $f(t)$, and cumulative spike density, $F(t)$, for the whole interval (A and B), and then renormalized after a hypothesized spike occurring at 100 ms (C and D).

that the decoder update the model based on what has already been observed. One possibility is to apply equation (4.3) and assume that after observing k spikes, the probability of observing subsequent $n - k$ spikes is simply the original probability of observing n spikes. This requires some re-normalization of the spike count distribution, because when spike k is observed, the probability of observing less than k spikes becomes zero. It is also possible to change the spike count probability based on the amount of the total spike density concentrated after what has been observed. For example, if half of the spike density is gone, and we have observed only three spikes, the probability that the train will have 18 spikes is low.

This decoding scheme works instant-by-instant. Each change in the estimated stimulus probabilities is the result of observing whether or not a spike is fired during some time period. The same is true for changes in the various quantities in the model that are used to calculate the stimulus probabilities. The decoder does not see the future: it has no information about what will happen later in the train. Similarly, the decoder does not have any explicit knowledge about the past – how many spikes have already arrived, for example. Everything the decoder knows about the past is stored in the model parameters, which have been estimated from previous data. These stored parameter values are used to calculate stimulus probabilities and the probabilities of spikes given each stimulus. In a neural system, the equivalent of such parameters might be stored in the strength of synaptic connections, which will have been influenced by both genetics and experience.

This discussion assumes that only the spike count distribution will be adjusted. In principle, the spike density function could also be adjusted (beyond the necessary truncation as time passes), but that would require much greater quantities of data than are typically available. Furthermore, Oram et al. [25] provides evidence that trains generated without adjusting the spike density function have statistical characteristics that match observed data.

4.3   Simplifying the Order Statistic Model

Up to this point every step has been formally correct, given the assumptions that the spikes are stochastic samples from the rate function given the spike count distribution, and that the spike density for a given stimulus is the same in all trials, no matter how many spikes arrive. The count-weighted order statistic model is useful, but quite computationally intensive, because it requires calculating the order statistic for each count of interest. The only way to reduce this complexity is to introduce simplifying assumptions that allow some of the calculations to be done analytically. A computationally easy assumption is that a spike train is generated by a homogeneous Poisson process. In this case, the count-weighted sum of order statistics simplifies to give the expected exponential distribution.

An inhomogeneous Poisson process retains the Poisson assumption on spike counts, while allowing the spike density function to change over time. This can be converted to a homogeneous Poisson process using time rescaling [7, 43], and the resulting times converted back to "real" times. Even without converting to a homogeneous Poisson process, the Poisson distribution of spike counts that is part of even an inhomogeneous Poisson process simplifies calculations. It can be shown that for a Poisson process with time-varying mean rate $\lambda_{s,i} f_s(t)$, the probability that the first spike occurs at time j simplifies to

$$P(\tau_1 = j | s, \lambda_{s,i}) = \lambda_{s,i} f_s(j) e^{-\sum_{k=t_0}^{j-1} \lambda_{s,i} f_s(k)} \tag{4.4}$$

where $f_s(j)$ is the spike density function (normalized peristimulus time histogram, or normalized PSTH), $\lambda_{s,i}$ is a rate multiplier, s again indexes the stimuli and i indexes different Poisson means.

However, even an inhomogeneous Poisson process is not an adequate model for spike trains observed in many cortical areas. For one thing, in trains from many areas, the variance of the number of spikes elicited across presentations of a single stimulus is consistently greater than the mean (see figure 4.2B) [11, 15, 38, 44, 45]. This means that the spike trains could not have been generated by a Poisson process.

A mixture of Poisson processes will have a spike count described by a mixture of Poisson distributions. A model allowing a mixture of a few Poisson distributions adds substantial flexibility, while keeping the calculations reasonably simple. Almost all spike count distributions we have checked can be fit by one, two, or three Poisson distributions [47]. Intuitively, the approach is reasonable if we consider this a procedure to fit a smooth (not even necessarily unimodal) distribution. It does not represent a commitment to a multimodal mechanism; it is just a convenient computational approach for approximating over-dispersed distributions.

Equation (4.4) calculates the sum of count-specific first order statistics $P(t_1|s, n)$ for each n, weighted with the appropriate Poisson probabilities. Finally, we add the first order statistics for each mean rate $\lambda_{s,i}$, weighted by the probability $p(\lambda_{s,i}|s)$ of observing that rate:

$$P(\tau_1 = t_j|s) = \sum_i p(\lambda_{s,i}|s)P(\tau_1 = t_j|s, \lambda_{s,i}) \qquad (4.5)$$

These calculations are conceptually identical to those described in terms of order statistics in the previous section (and give identical results if the spike count distribution was that arising from the mixture of Poisson distributions). However, because sums across the counts in a Poisson distribution can be taken analytically, and spike count distributions are modeled using a mixture of only a few Poisson distributions [47], the calculations using a mixture of Poisson distributions are substantially faster. The speed-up comes because we calculate spike probabilities for only a few Poisson means, rather than for each possible spike count. Intuitively, this says that each train comes from one of a small number of Poisson processes (although we are not sure at the outset which one).

Calculating new order statistics after a spike arrives requires estimating the remaining spike count distribution $\tilde{p}_s(n)$ for each stimulus s (see equation (4.2)), or the Poisson means $\lambda_{s,i}$ and weights $p(\lambda_{s,i}|s)$ (see equation (4.5)). We can either estimate the parameters for each subinterval from the model used for the full interval, or we can broaden the model, independently measuring or estimating spike count distributions starting at a variety of times. The first option is preferable if achievable, both because it describes the data much more compactly and because it is usually easier to understand. In the order statistic formulation, however, the estimation is computationally expensive.

In the multiple Poisson formulation, calculating the necessary subinterval distributions is simpler: the rate function of a Poisson process on a subinterval is the original rate function restricted to that interval. The weights $p(\lambda_{s,i}|s)$ can be continuously updated using the Bayes Rule, because each weight is the probability with which we believe the spike train being decoded comes from the particular process. Because the Poisson processes differ only by a multiplier of the rate, our only evidence of which process the train comes from is the number of spikes we've seen. Thus we again apply the Bayes theorem:

$$p(\lambda_{s,i}|s)(j) = \frac{P(n(j)|s, \lambda_{s,i})p(\lambda_{s,i}|s)(0)}{\sum_i P(n(j)|s, \lambda_{s,i})p(\lambda_{s,i}|s)(0)} \tag{4.6}$$

where $p(\lambda_{s,i}|s)(0)$, the prior distribution, denotes the weights given the stimulus, in the case of a sensory neuron, at the beginning of the trial. Note again that the weights $p(\lambda_{s,i}|s)$ are stimulus-specific. It is also straightforward to update this distribution over time, rather than starting each time from the original distribution.

The decoding works instant-by-instant. In figure 4.7, we show decoding for two spike trains that decode correctly, one for stimulus 1, the bar at zero degree orientation, and one for stimulus 4, the bar at 67.5 degrees. The overall performance is quite good (figure 4.8). The prior probability of a stimulus is about 12.5 % (ignoring slight differences in the number of presentations of different stimuli). Finally, we ask how well each stimulus is decoded. In the example here, the 22.5 and 112.5 degree bars are not decoded at greater than chance probability (figure 4.9).

4.4   Discussion

Application of Bayes theorem provides a natural procedure for transforming knowledge about the response elicited by different stimuli into knowledge about the stimuli likely to have elicited an observed response. This requires accurately estimating the conditional probabilities of the response given different stimuli. This estimation problem is fraught with potential inaccuracies [23], but over the past several years, because experimentalists have become more familiar with these problems, they have made exceptional efforts to collect sufficient amounts of data to carry out these calculations.

The Bayesian approach has become a standard (but not the only [36, 32]) tool for making the transformation, and thus, making an estimate of the response. Several groups carry out such calculations [8, 19, 40, 48]. What distinguishes the different calculations are the response models that are used. Given the Bayesian framework, what remains is to determine is whether the response can be modeled with modest (experimentally obtainable) amounts of data. We make two simple, explicit statistical assumptions, that is, (1) spikes stochastically sample an underlying rate probability function (the spike density or peristimulus time histogram), and (2) with a distribution of samples given by the spike count distribution. Spike trains that are consistent with these assumptions can be modeled exactly. That is, if we assume that the neuronal action potentials can be treated as realizations of a point process that samples an underlying rate function in a stochastic manner, order statistics exactly describe the statistics of the trains.

We have, for computational convenience, chosen to approximate the exact order statistic model with the computational mixture of Poisson processes.

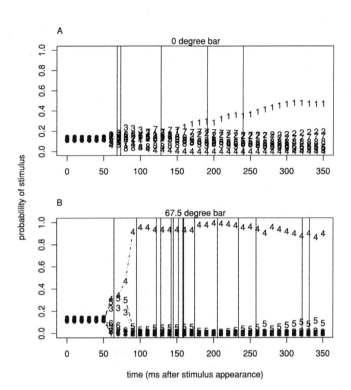

Figure 4.7 Decoding examples for two spike trains. (A). The decoder decodes this response elicited by the zero degree bar (stimulus #1), a low firing rate example, and after about 150 ms, it makes the correct choice of stimulus. The low firing rate examples will typically be decoded later, because there must be time to determine whether an early spike occurs. The lack of spikes plays a big role in this decoding. (B). This response here was elicited by the 67.5 degree bar (stimulus #4), the highest firing rate. The first spike (at about 60 ms) begins the separation from the low firing rate examples. Then the response starts to separate the high firing examples, which is basically finished by the second spike. The rest of the spikes just keep the confidence level for the decoding at a high level. Spike times are shown by vertical lines.

This is no longer exact, but as long as the spike count distribution can be fit by a mixture of Poisson processes (and for our data, that seems to work well with only a few Poisson distributions), decoding from this approximate order statistic model can be accomplished in nearly real time on even small computers: as computers become faster, this approximation might not needed, but for the present it is convenient. The formulation above points out that no matter what model is chosen for spike generation, the data collected can be used to estimate the stimulus (experimental condition) given the response.

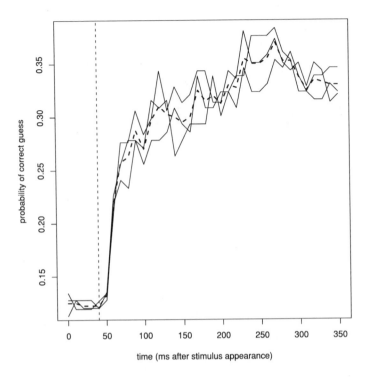

Figure 4.8 Overall decoding performance for the illustrated neuron. The decoder carried out three splits of the data (performance shown by each of the solid lines). The average decoding performance is shown by the dashed line. The vertical line is at 40 ms to make comparison to the data in figure 4.1 easier. The decoding is at the random level ($\sim$12.5%) until just after 50 ms, when decoding rises quickly. In this example most of the decoding is related to the time of the first spike or two, but the decoding does continue to improve until about 250 ms after stimulus appearance.

The approach we have taken is similar in the assumption of stochasticity of spike occurrence to the approach taken by Brown and colleagues, who use models based on the interval distributions, where they use the conditional intensity function for the interval distribution [3, 4, 14, 26, 39]. Their approach was developed for situations in which there are long trials, or perhaps no trials, such as a rat running in a maze. They are able to estimate the rat's location quite accurately using the conditional intensity function. Recent work includes estimation of the effect on one neuron's firing of firing by other neurons [39].

Another interesting hypothesis about how the responses of multiple neurons might be combined arises from the observation that certain judgments, for example whether a flashed stimulus presents an animal or not, can be made

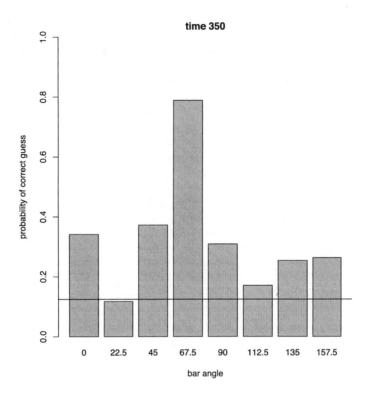

Figure 4.9 The probability of guessing correctly stimulus-by-stimulus at the end of the analysis window, 350 ms after stimulus appearance. One stimulus, the 67.5 degree bar, is decoded with a very high probability. Two stimuli have no greater than chance (binomial test) probability of being correctly decoded.

extremely quickly. Based on this, it has been suggested that the recruitment order of the neurons in a population, i.e., the relative latencies of responses across neurons, might carry a lot of the information about a stimulus [31, 37]. Recently, Johansson and Birznieks showed experimentally that recruitment order carries information about tactile stimuli in the human median nerve [18]. The recruitment order hypothesis is easiest to apply in areas in which there is no significant ongoing activity and latency can be defined as the time of the first spike after stimulus presentation. In areas of the brain, such as area TE, in which there is substantial and spontaneous ongoing activity, there is no clear first spike in a response, and, therefore, latency must be determined using statistical methods.

Above we have only concerned ourselves with a logical aspect of this process – what are the messages being carried by single neuronal responses. We have ignored an important aspect of neural responses: what are the possible mechanisms for interpreting or using the responses? For example, in many instances it is likely that spikes arriving close together in time are weighted more heavily than their simple sum would predict [6, 33]. Here we have considered the interpretation of single neuronal spike trains as a decoding problem, but, in reality information is distributed across many neurons, and there is no explicit decoder. The true goal is to understand the impact of multiple spike trains on their targets through the biophysical mechanisms in the synaptic machinery. Experiments in some invertebrates take advantage of the near identity of neurons and connections among neurons from one individual to the next to investigate these mechanisms [17]. Indeed, in these systems the variations among individuals are of great interest. In vertebrates, the connections among neurons are not the same across individuals.

While interesting theoretical work is being done on how population codes might work [28, 27, 34], so far we do not have the ability to record both the inputs and outputs of local circuitry in vertebrates. True understanding of population codes may require new experimental techniques for such recordings.

Acknowledgements

This research was supported in part by the Intramural Research Program of NIMH/NIH.

References

[1] Arnold BC, Balakrishnan N, Nagaraja HN (1992) *A First Course in Order Statistics*. New York: Wiley.

[2] Bair W, Koch C (1996) Temporal precision of spike trains in extrastriate cortex of the behaving macaque monkey. *Neural Computation*, 8:1185-1202.

[3] Barbieri R, Frank LM, Nguyen DP, Quirk MC, Solo V, Wilson MA, Brown EN (2004) Dynamic analyses of information encoding in neural ensembles. *Neural Computation*, 16:277-307.

[4] Barbieri R, Wilson MA, Frank LM, Brown EN (2005) An analysis of hippocampal spatio-temporal representations using a Bayesian algorithm for neural spike train decoding. *IEEE Transaction on Neural Systems and Rehabilitation Engineering*, 13:131-136.

[5] Barlow HB (1972) Single units and sensation: a neuron doctrine for perceptual psychology? *Perception*, 1:371-394.

[6] Brenner N, Strong SP, Koberle R, Bialek W, de Ruyter van Steveninck RR (2000) Synergy in a neural code. *Neural Computation*, 12:1531-1552.

[7] Brown EN, Barbieri R, Ventura V, Kass RE, Frank LM (2002) The time-rescaling theorem and its application to neural spike train data analysis. *Neural Computation*, 14:325-346.

[8] Brown EN, Frank LM, Tang D, Quirk MC, Wilson MA (1998) A statistical paradigm for neural spike train decoding applied to position prediction from ensemble firing patterns of rat hippocampal place cells. *Journal of Neuroscience*, 18:7411-7425.

[9] Buracas GT, Zador AM, DeWeese MR, Albright TD (1998) Efficient discrimination of temporal patterns by motion-sensitive neurons in primate visual cortex. *Neuron*, 20:959-969.

[10] David HA, Nagaraja HN (2003) *Order Statistics*, 3rd edition. New York: Wiley-Interscience.

[11] Dean AF (1981) The variability of discharge of simple cells in the cat striate cortex. *Experimental Brain Research*, 44:437-440.

[12] Eckhorn R, Popel B (1974) Rigorous and extended application of information theory to the afferent visual system of the cat. I. Basic concepts. *Kybernetik*, 16:191-200.

[13] Eckhorn R, Popel B (1975) Rigorous and extended application of information theory to the afferent visual system of the cat. II. Experimental results. *Biological Cybernetics*, 17:71-77.

[14] Eden UT, Frank LM, Barbieri R, Solo V, Brown EN (2004) Dynamic analysis of neural encoding by point process adaptive filtering. *Neural Computation*, 16:971-998.

[15] Gawne TJ, Kjaer TW, Richmond BJ (1996) Latency: another potential code for feature binding in striate cortex. *Journal of Neurophysiology*, 76:1356-1360.

[16] Gershon ED, Wiener MC, Latham PE, Richmond BJ (1998) Coding strategies in monkey V1 and inferior temporal cortices. *Journal of Neurophysiology*, 79:1135-1144.

[17] Jacobs GA, Theunissen FE (2000) Extraction of sensory parameters from a neural map by primary sensory interneurons. *Journal of Neuroscience*, 20:2934-2943.

[18] Johansson RS, Birznieks I (2004) First spikes in ensembles of human tactile afferents code complex spatial fingertip events. *Nature Neuroscience*, 7:170-177.

[19] Kass RE, Ventura V, Brown EN (2005) Statistical issues in the analysis of neuronal data. *Journal of Neurophysiology*, 94:8-25.

[20] Loader C (1999) *Local Regression and Liklihood*. New York: Springer-Verlag.

[21] Mainen ZF, Sejnowski TJ (1995) Reliability of spike timing in neocortical neurons. *Science*, 268:1503-1506.

[22] McClurkin JW, Gawne TJ, Optican LM, Richmond BJ (1991) Lateral geniculate neurons in behaving primates. II. Encoding of visual information in the temporal shape of the response. *Journal of Neurophysiology*, 66:794-808.

[23] Optican LM, Gawne TJ, Richmond BJ, Joseph PJ (1991) Unbiased measures of transmitted information and channel capacity from multivariate neuronal data. *Biological Cybernetics*, 65:305-310.

[24] Optican LM, Richmond BJ (1987) Temporal encoding of two-dimensional patterns by single units in primate inferior temporal cortex. III. Information theoretic analysis. *Journal of Neurophysiology*, 57:162-178.

[25] Oram MW, Wiener MC, Lestienne R, Richmond BJ (1999) Stochastic nature of precisely timed spike patterns in visual system neuronal responses. *Journal of Neurophysiology*, 81:3021-3033.

[26] Pillow JW, Paninski L, Uzzell VJ, Simoncelli EP, Chichilnisky EJ (2005) Prediction and decoding of retinal ganglion cell responses with a probabilistic spiking model. *Journal of Neuroscience*, 25:11003-11013.

[27] Pouget A, Dayan P, Zemel RS (2003) Inference and computation with population codes. *Annual Review of Neuroscience*, 26:381-410.

[28] Pouget A, Zhang K, Deneve S, Latham PE (1998) Statistically efficient estimation using population coding. *Neural Computation,* 10:373-401.

[29] Richmond BJ, Optican LM, Podell M, Spitzer H (1987) Temporal encoding of two-dimensional patterns by single units in primate inferior temporal cortex. I. Response characteristics. *Journal of Neurophysiology,* 57:132-146.

[30] Richmond BJ, Optican LM, Spitzer H (1990) Temporal encoding of two-dimensional patterns by single units in primate primary visual cortex. I. Stimulus-response relations. *Journal of Neurophysiology,* 64:351-369.

[31] Rousselet GA, Fabre-Thorpe M, Thorpe SJ (2002) Parallel processing in high-level categorization of natural images. *Nature Neuroscience,* 5:629-630.

[32] Sanchez JC, Erdogmus D, Nicolelis MA, Wessberg J, Principe JC (2005) Interpreting spatial and temporal neural activity through a recurrent neural network brain-machine interface. *IEEE Transactions of Neural Systems and Rehabilitation Engineering,* 13:213-219.

[33] Segundo JP, Moore GP, Stensaas LJ, Bullock TH (1963) Sensitivity of neurones in Aplysia to temporal pattern of arriving impulses. *Journal of Experimental Biology,* 40:643-667.

[34] Series P, Latham PE, Pouget A (2004) Tuning curve sharpening for orientation selectivity: coding efficiency and the impact of correlations. *Nature Neuroscience,* 7:1129-1135.

[35] Strong SP, de Ruyter van Steveninck R, Bialek W, Koberle R (1998) On the application of information theory to neural spike trains [in process citation]. Pac Symp Biocomput 621-632.

[36] Taylor DM, Tillery SI, Schwartz AB (2002) Direct cortical control of 3D neuroprosthetic devices. *Science,* 296:1829-1832.

[37] Thorpe SJ (1990) Spike arrival times: A highly efficient coding scheme for neural networks. In Eckmiller R, Hartmann G, Hauske G, eds., *Parallel Processing in Neural Systems and Computers,* pages 91-94, Amsterdam, The Netherlands: Elsevier.

[38] Tolhurst DJ, Movshon JA, Dean AF (1983) The statistical reliability of signals in single neurons in cat and monkey visual cortex. *Vision Research,* 23:775-785.

[39] Truccolo W, Eden UT, Fellows MR, Donoghue JP, Brown EN (2005) A point process framework for relating neural spiking activity to spiking history, neural ensemble, and extrinsic covariate effects. *Journal of Neurophysiology,* 93:1074-1089.

[40] Ventura V, Cai C, Kass RE (2005) Statistical assessment of time-varying dependency between two neurons. *Journal of Neurophysiology,* 94:2940-2947.

[41] Victor JD, Purpura KP (1996) Nature and precision of temporal coding in visual cortex: a metric- space analysis. *Journal of Neurophysiology,* 76:1310-1326.

[42] Werner G, Mountcastle VB (1965) Neural activity in mechanoreceptive cutaneous afferents: stimulus-response relations, Weber functions, and information transmission. *Journal of Neurophysiology,* 28:359-397.

[43] Wiener MC (2003) An adjustment to the time-rescaling method for application to short-trial spike train data. *Neural Computation,*15:2565-2576.

[44] Wiener MC, Richmond BJ (1998) Using response models to study coding strategies in monkey visual cortex. *Biosystems,* 48:279-286.

[45] Wiener MC, Richmond BJ (1999) Using response models to estimate channel capacity for neuronal classification of stationary visual stimuli using temporal coding. *Journal of Neurophysiology*, 82:2861-2875.

[46] Wiener MC, Richmond BJ (2002) Model based decoding of spike trains. Biosystems 67:295-300.

[47] Wiener MC, Richmond BJ (2003) Decoding spike trains instant by instant using order statistics and the mixture-of-Poissons model. *Journal of Neuroscience*, 23:2394-2406.

[48] Wu W, Gao Y, Bienenstock E, Donoghue JP, Black MJ (2006) Bayesian population decoding of motor cortical activity using a Kalman filter. *Neural Computation*, 18:80-118.

5   Bayesian Treatments of Neuroimaging Data

Will Penny and Karl Friston

5.1   Introduction

In this chapter we discuss the application of Bayesian methods to neuroimaging data. This includes data from positron emission tomography (PET), functional magnetic resonance imaging (fMRI), electroencephalography (EEG), and magnetoencephalography (MEG). We concentrate on fMRI but the concepts, methodologies, and modeling approaches apply to all modalities.

A general issue in the analysis of brain imaging data is the relationship between the neurobiological hypothesis one posits and the statistical models adopted to test that hypothesis. One key distinction is between functional specialization and integration.

Briefly, fMRI was originally used to provide functional maps showing which regions are specialized for specific functions, a classic example being the study by Zeki et al. [27] who identified V4 and V5 as being specialized for the processing of color and motion, respectively. More recently, these analyses have been augmented by functional integration studies, which describe how functionally specialized areas interact and how these interactions depend on changes of context. A recent example is the study by Buchel et al. [1] who found that the success with which a subject learned an object-location association task was correlated with the coupling between regions in the dorsal and ventral visual streams.

Functionally specialized brain responses are typically characterized using the general linear model (GLM). An fMRI data set comprises a time series of volumetric data. In "mass-univariate" approaches GLMs are fitted to fMRI time series at each voxel (volume element), resulting in a set of voxel-specific parameters. These parameters are then used to form posterior probability maps (PPMs) that characterize regionally specific responses to experimental manipulation. Figure 5.5, for example, shows a PPM highlighting regions that are sensitive to visual motion stimuli.

Analyses of functional integration are implemented using multivariate approaches that examine the changes in multiple brain areas induced by experi-

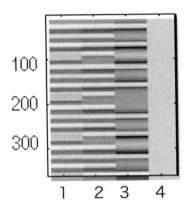

Figure 5.1 Design matrix for study of attention to visual motion. The four columns correspond to "Photic" stimulation, "Motion", "Attention", and a constant. There are as many rows in the design matrix as there are time points in the imaging time series. For this data set there are 360 images. The first three columns in the design matrix were formed by representing the experimental condition using a boxcar regressor and then convolving with a canonical hemodynamic response function (see figure 5.2).

mental manipulation. Although there a number of methods for doing this we focus on a recent approach called dynamic causal modeling (DCM).

This chapter is structured as follows. Section 5.2 introduces an fMRI data set that is analyzed in later sections. Section 5.3 describes the GLM and section 5.4 describes Bayesian estimation procedures for GLMs and extensions for nonlinear models. Section 5.5 describes PPM for making inferences about functional specialization, and section 5.6 describes DCM for making inferences about functional integration.

5.2   Attention to Visual Motion

This section describes a data set that will be analyzed using PPMs and DCMs. Subjects were studied with fMRI under identical stimulus conditions (visual motion subtended by radially moving dots) while manipulating the attentional component of the task (detection of velocity changes).

The data were acquired from normal subjects at 2 Tesla using a Magnetom VISION (Siemens, Erlangen, Germany) whole-body MRI system, equipped with a head volume coil. Contiguous multislice T2*-weighted fMRI images were obtained with a gradient echo-planar sequence (TE = 40 ms, TR = 3.22 seconds, matrix size = 64 x 64 x 32, voxel size 3 x 3 x 3 mm).

Each subject had four consecutive 100-scan sessions comprising a series of ten scan blocks under five different conditions: D F A F N F A F N S. The first condition (D) was a dummy condition to allow for magnetic saturation effects.

F (Fixation) corresponds to a low-level baseline where the subjects viewed a fixation point at the center of a screen.

In condition A (Attention) subjects viewed 250 dots moving radially from the center at 4.7 degrees per second and were asked to detect changes in radial velocity (which did not actually occur). This attentional manipulaton was validated post hoc using psychophysics and the motion aftereffect. In condition N (No attention) the subjects were asked simply to view the moving dots. In condition S (Stationary) subjects viewed stationary dots. The order of A and N was swapped for the last two sessions. In all conditions subjects fixated the center of the screen.

In a prescanning session the subjects were given five trials with five speed changes (reducing to 1%). During scanning there were no speed changes and no overt response was required in any condition. In this chapter we analyze data from the first subject.

For the purpose of the analyses in this chapter the above experimental conditions were formulated using the following factors or causes. "Photic" stimulation comprised the $\{A, B, S\}$ conditions, "motion" comprised the $\{N, A\}$ conditions and "Attention" comprised the A condition. These three variables are encoded into the design matrix in figure 5.1. The relative contribution of each of these variables can be assessed using standard least squares or Bayesian estimation. Classical inferences about these contributions are made using T or F statistics, depending upon whether one is looking at a particular linear combination (e.g. a subtraction), or all of them together. Bayesian inferences are based on the posterior or conditional probability that the contribution exceeded some threshold, usually zero.

5.3   The General Linear Model

The general linear model is an equation that expresses an observed response variable y in terms of a linear combination of explanatory variables X:

$$y = X\beta + e, \tag{5.1}$$

where y is a $T \times 1$ vector comprising responses at, e.g. T time points, X is a $T \times K$ design matrix, β is a vector of regression coefficients, and e is a $T \times 1$ error vector.

The general linear model is variously known as "analysis of covariance" or "multiple regression analysis" and subsumes simpler variants, like the "T test" for a difference in means, to more elaborate linear convolution models such as finite impulse response (FIR) models. The matrix X that contains the explanatory variables (e.g. designed effects or confounds) is called the design matrix.

Each column of the design matrix corresponds to some effect one has built into the experiment or that may confound the results. These are referred to as explanatory variables, covariates, or regressors. The design matrix can contain both covariates and indicator variables. Each column of X has an associated unknown parameter. Some of these parameters will be of interest, e.g. the effect of a particular sensorimotor or cognitive condition or the regression coefficient of hemodynamic responses on reaction time. The remaining parameters will be of no interest and pertain to confounding effects, e.g. the effect of being a particular subject.

A standard method for neuroimaging analysis is the mass-univariate approach [12] where GLMs are fitted to each voxel. This allows one to test for the same effects at each point in the brain. Due primarily to the presence of aliased biorhythms and unmodeled neuronal activity in fMRI, the errors in the GLM will be temporally autocorrelated. The general linear model can accommodate this as shown in section 5.4.

5.3.1   Contrasts

To assess effects of interest that are spanned by one or more columns in the design matrix one uses a contrast (i.e., a linear combination of parameter estimates). An example of a contrast weight vector would be [-1 1 0 0.....] to compare the difference in responses evoked by two conditions, modeled by the first two condition-specific regressors in the design matrix. Sometimes several contrasts of parameter estimates are jointly interesting. For example, when using polynomial or basis function expansions of some experimental factor. In these instances, a matrix of contrast weights is used that can be thought of as a collection of effects that one wants to test together. Such a contrast may look like

$$c^T = \begin{bmatrix} -1 & 0 & 0 & 0 & \cdot & \cdot & \cdot \\ 0 & 1 & 0 & 0 & \cdot & \cdot & \cdot \end{bmatrix}, \tag{5.2}$$

which would test for the significance of the first or second parameter estimates. The fact that the first weight is -1 as opposed to 1 has no effect on the test because F statistics are based on sums of squares [7]. .

5.3.2   Temporal Basis Functions

Functional MRI using blood oxygen level dependent (BOLD) contrast provides an index of neuronal activity indirectly via changes in blood oxygenation levels. This relationship can be characterized using temporal basis functions as shown in figure 5.2.

For a given impulse of neuronal activity the fMRI signal peaks some 4-6 seconds later, then after 10 seconds or so drops below zero and returns to baseline after 20 to 30 seconds. This response varies from subject to subject and from voxel to voxel and this variation can be captured using temporal basis functions. In [13] the form of the hemodynamic impulse response function (HRF) was estimated using a least squares deconvolution and a time invariant model, where evoked neuronal responses are convolved with the HRF to give the measured hemodynamic response. This simple linear framework is the cornerstone for making statistical inferences about activations in fMRI with the GLM. An impulse response function is the response to a single impulse, measured at a

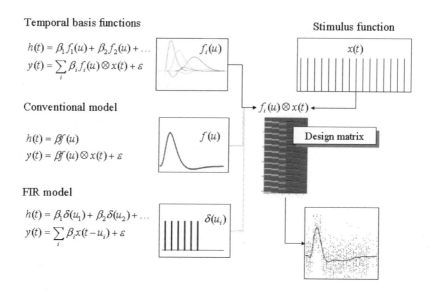

Temporal basis functions

$$h(t) = \beta_1 f_1(u) + \beta_2 f_2(u) + \dots$$
$$y(t) = \sum_i \beta_i f_i(u) \otimes x(t) + \varepsilon$$

$f_i(u)$

Stimulus function

$x(t)$

Conventional model

$$h(t) = \beta f(u)$$
$$y(t) = \beta f(u) \otimes x(t) + \varepsilon$$

$f(u)$

$f_i(u) \otimes x(t)$

Design matrix

FIR model

$$h(t) = \beta_1 \delta(u_1) + \beta_2 \delta(u_2) + \dots$$
$$y(t) = \sum_i \beta_i x(t - u_i) + \varepsilon$$

$\delta(u_i)$

Figure 5.2   Temporal basis functions offer useful constraints on the form of the estimated response that retain (i) the flexibility of finite impulse response (FIR) models and (ii) the efficiency of single regressor models. The specification of these models involves setting up stimulus functions x(t) that model expected neuronal changes, e.g., boxcars of epoch-related responses or spikes (delta functions) at the onset of specific events or trials. These stimulus functions are then convolved with a set of basis functions of peristimulus time u, that model the HRF, in some linear combination. The ensuing regressors are assembled into the design matrix. The basis functions can be as simple as a single canonical HRF (middle), through to a series of delayed delta functions (bottom). The latter case corresponds to a FIR model and the coefficients constitute estimates of the impulse response function at a finite number of discrete sampling times. Selective averaging in event-related fMRI [4] is mathematically equivalent to this limiting case.

series of times after the input. It characterizes the input-output behavior of the system (i.e. voxel) and places important constraints on the sorts of inputs that will excite a response. The HRFs, estimated in [13] resembled a Poisson or gamma function, peaking at about 5 seconds.

The basic idea behind temporal basis functions is that the hemodynamic response induced by any given trial type can be expressed as the linear combination of several basis functions of peristimulus time. As shown in figure 5.2, the convolution model for fMRI responses takes a stimulus function encoding the supposed neuronal responses and convolves it with an HRF to give a regressor that enters into the design matrix. When using basis functions, the stimulus function is convolved with all the basis functions to give a series of regressors. The associated parameter estimates are the coefficients or weights that determine the mixture of basis functions that best models the HRF for the trial type and voxel in question. We find the most useful basis set to be a canonical HRF and its derivatives with respect to the key parameters that determine its form (e.g. latency and dispersion) [16]. This is known as an informed basis set. The nice thing about this approach is that it can partition differences among evoked responses into differences in magnitude, latency, or dispersion, that can be tested for using specific contrasts [9].

Temporal basis functions are important because they enable a graceful transition between conventional multilinear regression models with one stimulus function per condition and FIR models with a parameter for each time point following the onset of a condition or trial type. Figure 5.2 illustrates this graphically (see figure legend).

In summary, temporal basis functions offer useful constraints on the form of the estimated response that retain (i) the flexibility of FIR models and (ii) the efficiency of single regressor models. The advantage of using several temporal basis functions (as opposed to an assumed form for the HRF) is that one can model voxel-specific forms for hemodynamic responses and formal differences (e.g. onset latencies) among responses to different sorts of events. The advantages of using an informed basis set over FIR models are that (i) the parameters are estimated more efficiently and (ii) stimuli can be presented at any point in the interstimulus interval. The latter is important because time-locking stimulus presentation and data acquisition give a biased sampling over peristimulus time and can lead to differential sensitivities, in multislice acquisition, over the brain.

5.4   Parameter Estimation

This section describes how the parameters of GLMs can be estimated using maximum likelihood and Bayesian approaches. We also show how the Bayesian approach can be applied to nonlinear models.

5.4.1   Maximum Likelihood

In what follows, $N(x; m, \Sigma)$ specifies a multivariate Gaussian distribution over x with mean m and covariance Σ. The likelihood specified by the GLM described in the previous section is given by

$$p(y|\beta) = N(y; X\beta, C_e), \tag{5.3}$$

where C_e is an error covariance matrix. The maximum-likelihood (ML) estimator is given by [25]:

$$\hat{\beta}_{ML} = \left(X^T C_e^{-1} X\right)^{-1} X^T C_e^{-1} y \tag{5.4}$$

This estimator is suitable for fMRI where the temporal autocorrelation in the errors is specified by the matrix C_e. For the moment we consider that C_e is known, although in section 5.4.3 we show how it can be estimated. For other modalities $C_e = \sigma^2 I$ often suffices. The ML estimate then reduces to the ordinary least squares (OLS) estimator

$$\hat{\beta}_{OLS} = \left(X^T X\right)^{-1} X^T y \tag{5.5}$$

5.4.2   Bayes Rule for GLMs

The Bayesian framework allows us to incorporate our prior beliefs about parameter values. This allows one to combine information from multiple modalities or to implement soft neurobiological constraints.

There are many examples of this. In fMRI, the search for activations can be restricted to regions thought to be gray matter as identified from structural MRI [17]. In EEG source localization, source orientations can be softly constrained to be perpendicular to the structural MRI estimates of the cortical surface [24]. More challengingly, estimation of neuronal activity can be based on simultaneously acquired EEG and fMRI [19].

In the context of dynamic causal models, described in section 5.7, parameter estimation can be constrained by neurophysiological data. Hemodynamic transit times, for example, can be constrained to realistic values and parameters governing neuronal dynamics can be constrained to give rise to stable dynamical systems.

If our beliefs can be specified using the Gaussian distribution

$$p(\beta) = N(\beta; \mu_p, C_p), \tag{5.6}$$

where μ_p is the prior mean and C_p is the prior covariance, then the posterior distribution is [18]

$$p(\beta|Y) = N(\beta; \mu, C), \tag{5.7}$$

where

$$\begin{aligned} C^{-1} &= X^T C_e^{-1} X + C_p^{-1} \\ \mu &= C(X^T C_e^{-1} y + C_p^{-1} \mu_p). \end{aligned} \tag{5.8}$$

The posterior precision, C^{-1}, is equal to the sum of the prior precision plus the data precision. The posterior mean, μ, is given by the sum of the prior mean plus the data mean, but where each is weighted according to its relative precision. In the absence of prior information, i.e. $C_p^{-1} = 0$, the above estimate reduces to the ML estimate.

Bayes rule is illustrated for GLMs with two regression coefficients in figure 5.3. The figure shows an example where the prior is centered at zero. This is known as a shrinkage prior because parameter estimates are shrunk toward zero. The figure shows that the shrinkage is greater for β_2, the parameter about which the data are less informative.

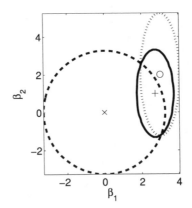

Figure 5.3 Bayesian estimation for GLMs with two parameters. The prior (dashed line) has mean $\mu_p = 0$ (cross) and precision $C_p^{-1} = \mathrm{diag}([1, 1])$. The likelihood (dotted line) has mean $X^T y = [3, 2]^T$ (circle) and precision $(X^T C_e^{-1} X)^{-1} = \mathrm{diag}([10, 1])$. The posterior (solid line) has mean $\mu = [2.73, 1]^T$ (cross) and precision $C^{-1} = \mathrm{diag}([11, 2])$. In this example, the measurements are more informative about β_1 than β_2. This is reflected in the posterior distribution.

5.4.3   Variance Components

It is also possible to compute the probability of the data after integrating out the dependence on model parameters

$$p(y) = \int p(y|\beta)p(\beta)d\beta \tag{5.9}$$

This is known as the model evidence.

Bayesian estimation as described in the previous section assumed that we knew the prior covariance, C_p, and error covariance, C_e. This information is, however, rarely available. In [15] a parametric empirical Bayesian (PEB) framework was developed in which these covariances are expressed as

$$C_p = \sum_i \lambda_i Q_i \tag{5.10}$$

$$C_e = \sum_j \lambda_j Q_j,$$

where Q_i and Q_j are known "covariance components" and λ_i, λ_j are hyperparameters that can be set so as to maximize the evidence. For example, Q_j can be set up to describe the temporal autocorrelations that are typically observed in fMRI [10]. This algorithm is used in the estimation of PPMs (see section 5.5).

If the priors are correct, then Bayesian estimation is more accurate than ML estimation [3]. But in general it is not possible to ensure that the "correct" priors are used. We can, however, use the best prior in a family of priors by using the PEB approach described above. It is also possible to compare different families of priors using Bayesian model comparison based on the model evidence [20, 21].

5.4.4 Nonlinear Models

For nonlinear models,

$$y = b(\theta) + e, \tag{5.11}$$

where $b(\theta)$ is a nonlinear function of parameter vector θ, the PEB framework can be applied by locally linearizing the nonlinearity, about a "current" estimate μ_i, using a first-order Taylor series expansion

$$b(\theta) = b(\mu_i) + \frac{\partial b(\mu_i)}{\partial \theta}(\theta - \mu_i) \tag{5.12}$$

Substituting this into equation (5.11) and defining $r \equiv y - b(\mu_i)$, $J \equiv \frac{\partial b(\mu_i)}{\partial \theta}$ and $\Delta\theta \equiv \theta - \mu_i$ gives

$$r = J\Delta\theta + e, \tag{5.13}$$

which now conforms to a GLM (cf. equation (5.1)). The prior, likelihood and posterior are now given by

$$
\begin{aligned}
p(\Delta\theta) &= \mathsf{N}(\Delta\theta; \mu_p - \mu_i, C_p) \\
p(r|\Delta\theta) &= \mathsf{N}(r; J\Delta\theta, C_e) \\
p(\Delta\theta|r) &= \mathsf{N}(\Delta\theta; \Delta\mu, C_{i+1}).
\end{aligned}
\tag{5.14}
$$

The quantities $\Delta\mu$ and C_{i+1} can be found using the result for the linear case (substitute r for Y and J for X in equation 5.8). If we define our "new" parameter estimate as $\mu_{i+1} = \mu_i + \Delta\mu$, then

$$
\begin{aligned}
C_{i+1}^{-1} &= J^T C_e^{-1} J + C_p^{-1} \\
\mu_{i+1} &= \mu_i + C_{i+1}(J^T C_e^{-1} r + C_p^{-1}(\mu_p - \mu_i)).
\end{aligned}
\tag{5.15}
$$

This update is applied recursively. It can also be combined with hyperparameter estimates, to characterize C_p and C_e, as described in the previous section and in [8]. This algorithm is used to estimate parameters of dynamic causal models (see section 5.6). In this instance $b(\theta)$ corresponds to the integration of a dynamic system or, equivalently, a convolution operator.

5.5 Posterior Probability Mapping

The dominant paradigm for the analysis of neuroimaging data to date has been statistical parametric mapping [12, 7]. This is a mass-univariate approach in which GLMs are fitted at each voxel using ML or OLS estimators. Contrasts of parameter estimates are then used to make maps of statistical parameters (e.g. T or F values) that quantify effects of interest. These maps are then thresholded using random field theory (RFT)[7] to correct for the multiple statistical tests made over the image volume.

The RFT correction is important as it protects against false-positive inferences. A naive or "uncorrected p-value" of 0.05, used with images containing 100,000 voxels, will lead to SPMs containing on average 5,000 false-positives. This is clearly too liberal. RFT protects instead against family-wise errors (FWEs) where the "family" is the set of voxels in an image. An FWE rate or "corrected p-value" of 0.05 implies on average only a single error in 20 SPMs. This much more conservative criterion has become a standard in the analysis of PET and fMRI data.

Despite its success, statistical parametric mapping has a number of fundamental limitations. In SPM the p-value, ascribed to a particular effect, does not reflect the likelihood that the effect is present but simply the probability of getting the observed data in the effect's absence. If sufficiently small, this p-value can be used to reject the null hypothesis that the effect is negligible. There are several shortcomings of this classical approach.

Firstly, one can never reject the alternate hypothesis (i.e. say that an activation has not occurred) because the probability that an effect is exactly zero is itself zero. This is problematic, for example, in trying to establish double dissociations or indeed functional segregation; one can never say one area responds to color but not motion and another responds to motion but not color.

Secondly, because the probability of an effect being zero is vanishingly small, given enough scans or subjects one can always demonstrate a significant effect at every voxel. This fallacy of classical inference is becoming relevant practically, with the thousands of scans entering into some fixed-effect analyses of fMRI data. The issue here is that a trivially small activation can be declared significant if there are sufficient degrees of freedom to render the variability of the activation's estimate small enough.

A third problem, that is specific to SPM, is the correction or adjustment applied to the p-values to resolve the multiple comparison problem. This has the somewhat nonsensical effect of changing the inference about one part of the brain in a way that is contingent on whether another part is examined. Put simply, the threshold increases with search volume, rendering inference very sensitive to what that inference encompasses. Clearly the probability that any voxel has activated does not change with the search volume and yet the classical p-value does.

All these problems would be eschewed by using the probability that a voxel had activated, or indeed its activation was greater than some threshold. This sort of inference is precluded by classical approaches, which simply give the likelihood of getting the data, given no activation. What one would really like is the probability distribution of the activation given the data. This is the posterior probability used in Bayesian inference.

The posterior distribution requires both the likelihood, afforded by assumptions about the signal and distribution of errors, and the prior probability of activation. These priors can enter as known values or can be estimated from the data. To date, two types of prior have been advocated for fMRI. A global shrinkage prior [14], which for the ith voxel and jth regression coefficient is given by

$$p(\beta_{ij}) = \mathsf{N}(\beta_{ij}; 0, \sigma_j^2), \tag{5.16}$$

where σ_j^2 quantifies the effect variability over the brain. This prior encodes a belief that every region of the brain is activated in every task but to a greater or lesser degree. More recently gaussian markov random field (GMRF) priors have been proposed [23]. These can be written

$$p(\beta_{ij}) = \mathsf{N}(\beta_{ij}; \sum_{k \in N_i} a_k \beta_{kj}, \sigma_j^2), \tag{5.17}$$

where N_i defines a set of voxels in the neighborhood of voxel i and a_k are spatial weighting coefficients. This encourages parameter estimates to be similar to those at nearby voxels. These priors provide an adaptive spatial regularization that renders the resulting Bayesian inference more sensitive than the equivalent classical inference [23].

5.5.1 Attention to Visual Motion

In this section we compare Bayesian and classical inference using PPMs and SPMs based on real data. These data were analyzed using a conventional SPM procedure [7, 12] and the PEB approach (using global shrinkage priors) described in the previous section. Inference in PPMs is based on the posterior distribution of effect sizes, which is shown for a single voxel in figure 5.4. This collection of posterior distributions can be turned into a PPM by specifying (i) an effect-size threshold and (ii) a probability threshold [14]. Here we used an effect-size threshold of 0.7% of whole-brain mean, and a probability threshold of 0.95.

The SPM and PPM for these data are presented in figures 5.5 and 5.6. We used a contrast that tested for the effect of visual motion above and beyond that due to photic stimulation with stationary dots, i.e. $c^T = [0100]$ (cf. the design matrix in figure 5.1). These effects are restricted to visual and extrastriate cortex involved in motion processing.

The difference between the PPM and SPM is immediately apparent on inspection of figure 5.6. The critical thing to note is that the SPM identifies a smaller number of voxels than the PPM. Indeed the SPM appears to have missed a critical and bilaterally represented part of the V5 complex (circled cluster on the PPM in the right panel of figure 5.6). The SPM is more conservative because the correction for multiple comparisons in these data is very severe, rendering classical inference relatively insensitive. It is interesting to note that dynamic motion in the visual field has such widespread (if small) effects at a hemodynamic level.

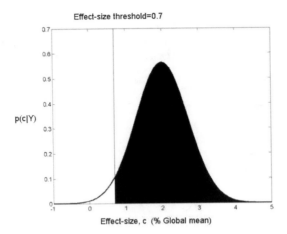

Figure 5.4   Posterior distribution of effect size at a particular voxel. The shaded area gives the posterior probability that the effect size is larger than the chosen threshold of 0.7%. For this voxel, this probability is 0.967. This is larger than the probability threshold 0.95 so this voxel would appear in the PPM shown in figure 5.5.

5.6   Dynamic Causal Modeling

Dynamic causal modeling (DCM) is used to make inferences about functional integration and has been formulated for the analysis of fMRI time series in [11]. The term "causal" in DCM arises because the brain is treated as a deterministic dynamical system in which external inputs cause changes in neuronal activity which in turn cause changes in the resulting BOLD signal that is measured with fMRI. This is to be contrasted with a conventional GLM where there is no explicit representation of neuronal activity. The second main difference to the GLM is that DCM allows for interactions between regions. Of course, it is this interaction which is central to the study of functional integration.

Current DCMs for fMRI comprise a bilinear model for the neurodynamics and an extended balloon model for the hemodynamics [2, 8]. The neurodynamics are described by the multivariate differential equation

$$\dot{z} = \left(A + \sum_i u_i B_i \right) z + Cu, \tag{5.18}$$

where z is a vector of neuronal activity, $\dot{z}$ denotes the time derivative, and u is a vector of experimental stimuli. This is known as a bilinear model because the dependent variable, $\dot{z}$, is linearly dependent on the product of u_i and z. That u_i and z combine in a multiplicative fashion endows the model with "nonlinear"

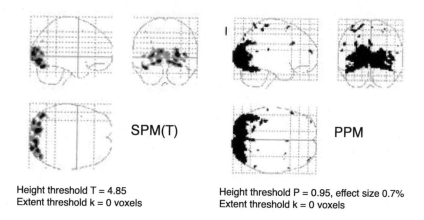

Height threshold T = 4.85
Extent threshold k = 0 voxels

Height threshold P = 0.95, effect size 0.7%
Extent threshold k = 0 voxels

Figure 5.5 Maximum intensity projections (MIPs) of SPM (left) and PPM (right) for the fMRI study of attention to visual motion. The SPM uses a threshold corrected for multiple comparisons at p = 0.05. The PPM uses an effect-size threshold of 0.7% and a probability threshold of 0.95.

dynamics that can be understood as a nonstationary linear system that changes according to experimental manipulation u. Importantly, because u is known, parameter estimation is relatively simple.

Connectivity in DCM is characterized by a set of "intrinsic connections", A, that specify which regions are connected and whether these connections are unidirectional or bidirectional. We also define a set of input connections, C, that specify which inputs are connected to which regions, and a set of modulatory or bilinear connections, B, that specify which intrinsic connections can be changed by which inputs. The overall specification of input, intrinsic, and modulatory connectivity comprise our assumptions about model structure. This in turn represents a scientific hypothesis about the structure of the large-scale neuronal network mediating the underlying sensorimotor or cognitive function.

In DCM, neuronal activity gives rise to fMRI activity by a dynamic process described by an extended balloon model for each region or node. This involves a set of hemodynamic state variables, state equations, and hemodynamic parameters, h. In brief, for the ith region, neuronal activity z_i causes an increase in the vasodilator signal s_i that is subject to autoregulatory feedback. Inflow f_i responds in proportion to this signal with concomitant changes in blood vol-

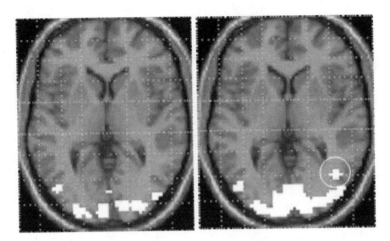

Figure 5.6 Overlays for SPM (left) and PPM (right) for the fMRI study of attention to visual motion, showing axial slices at $z = 3$ mm through extrastriate cortex. The thresholds are the same as those used in the MIPs in figure 5.5

ume v_i and deoxyhemoglobin content q_i.

$$
\begin{aligned}
\dot{s}_i &= z_i - \kappa_i s_i - \gamma_i(f_i - 1) \\
\dot{f}_i &= s_i \\
\tau_i \dot{v}_i &= f_i - v_i^{1/\alpha} \\
\tau_i \dot{q}_i &= f_i \frac{E(f_i, \rho_i)}{\rho_i} - v_i^{1/\alpha} \frac{q_i}{v_i}
\end{aligned}
\tag{5.19}
$$

Outflow is related to volume $f_{out} = v^{1/\alpha}$ through Grubb's exponent α [11]. The oxygen extraction is a function of flow $E(f, \rho) = 1 - (1 - \rho)^{1/f}$ where ρ is resting oxygen extraction fraction. The BOLD signal is then taken to be a static nonlinear function of volume and deoxyhemoglobin content [11].

Together these equations describe a nonlinear hemodynamic process that may be regarded as a biophysically informed generalization of the linear convolution models used in the GLM. This process converts neuronal activity in the ith region z_i to the hemodynamic response. Full details are given in [8, 11].

Fitting a DCM to fMRI time series Y involves the following steps. Firstly, the parameters $\theta = \{A, B, C, h\}$ are initialized by setting them to their prior values. These priors incorporate biophysical and dynamic constraints. The neurodynamic (equation (5.18)) and hemodynamic processes (equation (5.19)) are numerically integrated to obtain a predicted fMRI time series. This integration is efficient because most fMRI experiments employ input vectors that are highly sparse by experimental design. The parameters θ are then updated using the PEB algorithm described in section 5.4.4. The PEB and integration steps are iterated until convergence. Inferences about connections can then be made from the posterior density $p(\theta|Y)$.

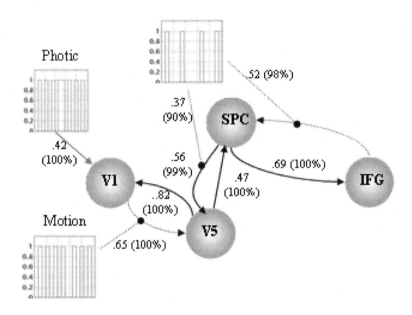

Figure 5.7 DCM for the fMRI study of attention to visual motion. The most interesting aspects of this connectivity involve the role of motion and attention in exerting bilinear effects. Critically, the influence of motion is to enable connections from V1 to the motion-sensitive area V5. The influence of attention is to enable backward connections from the inferior frontal gyrus (IFG) to the superior parietal cortex (SPC). Furthermore, attention increases the influence of SPC on V5. Dotted arrows connecting regions represent significant bilinear effects in the absence of a significant intrinsic coupling. Numbers in brackets represent the posterior probability, expressed as a percentage, that the effect size is larger than 0.17. This cutoff corresponds to a time constant of 4 seconds or less - in DCM stronger effects have faster time constants.

5.6.1   Attention to Visual Motion

We now return to the attention to visual motion study so as to make inferences about functional integration. Firstly a number of regions were selected. These were located in primary visual cortex V1, motion-sensitive area V5, superior parietal cortex, (SPC), and (inferior frontal gyrus), IFG. These regions were based on maxima from conventional SPMs testing for the effects of photic stimulation, motion, and attention. The DCM was set up as shown in figure 5.7. Regional time courses were taken as the first eigenvariate of 8 mm spherical volumes at each location. This eigenvariate approach was used so as to obtain a single representative time series from the cluster of active voxels in each region and was implemented using a singular value decomposition (SVD)

The inputs, in this example, comprise one sensory perturbation and two contextual inputs. The sensory input was simply the presence of photic stimulation and the first contextual one was presence of motion in the visual field. The second contextual input, encoding attentional set, was unity during attention to speed changes and zero otherwise. The outputs corresponded to the four regional eigenvariates. The intrinsic connections were constrained to conform to a hierarchical pattern in which each area was reciprocally connected to its supraordinate area. Photic stimulation entered at, and only at, V1. The effect of motion in the visual field was modeled as a bilinear modulation of the V1 to V5 connectivity and attention was allowed to modulate the backward connections from IFG and SPC.

The results of the DCM are shown in figure 5.7. Of primary interest here is the modulatory effect of attention that is expressed in terms of the bilinear coupling parameters for this third input. As hoped, we can be highly confident that attention modulates the backward connections from IFG to SPC and from SPC to V5. Indeed, the influences of IFG on SPC are negligible in the absence of attention (dotted connection in figure 5.7). It is important to note that the only way that attentional manipulation could affect brain responses was through this bilinear effect. Attention-related responses are seen throughout the system. This attentional modulation is accounted for by changing just two connections. This change is, presumably, instantiated by instructional set at the beginning of each epoch.

This analysis also illustrates how functional segregation is modeled in DCM. Here one can regard V1 as "segregating" motion from other visual information and distributing it to the motion-sensitive area V5. This segregation is modeled as a bilinear "enabling" of V1 to V5 connections when, and only when, motion is present. Note that in the absence of motion the intrinsic V1 to V5 connection was trivially small (in fact the posterior mean was -0.04). The key advantage of entering motion through a bilinear effect, as opposed to a direct effect on V5, is that we can finesse the inference that V5 shows motion-selective responses with the assertion that these responses are mediated by afferents from V1. The two bilinear effects above represent two important aspects of functional integration that DCM was designed to characterize.

Finally, we note that the inferences we have made are dependent on the particular model we have chosen, that is, the pattern of intrinsic and modulatory connectivity. As alluded to in section 5.4.3, it is possible to compare models using Bayesian model comparison based on the model evidence. This has been implemented for DCMs applied to these data and resulted in two main findings [21]. Firstly, models with reciprocal connections between hierarchical areas are favored over models with purely feedforward connections or models with a full connectivity. Secondly, attentional effects are best explained by modulation of forward rather than backward connections.

5.7 Discussion

This chapter has described the application of Bayesian methods to neuroimaging data. A key issue we have addressed is the relationship between the neurobiological hypothesis one posits and the statistical models adopted to test that hypothesis.

Historically, the focus of neuroimaging analysis has been the identification of regions that are specialized for certain functions. More recently these approaches have been augmented with multivariate approaches that describe imaging data in terms of distributed network models [22].

Ideally one would like to take neural network models defined by computational neuroscientists and use imaging data to estimate unknown parameters. While this is some way off steps are nevertheless being made to close the gap. A key step in this direction is the development of the DCM framework. This is currently being extended to explain event-related potentials derived from EEG/MEG data. The underlying neuronal models contain excitatory and inhibitory parameters that govern the dynamics of neuronal masses [6]. These parameters are estimated using the PEB framework described in this chapter.

This illustrates a key point that guides the development of our methodologies. As our models become more realistic and therefore complex they need to be constrained in some way and a simple and principled way of doing this is to use priors in a Bayesian context.

Due to the concise nature of this review we have been unable to cover a number of important topics in the analysis of imaging data.

The first is the use of spatial "preprocessing" methods to remove the effects of motion, and to spatially normalize data to transform it into a standard anatomical space. This is necessary so that regionally specific effects can be reported in a frame of reference that can be related to other studies. It is also necessary for analyses of group data. These methods adopt Bayesian paradigms to constrain the estimated transformations. Further details can be found in [7].

The second area is multimodal integration. We have also applied the PEB framework described in this chapter to the problem of source localization in EEG/MEG [24]. See also [26] for a recent approach using variational Bayes (VB). We, and many others (see e.g. [5]), are currently developing models that will integrate information from EEG, to find out primarily when activations occur, with information from fMRI/MRI, to find out where activations occur. This is an exciting area that would significantly strengthen the bridge between modalities in imaging neuroscience and our understanding of the neurobiology underlying cognitive processing.

References

[1] Buchel C, Coull JT, Friston KJ (1999) The predictive value of changes in effective connectivity for human learning. *Science*, 283:1538–1541.

[2] Buxton RB, Wong EC, Frank LR (1998) Dynamics of blood flow and oxygenation changes during brain activation: The Balloon Model. *Magnetic Resonance in Medicine*, 39:855–864.

[3] Copas JB (1983) Regression prediction and shrinkage. *Journal of the Royal Statistical Society Series B*, 45:311–354.

[4] Dale A, Buckner R (1997) Selective averaging of rapidly presented individual trials using fMRI. *Human Brain Mapping*, 5:329–340.

[5] Dale AM, Sereno MI (1993) Improved localisation of cortical activity by combining EEG and MEG with MRI cortical surface reconstruction. *Journal of Cognitive Neuroscience*, 5:162–176.

[6] David O, Friston KJ (2003) A neural mass model for MEG/EEG: coupling and neuronal dynamics. *NeuroImage*, 20(3):1743–1755.

[7] Frackowiak RSJ, Friston KJ, Frith C, Dolan R, Price CJ, Zeki S, Ashburner J, Penny WD (2003) *Human Brain Function*, 2nd edition. New York: Academic Press.

[8] Friston KJ (2002) Bayesian estimation of dynamical systems: an application to fMRI. *NeuroImage*, 16:513–530.

[9] Friston KJ, Fletcher P, Josephs O, Holmes AP, Rugg MD, Turner R (1998) Event-related fMRI: characterizing differential responses. *NeuroImage*, 7:30–40.

[10] Friston KJ, Glaser DE, Henson RNA, Kiebel SJ, Phillips C, Ashburner J (2002) Classical and Bayesian inference in neuroimaging: applications. *NeuroImage*, 16:484–512.

[11] Friston KJ, Harrison L, Penny WD (2003) Dynamic causal modelling. *NeuroImage*, 19(4):1273–1302.

[12] Friston KJ, Holmes AP, Worsley KJ, Poline JB, Frith C, Frackowiak RSJ (1995) Statistical parametric maps in functional imaging: a general linear approach. *Human Brain Mapping*, 2:189–210.

[13] Friston KJ, Jezzard P, Turner R (1994) Analysis of functional MRI time-series. *Human Brain Mapping*, 1:153–171.

[14] Friston KJ, Penny WD (2003) Posterior probability maps and SPMs. *NeuroImage*, 19(3):1240–1249.

[15] Friston KJ, Penny WD, Phillips C, Kiebel SJ, Hinton G, Ashburner J (2002) Classical and Bayesian inference in neuroimaging: theory. *NeuroImage*, 16:465–483.

[16] Henson RNA, Rugg MD, Friston KJ (2001) The choice of basis functions in event-related fMRI. *NeuroImage*, 13(6):127, June. Supplement 1.

[17] Kiebel SJ, Goebel R, Friston KJ (2000) Anatomically informed basis functions. *NeuroImage*, 11(6):656–667.

[18] Lee PM (1997) *Bayesian Statistics: An Introduction*, 2nd edition. London: Arnold.

[19] Melie-Garcia L, Trujillo-Barreto N, Martinez-Montes E, Valdes-Sosa P (1999) A symmetrical Bayesian model for fMRI and EEG/MEG neuroimage fusion. *International Journal of Biolelectromagnetism*, 3(1).

[20] Penny WD, Flandin G, Trujillo-Bareto N (2007) Bayesian comparison of spatially regularised general linear models. *Human Brain Mapping*, 28(4):275-293.

[21] Penny WD, Stephan KE, Mechelli A, Friston KJ (2004) Comparing dynamic causal models. *NeuroImage*, 22(3):1157–1172.

[22] Penny WD, Stephan KE, Mechelli A, Friston KJ (2004) Modelling functional integration: a comparison of structural equation and dynamic causal and models. *NeuroImage*, 23:264-274.

[23] Penny WD, Trujillo-Barreto N, Friston KJ (2005) Bayesian fMRI time series analysis with spatial priors. *NeuroImage*, 24(2):350–362.

[24] Phillips C, Rugg MD, Friston KJ (2002) Systematic regularization of linear inverse solutions of the EEG source localization problem. *NeuroImage*, 17(1):287–301.

[25] Rao CR, Toutenberg H (1995) *Linear Models: Least Squares and Alternatives*. New York: Springer-Verlag.

[26] Sato M, Yoshioka T, Kajiwara S, Toyoma K, Goda N, Doya K, Kawato (2004) Hierarchical Bayesian estimation for MEG inverse problem. *Neuroimage*, 23:806–826.

[27] Zeki S, Lueck CJ, Friston KJ, Kennard C, Watson JD, Frackowiak RS (1991) A direct demonstration of functional specialization in human visual cortex. *Journal of Neuroscience*, 11(3):641–649.

PART III

Making Sense of the World

6 Population Codes

Alexandre Pouget and Richard S. Zemel

6.1 Introduction

Many variables in the brain are encoded with what are known as population codes. The representation of the orientation of visual contours provides a classic example of a population code [22]. Figure 6.1 shows an (idealized) example of the tuning curves of a population of orientation-tuned cells in V1 in response to visual contours of different orientations, presented at the best position on the retina. These can be roughly characterized as bell-shaped curves, which we denote as $f_i(s)$, where i is an index over neurons and s is the encoded variable, such as the orientation of the edge in the receptive field. Each tuning curve is characterized by the location of its peak, also known as the preferred orientation (denoted s_i). In a cortical hypercolumn, the preferred orientations are spread approximately evenly along a circle, so that all orientations are represented equally well. The highlighted cell in figure 6.1 has preferred orientation s_i=90 degrees.

Evidence exists for this form of coding at the sensory input areas of the brain (e.g., retinotopic and tonotopic maps), as well as at the motor output level, and in many other intermediate neural processing areas, including superior colliculus neurons encoding saccade direction [24], higher visual area MT neurons responding to local velocity [25], adjacent area MST neurons sensitive to global motion parameters [17], inferotemporal (IT) neurons responding to human faces [31], hippocampal place cells responding to the location of a rat in an environment [26], and cells in primary motor cortex of a monkey responding to the direction it is to move its arm [13].

A major focus of theoretical neuroscience has been understanding how populations of neurons *encode* information about single variables and how this information can be *decoded* from the population activity. This is the focus of the first part of this chapter. Recently, several studies have also considered how neuronal populations may offer a rich representation of such things as *uncertainty* or probability distribution over the encoded stimulus, and what computational advantages (or disadvantages) such schemes have. These approaches

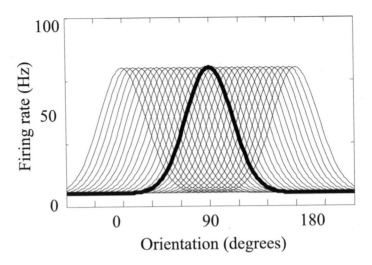

Figure 6.1 Homogeneous population code. Bell-shaped tuning functions $f_i(s)$ for a collection of idealized model V1 neurons as a function of angle s (and at a given stimulus contrast). The thick line shows a cell's Gaussian tuning function, with preferred value $s_i = 90$ degrees and standard deviation of $\sigma = 15$ degrees plus a baseline activity of 5 Hz.

are reviewed in the second half of this chapter.

6.2 Coding and Decoding

We start by reviewing the standard approach to coding and decoding, using orientation selectivity as a case study.

The tuning curves shown in figure 6.1 only specify the mean activity of a neuron as a function of the orientation of the contour, where the activity is typically the number of spikes, or alternatively the number of spikes per second, also known as the firing rate (to simplify this discussion, we consider that the number of spikes are always measured over a 1 second time interval, such that spike counts and rates are always equal). On any given trial, however, the actual number of spikes r_i is not exactly equal to what the tuning curve, $f_i(s)$, predicts because neural activity in the cortex is variable. In other words, r_i is a random quantity (called a random variable) with mean $\langle r_i \rangle = f_i(s)$ (using $\langle g \rangle$ to indicate averaging over the randomness). We mostly consider in this chapter the simplest model of this for which the number of spikes r_i has a Poisson distribution (see, chapter 1, table 1.2). We also assume that we are dealing with a population of N neurons with independent noise. We use bold letter **r** to indicate a vector whose components are the individual spike counts (r_i); the probability $p(\mathbf{r}|s)$ of spike counts is given by:

$$p(\mathbf{r}|s) = \prod_{i=1}^{N} p(r_i|s) = \prod_{i=1}^{N} \frac{f_i(s)^{r_i} e^{-f_i(s)}}{r_i!} \tag{6.1}$$

For this distribution, the variance is equal to the mean, which is indeed a good approximation to the noise found in the nervous system (see, for instance, [46, 39, 15]). In this chapter, we also restrict our discussion to rate-based descriptions, ignoring the details of precise spike timing.

Equation (6.1) is called an *encoding* model of orientation, specifying how orientation information is encoded in the population response. One natural question is to ask how orientation s can be read out of, i.e., decoded from the noisy spike counts $\mathbf{r}$. Decoding can be used as a computational tool, for instance, to assess the fidelity with which the population manages to code for the stimulus, or (at least a lower bound to) the *information* contained in the activities [6, 34]. However, decoding is not an essential neurobiological operation, as there is almost never a reason to decode the stimulus explicitly. Rather, the population code is used to support computations involving s, whose outputs are represented in the form of yet more population codes over the same or different collections of neurons [50, 10, 4, 33]. In this chapter, we consider the narrower, but still important, computational question of extracting approximations $\hat{s}(r)$ to s.

6.2.1 Population Vector

A simple heuristic method for decoding orientation, or any periodic variable, is to say that cell i "votes" for a vector, $\mathbf{c}_i$, pointing in the direction of its preferred orientation s_i with a strength determined by its activity r_i. Then, the *population vector*, $\hat{\mathbf{c}}$, is computed by pooling all votes [13], and an estimate $\hat{s}_{\text{PV}}(r)$ can be derived from the direction of $\hat{\mathbf{c}}$

$$\begin{aligned} \hat{\mathbf{c}} &= \sum_{i=1}^{N} \frac{r_i \mathbf{c}_i}{\sum_{j=1}^{N} r_j} \\ \hat{s}_{\text{PV}}(\mathbf{r}) &= \text{direction}(\hat{\mathbf{c}}) \end{aligned} \tag{6.2}$$

This estimator will only work for periodic variables, although variations exist for nonperiodic variables as well [41, 14]. The main problem with the population vector method is that it is not sensitive to the noise process that generates the actual rates r_i from the mean rates $f_i(s)$ (equation (6.1)). As a result, it tends to produce large errors.

Those errors can be quantified in several ways. One popular approach entails computing the mean and standard deviation of the estimator over many trials in which the value of s was maintained constant. Ideally, the mean should be as close as possible to the true value of s on these trials. The difference between the mean of the estimate and the true value is called the *bias*, and the estimator is said to be unbiased when the bias is equal to zero. Likewise, the *variance* of the estimator should be as small as possible, that is, if the same stimulus s is presented over many trials, it is best to have as little variability as possible in the estimates. As we will see, it is possible to compute a lower bound on the standard deviation of an unbiased estimator, known as the Cramér-Rao bound [28]. The best estimators are the ones which reach this bound.

This is not the case for the population vector estimator, which is often biased and whose standard deviation is generally well above the Cramér-Rao bound [41]. Nevertheless, it can perform reasonably well in some situations, as demonstrated in particular by Georgopoulos et al. [13].

6.2.2   Maximum Likelihood Estimator

A particularly important estimator is the *maximum likelihood* estimator (section 1.4.1) [28]. This starts from the full probabilistic encoding model, which, by taking into account the noise corrupting the activities of the neurons, specifies the probability $p(\mathbf{r}|s)$ of observing activities $\mathbf{r}$ if the stimulus is s. For the Poisson encoding model, this *likelihood* is given by equation (6.1).

Values of s for which $p(\mathbf{r}|s)$ is high are orientations which are likely to have produced the observed activities $\mathbf{r}$; values of s for which $p(\mathbf{r}|s)$ is low are unlikely. The maximum likelihood estimate $\hat{s}_{ML}(\mathbf{r})$ is the value that maximizes $p(\mathbf{r}|s)$:

$$\hat{s}_{ML}(\mathbf{r}) = \arg\max_{s} p(\mathbf{r}|s) \qquad (6.3)$$

For a large number of neurons with independent noise, the maximum likelihood estimator can be shown to be unbiased and has minimal variance (see section 6.2.4) [29, 38]. This method is therefore optimal in this case. In general, even when these conditions are not met, maximum likelihood outperforms the population vector estimator.

However, there is a cost. This method requires that we estimate the likelihood function $p(\mathbf{r}|s)$. Looking at equation (6.1), one can see that, when the noise is independent and Poisson, we need to know the tuning curves $f_i(s)$ to estimate $p(\mathbf{r}|s)$. By contrast, the population vector only needs estimates of the preferred orientations, s_i, i.e., the orientation corresponding to the peak of the tuning curves. Clearly, estimating s_i can be done with a lot less data than are needed to estimate the full tuning curves. This is an important issue in many experiments because data tend to be very limited. The maximum likelihood approach can be used even with a small set of data, but if the estimate of $f_i(s)$ is poor, the performance of the estimator will suffer. In particular, it is no longer guaranteed to outperform the population vector estimator.

6.2.3   Bayesian Estimates

The final class of estimators we review are called *Bayesian* estimates (see, chapter 1, section 1.4.3). They combine the likelihood $p(\mathbf{r}|s)$ with any prior information about the stimulus s (for instance, that horizontal and vertical orientation are more likely in man-made environments like houses) to produce a *posterior* distribution $p(s|\mathbf{r})$ [12, 36]:

$$p(s|\mathbf{r}) = \frac{p(\mathbf{r}|s)\,p(s)}{p(\mathbf{r})} \tag{6.4}$$

When the prior distribution $p(s)$ is uniform, that is, when there is no specific prior information about s, this is a renormalized version of the likelihood, where the renormalization ensures that it is a proper probability distribution (i.e., integrates to 1). The posterior distribution summarizes everything that the neural activity and any prior information have to say about s, and so is the most complete basis for decoding. Bayesian inference proceeds using a *loss* function L($s\prime,s$), which indicates the cost of reporting $s\prime$ when the true value is s; it is optimal to decode to the value $\hat{s}(\mathbf{r})$ that minimizes the cost, averaged over the posterior distribution [7].

In most situations, the Bayesian and maximum likelihood decoding typically outperform the population vector approach by a rather large margin [52]. In general, the greater the number of cells, the greater the accuracy with which the stimulus can be decoded by any method, since more cells can provide more information about s. However, this conclusion does depend on the way, if at all, that the noise corrupting the activity is correlated between the cells [42, 27, 1, 49, 43, 48], and the way that information about these correlations is used by the decoders.

6.2.4 Assessing the Quality of an Estimator: Fisher information

As we have discussed, the quality of an estimator can be assessed by computing the absolute value of the bias and the variance of the estimator. The best estimators are the ones minimizing these two measures. For simplicity, we will assume that we are dealing with unbiased estimators, in which case the main factor is the variance of the estimator (the best estimators are often close to being unbiased when using large neuronal populations). For unbiased estimators, it is possible to derive a lower bound, also known as the Cramér-Rao bound, on the variance of any estimator [28]. This bound is related to a quantity known as Fisher information, $I_F(s)$: Specifically, the variance, σ_s^2, of any unbiased estimator of s is such that

$$\sigma_s^2 \geq \frac{1}{I_F(s)}, \tag{6.5}$$

where Fisher information is defined as

$$I_F(s) = -\left\langle \frac{\partial^2 \ln p(\mathbf{r}|s)}{\partial s^2} \right\rangle, \tag{6.6}$$

where the brackets indicate an average over values of $\mathbf{r}$. Therefore, if Fisher information is large, the best decoder will recover s with a small variance, that is to say with a high accuracy. In the case of independent Poisson noise, the variance of the maximum likelihood estimator reaches the Cramér-Rao bound (that is, equation (6.5) becomes an equality) as the number of neurons grows to infinity [30, 38]. It is therefore the optimal estimator in this situation.

Another approach to quantify the quality of an estimator would be to compute the amount by which s must be changed in order to detect the change reliably (say 80% of the time) from observation of the spike counts, $\mathbf{r}$. If this change, δs, is small, one can conclude that the neural code contains a lot of information about s. In psychophysics, δs is known as the discrimination threshold of an ideal observer of $\mathbf{r}$ [18]. Interestingly, δs is inversely proportional to Fisher information. This makes sense because if Fisher information is large, the variance of the best estimator is small, and therefore, it is possible to detect small changes in s.

The relationship between Fisher information and discrimination threshold is one of the appealing properties of Fisher information. It allows us to establish a direct link between the quality of a neural code and behavioral performance. Another advantage is that it can be used to identify which aspects of a neural code have the highest impact of information content (and therefore, behavioral performance). For instance, in the case of a population of N neurons with independent Poisson noise, one can compute Fisher information explicitly from equation (6.6):

$$I_F\left(s\right) = \sum_{i=1}^{N} \frac{f_i'\left(s\right)^2}{f_i\left(s\right)}, \tag{6.7}$$

where $f_i'\left(s\right)$ is the derivative (or slope) of the tuning curve. The denominator in equation 5 is the variance of the noise corrupting the responses, which in the case of Poisson noise, happens to equal the mean, which is why $f_i\left(s\right)$ appears in the denominator.

Equation (6.7) shows that Fisher information decreases as the variance of the noise increases, which seems intuitively correct. Perhaps more surprisingly, information grows with the slope of the tuning curves: the steeper the side of the tuning curves, the more information in the population. This means that at the peak of the tuning curve, where the tuning curve flattens out, and hence where the derivative is equal to zero, a neuron conveys no Fisher information about s. This implies that the neurons firing the most in response to a stimulus are not the most informative ones. Instead, the most informative neurons are the ones firing at intermediate values, where the slope of the tuning curve reaches its maximum.

6.3   Representing Uncertainty with Population Codes

In the previous section we reviewed the standard view of population codes. In this view, the information conveyed by the population has associated uncertainty due to noisy neural activities, and this inherent uncertainty can be seen as a nuisance with respect to decoding the responses. Recently, however, an alternative view has emerged, in which the uncertainty in the encoded variables is seen as desirable. In many situations, there is inherent uncertainty in the variable. For example, many experiments support the idea that perception is a result of a statistical inference process [23]. One example is demonstrations of how the perceived speed of a grating increases with contrast [45, 44, 5]. This effect is easy to explain within a probabilistic framework. The idea is that the nervous system seeks the posterior distribution of velocity given the image sequence, obtained through Bayes rule.

In another experiment, subjects were asked to judge the height of a bar, which they could see and touch [11]. They viewed a stimulus consisting of many dots, displayed as if glued to the surface of the bar. To make the task harder, each dot was moved in depth away from the actual depth of the bar, according to a noise term drawn from a Gaussian distribution. As the width of the noise distribution was increased, subjects found it harder to estimate the height of the bar accurately. Then haptic information about the height was also provided through a force-feedback robot, allowing subjects the chance to integrate it with the variably uncertain visual information. Ernst and Banks reported that humans behave as predicted by Bayes law in combining these two information sources, taking into account the reliability of the two different cues[12].

This and many other psychophysical experiments suggest that the human brain somehow represents and manipulates uncertain information, which can be described in terms of probability distributions. In addition, from a computational standpoint, preserving and utilizing the full information contained in the posterior distribution $P(s|\mathbf{r})$ over a stimulus given neural responses, is of crucial importance. We use the term *distributional population codes* for population code representations of such probability distributions. The task of representing distributions can be seen as involving two spaces: an *explicit* space of neural activities, and an *implicit* space in which a probability distribution over the random variable is associated with the neurons. The random variable could be a continuous variable, such as the orientation of a bar, or a discrete variable, such as the reported information in a two-alternative forced choice task. Several schemes have been proposed for encoding and decoding a probability distribution over a random variable in populations of neurons. Here we briefly review some of the main types of such proposals.

6.3.1 Direct Encoding

Perhaps the simplest method of representing a distribution is when the neural activity corresponds directly to the probability. For example, if the random variable s can take on two values, with probability p = $P(s_1)$ and 1-p = $P(s_2)$, then two neurons a and b could represent p by some simple function of their activities: p could be the difference in the spike counts of neurons a and b, or log p could be the ratio of spike counts [16, 9]. Alternatively, the spike counts of neurons a and b could be seen as samples drawn from $P(s_1)$ and $P(s_2)$, respectively [21]. These systems can be generalized readily to variables that take on multiple discrete values [33].

Weiss and Fleet [47] took this direct encoding a step further, suggesting a probabilistic interpretation of a standard model, the motion-energy filter model, which is one of the most popular accounts of motion processing in the visual system [2]. Under their interpretation, the activity of a neuron tuned to preferred velocity v (ignoring its other preferences for retinal location, spatial frequency, etc.) is viewed as reporting the logarithm of the likelihood function of the image I given the motion, $\log P(I|bfv)$. This suggestion is intrinsically elegant, providing a statistical interpretation for conventional filter theory, and thereby suggesting a *constructive* mechanism, whereby neural activities come to represent distributions. Further, in the case that there is only a single motion in the image, decoding only involves the simple operation of (summing and) exponentiating to find the full likelihood. A variety of schemes for computing based on the likelihood are made readily possible by this scheme, although some of these require that the likelihood only have one peak for them to work.

6.3.2   Probabilistic Population Codes

A second distributional population coding scheme is closely related to the Bayesian decoder described in section 6.2.3 above. When a Bayesian approach is used to decode a population pattern of activity (equation (6.4)), the result is a posterior distribution $p(s|r)$ over the stimulus [12, 36]. This decoding method effectively interprets the population activity as a code for the probability distribution, $p(s|r)$, hence the name probabilistic population codes.

If the noise in the response of neurons in a large population is assumed to be independent, the law of large numbers dictates that this posterior distribution converges to a Gaussian [28]. Like any Gaussian distribution, it is fully characterized by its mean and standard deviation. The mean of this posterior distribution is controlled by the position of the noisy hill of activity. If the noisy hill is centered around a different stimulus value, so will be the posterior distribution. When the noise is independent and follows a Poisson distribution, the standard deviation of the posterior distribution is controlled by the amplitude of the hill. These effects are illustrated in figure 6.2.

Under this interpretation, there is a direct relationship between the gain of the population activity and the standard deviation of the posterior distribution. In other words, this scheme predicts that when the uncertainty of a stimulus increases, the gain of the population code encoding this stimulus should go down. This is indeed what happens with contrast: as the contrast of an oriented grating is decreased, which effectively increases the uncertainty about its orientation, the response of orientation-selective neurons decreases [37].

In its more general version, and in particular for correlated Poisson-like variability, this type of code can be used to encode any probability distribution, not just Gaussians. Indeed, if neurons are correlated, the law of large numbers no longer applies, which implies that the posterior distribution can take any form.

One of the advantages of this approach is that, with Poisson like variability, many Bayesian inferences reduce to simple sums of firing rates [32]. By

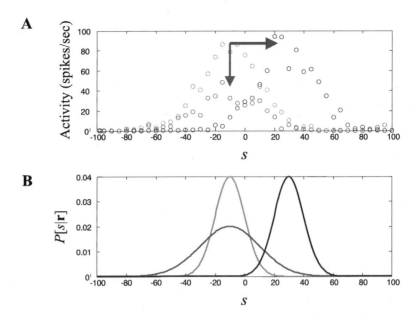

Figure 6.2   A. Population patterns of activity from a population of neurons with tuning curves as in figure 6.1, corrupted by Poisson noise. B. Posterior probability distributions obtained with a Bayesian decoder (equation 6.2) applied to the patterns in A. When the pattern of activity is simply translated (*blue arrow*), the peak of the distribution translates by the same amount and the width remains the same (*green* versus *blue curve* in *lower* panel). When the gain of the population activity decreases (*red arrow*), the posterior distribution widens (*green* vs. *red curves* in *bottom* panel) (see color insert).

Poisson-like variability, we mean variability of the type:

$$p(\mathbf{r}|s,g) = \phi(\mathbf{r},g) \exp\left(-(\Sigma^{-1}\mathbf{f}'(s)) \cdot \mathbf{r}\right), \tag{6.8}$$

where $\phi(\mathbf{r},g)$ is some arbitrary function, $\mathbf{f}'(s)$ are the derivatives of the tuning curves with respect to s, g is the gain of the population activity $\mathbf{r}$, and Σ is the covariance matrix of $\mathbf{r}$. As a special case, this equation includes distributions in which neurons are correlated and their mean activity scale with the variance, as seen in cortex. These distributions turn Bayesian inference into sums when the Bayesian inference involves a product of probability distributions. Indeed, if we multiply two distributions of the form shown in equation (6.8), the product of the exponential of the rates will yield an exponential of the sum of the rates.

6.3.3   Convolution Encoding

An alternative form of distributional population coding involves a Bayesian formulation of the representation of any form of posterior distribution $p(s|\mathbf{I})$

over the sensory input s given the encoded variable I. These coding schemes therefore are particularly suitable for a non-Gaussian distribution $p(s|\mathbf{I})$, which cannot be characterized by a few parameters such as its mean and variance. One possibility inspired by the encoding of nonlinear functions is to represent the distribution using a *convolution code*, obtained by convolving the distribution with a particular set of *kernel functions*.

The canonical kernel is the sine, as used in Fourier transforms. Most nonlinear functions of interest can be recovered from their Fourier transforms, which implies that they can be characterized by their Fourier coefficients. To specify a function with infinite accuracy one needs an infinite number of coefficients, but for most practical applications, a few coefficients suffice. One could therefore use a large neuronal population of neurons to encode any function by devoting each neuron to the encoding of one particular coefficient. The activity of neuron i is computed by taking the dot product between a sine function assigned to that neuron and the function being encoded (as is done in a Fourier transform).

Many other kernel functions may be used for convolution codes. For instance, one could use Gaussian kernels, in which case the activity of the neurons is obtained through:

$$f_i\left(p\left(s|\mathbf{I}\right)\right) = \int ds \exp\left(-\frac{(s-s_i)^2}{2\sigma_i^2}\right) p\left(s|\mathbf{I}\right). \tag{6.9}$$

Gaussian kernels are usually better than sine kernels for learning and computation when the distributions are concentrated around one or a small number of values. If a large population of neurons is used, and their Gaussian kernels are translated copies of one another, equation (6.9) becomes a discrete convolution. In other words, the pattern of activity across the neuronal population is simply the original distribution, filtered by a Gaussian kernel.

Note that when there is no uncertainty associated with encoded variable I, i.e., the encoded probability distribution is a Dirac function, $p(s|\mathbf{I}) = \delta(s,s^*)$, equation (6.9) reduces to:

$$f_i\left(p\left(s|\mathbf{I}\right)\right) = \exp\left(-\frac{(s^*-s_i)^2}{2\sigma_i^2}\right) \tag{6.10}$$

This is simply the equation for the response to orientation s^* of a neuron with a Gaussian tuning curve centered on s_i. In other words, the classical framework we reviewed in the first half of this chapter is a subcase of this more general approach.

With the convolution code, one solution to decoding is to use *deconvolution*, a linear filtering operation which reverses the application of the kernel functions. There is no exact solution to this problem but a close approximation to the original function can be obtained by applying a bandpass filter which typically takes the form of a Mexican hat kernel. The problem with this approach is that it fails miserably when the original distribution is sharply peaked, such as a

Dirac function. Indeed, a bandpass filter cannot recover the high frequencies, which are critical for sharply peaked functions. Moreover, linear filters do not perform well in the realistic case of noisy encoding neurons.

An alternative to this linear decoding scheme for convolution codes is to adopt a probabilistic approach. For instance, given the noisy activity of a population of neurons, one should not try to recover the most likely value of s, but rather the most likely *distribution* over s, $p(s|\mathbf{I})$ [50]. This can be achieved using a nonlinear regression method such as the expectation-maximization (EM) algorithm [8].

One trouble with convolutional encoding (and indeed the other encodings that we have described) is that there is no systematic way of representing multiple values as well as uncertainty. For instance, a wealth of experiments on population coding is based on random dot kinematograms, for which some fraction of the dots move in randomly selected directions, with the rest (the *correlated* dots) moving in one particular direction, which is treated as the stimulus s^*. It is not obviously reasonable to treat this stimulus as a probability *distribution* $p(s|\mathbf{I})$ over a single direction s (with a peak at s^*), since, in fact, there is actual motion in many directions. Rather, the population should be thought of as encoding a weighting or multiplicity function $\rho(s)$, which indicates the strength of direction s in the stimulus. Sahani and Dayan [35] noted this problem, and suggested a variant of the convolution code, called the doubly distributional population code (DDPC), to cope with this issue.

6.3.4 Convolution Decoding

Anderson [3] took this approach a step further, making the seminal suggestion of convolutional *decoding* rather than convolutional encoding. In one version of this scheme, activity r_i of neuron i is considered to be a vote for a particular (usually probabilistic) decoding basis function $p_i(s)$. Then, the overall distribution decoded from $\mathbf{r}$ is

$$\hat{p}(s|\mathbf{I}) = \frac{\sum_i r_i p_i(s)}{\sum_j r_j}, \qquad (6.11)$$

The advantage of this scheme is the straightforward decoding model; one disadvantage is the difficulty of formulating an encoding model for which this decoder is the appropriate Bayes optimal approach. A second disadvantage of this scheme is shared with the linear deconvolution approach: it cannot readily recover the high frequencies that are important for sharply peaked distributions $p(s|\mathbf{I})$, which arise in the case of ample information in $\mathbf{I}$.

In the decoding schemes of both Anderson [3] and Zemel et al. [50] the key concept is to treat a population pattern of activity as a representation of a probability distribution, as opposed to a single value (as is done in the standard approach reviewed in the first section). To see the difference consider a situation in which the neurons are noise-free. If the population code is encoding a single value, we can now recover the value of s with absolute certainty. In the case of Anderson and Zemel et al., we can now recover the distribution, $p(s|\mathbf{I})$, with

absolute certainty. As discussed earlier, in many real-world situations $p(s|\mathbf{I})$ is
not a Dirac function, so optimal decoding recovers the distribution $p(s|\mathbf{I})$ with
absolute certainty, but the inherent uncertainty about s remains.

Another form of convolutional decoding is suggested by maximum entropy,
or random field approaches, such as the product of experts model [20], in
which the decoded distribution is a product of contributions of each neuron
(the *experts*) in the population:

$$p(s|\mathbf{r}) \propto \prod_i p_i(s)^{r_i} = \exp\left(\sum_i r_i \log p_i(s)\right) \tag{6.12}$$

Note that this scheme is similar to Anderson's convolution decoding scheme,
in that each neuron has a basis function associated with it, and the basis functions are combined linearly, weighted by the neural responses. Here, however,
the decoded distribution is not directly given by this weighted combination,
but instead is a normalized exponential of the sum. This allows for the recovery of highly peaked distributions, and natural formulations of operations
such as combining cues. Interestingly, this scheme is in fact identical to the
probabilistic population code approach described earlier, for the specific case
in which the noise is independent and Poisson. Indeed, in this case, the likelihood function used by the decoder takes the form shown in equation (6.1),
which can be reduced to equation (6.12).

This scheme can be extended to allow spikes to form a representation of a
temporally changing probability distribution [19]. In this approach, the basis
functions associated with each neuron include both a component relevant to
the underlying variable s, and a temporal component, and the log-linear combination is additive over previous spikes,

$$\log p(s(t)|\mathbf{r}(t)) = \sum_{\tau=0}^{t}\sum_i x_i(\tau)\phi_i(s, t - \tau), \tag{6.13}$$

where $x_i(\tau)$ is 1 if and only if neuron i spiked at time τ and $\phi_i(s, t - \tau)$ is a decoding temporal kernel function. This representation uses precise spike times
to code distributions over values. A problem with the model is that it is inherently a decoding model, specifying how spikes can be decoded to report the
distribution over s. How encoding should work is not clear, and Hinton and
Brown [19] and Smith and Lewicki [40] used an acausal scheme, positioning
spikes at time τ based on information about $p(s(t))$ where $t > \tau$. Zemel et
al. [51] proposed a recurrent network that learns the corresponding encoding
model, producing spikes in a causal manner so that the decoding model specified in equation (6.13) accurately represents the posterior distribution over s at
time t, based only on spikes at or before time t.

6.4   Conclusion

Population codes are coming of age as representational devices, in that there is a widely accepted standard encoding and decoding model together with a mature understanding of its properties. However, there remain many areas of active investigation. One particular one that we have highlighted is the way that uncertainty can be represented and manipulated in population codes. An important open question with respect to these models concerns how effectively they can represent time-varying inputs: most methods involve some form of spike counting, but when the stimulus is varying quickly with respect to the spiking process, then obtaining accurate counts is not feasible. An additional open question considers how they can be applied recursively, so that the same encoding and decoding schemes can apply at all levels in a network of population codes. Finally, as neurophysiological techniques improve to enable recording of responses in multiple populations simultaneously, questions concerning the information flow between populations can be addressed both theoretically and empirically.

References

[1] Abbott L, Dayan P (1999) The effect of correlated variability on the accuracy of a population code. *Neural Computation*, 11:91-101.

[2] Adelson EH, Bergen JR (1985) Spatiotemporal energy models for the perception of motion. *Journal of the Optical Society of America A*, 2:284-299.

[3] Anderson C (1994) Neurobiological computational systems. *In Computational Intelligence Imitating Life*, pages 213-222. New York: IEEE Press.

[4] Barber MJ, Clark JW, Anderson CH (2003) Neural representation of probabilistic information. *Neural Computation*, 15:1843-1864.

[5] Blakemore MR, Snowden RJ (1999) The effect of contrast upon perceived speed: a general phenomenon? *Perception*, 28:33-48.

[6] Borst A, Theunissen FE (1999) Information theory and neural coding. *Nature Neuroscience*, 2:947-957.

[7] DeGroot MH (1970) *Optimal Statistical Decisions*. New York: McGraw-Hill.

[8] Dempster AP, Laird NM, Rubin DB (1977) Maximum likelihood from incomplete data via the EM algorithm. *Journal of the Royal Statistical Society, B*, 39:1-38.

[9] Deneve S (2005) Bayesian inferences in spiking neurons. In *Neural Information Processing Systems*, Cambridge, MA: MIT Press.

[10] Deneve S, Latham P, Pouget A (1999) Reading population codes: a neural implementation of ideal observers. *Nature Neuroscience*, 2:740-745.

[11] Ernst MO, Banks MS (2002) Humans integrate visual and haptic information in a statistically optimal fashion. *Nature*, 415:429-433.

[12] Foldiak (1993) The "ideal homunculus": Statistical inference from neural population responses. In Eeckman F, Bower J, eds., *Computation and Neural Systems*, pages 55-60, Norwell, MA: Kluwer Academic Publishers.

[13] Georgopoulos A, Kalaska J, Caminiti R (1982) On the relations between the direction of two-dimensional arm movements and cell discharge in primate motor cortex. *Journal of Neuroscience*, 2:1527-1537.

[14] Georgopoulos A, Pellizer G, Poliakov A, Schieber M (1999) Neural coding of finger and wrist movements. *Journal of Computational Neuroscience*, 6:279-288.

[15] Gershon ED, Wiener MC, Latham PE, Richmond BJ (1998) Coding strategies in monkey V1 and inferior temporal cortices. *Journal of Neurophysiology*, 79:1135-1144.

[16] Gold JI, Shadlen MN (2001) Neural computations that underlie decisions about sensory stimuli. *Trends in Cognitive Sciences*, 5:10-16.

[17] Graziano MS, Andersen RA, Snowden RJ (1994) Tuning of MST neurons to spiral motions. *Journal of Neuroscience*, 14:54-67.

[18] Green DM, Swets JA (1966) *Signal Detection Theory and Psychophysics*. Los Altos, CA: Wiley.

[19] Hinton G, Brown A (2000) Spiking Boltzmann machines. In *Neural Information Processing Systems*, Cambridge, MA: MIT Press.

[20] Hinton GE (1999) Products of experts. In *Proceedings of the Ninth International Conference on Artificial Neural Networks*, pages 1-6, London: IEEE.

[21] Hoyer PO, Hyvarinen A (2003) Interpreting neural response variability as Monte Carlo sampling of the posterior. In *Neural Information Processing Systems* , volume 15, Cambridge, MA: MIT Press.

[22] Hubel D, Wiesel T (1962) Receptive fields, binocular interaction and functional architecture in the cat's visual cortex. *Journal of Physiology (London)*, 160:106-154.

[23] Knill DC, Richards W (1996) *Perception as Bayesian Inference*. New York: Cambridge University Press.

[24] Lee C, Rohrer WH, Sparks DL (1988) Population coding of saccadic eye movements by neurons in the superior colliculus. *Nature*, 332:357-360.

[25] Maunsell JHR, Van Essen DC (1983) Functional properties of neurons in middle temporal visual area of the macaque monkey. I. Selectivity for stimulus direction, speed, and orientation. *Journal of Neurophysiology*, 49:1127-1147.

[26] O'Keefe J, Dostrovsky J (1971) The hippocampus as a spatial map. Preliminary evidence from unit activity in the freely moving rat. *Brain Research*, 34:171-175.

[27] Oram M, Foldiak P, Perrett D, Sengpiel F (1998) The "Ideal Homunculus": decoding neural population signals. *Trends in Neurosciences*, 21:359-365.

[28] Papoulis A (1991) *Probability, Random Variables, and Stochastic Process*. New York: McGraw-Hill.

[29] Paradiso M (1988) A theory of the use of visual orientation information which exploits the columnar structure of striate cortex. *Biological Cybernetics*, 58:35-49.

[30] Paradiso MA, Carney T, Freeman RD (1989) Cortical processing of hyperacuity tasks. *Vision Research*, 29:247-254.

[31] Perrett DI, Smith PA, Potter DD, Mistlin AJ, Head AS, Milner AD, Jeeves MA (1985) Visual cells in the temporal cortex sensitive to face view and gaze direction. *Proceedings of the Royal Society of London. Series B: Biological Sciences*, 223:293-317.

[32] Pouget A, Latham PE (2005) Bayesian inference and cortical variability. In: *CoSyNe 2005*, Salt Lake City, www.cosyne.org.

[33] Rao RP (2004) Bayesian computation in recurrent neural circuits. *Neural Computation*, 16:1-38.

[34] Rieke F, Warland D, De Ruyter van Steveninck R, Bialek W (1999) *Exploring the Neural Code*. Cambridge, MA: MIT Press.

[35] Sahani M, Dayan P (2003) Doubly distributional population codes: simultaneous representation of uncertainty and multiplicity. *Neural Computation*, 15:2255-2279.

[36] Sanger T (1996) Probability density estimation for the interpretation of neural population codes. *Journal of Neurophysiology*, 76:2790-2793.

[37] Sclar G, Freeman R (1982) Orientation selectivity in the cat's striate cortex is invariant with stimulus contrast. *Experimental Brain Research*, 46:457-461.

[38] Seung H, Sompolinsky H (1993) Simple model for reading neuronal population codes. *Proceedings of the National Academy of Sciences of the United States of America*, 90:10749-10753.

[39] Shadlen M, Britten K, Newsome W, Movshon T (1996) A computational analysis of the relationship between neuronal and behavioral responses to visual motion. *Journal of Neuroscience*, 16:1486-1510.

[40] Smith E, Lewicki MS (2005) Efficient coding of time-relative structure using spikes. *Neural Computation*, 17:19-45.

[41] Snippe HP (1996) Parameter extraction from population codes: a critical assessment. *Neural Computation*, 8:511-529.

[42] Snippe HP, Koenderink JJ (1992) Information in channel-coded systems: correlated receivers. *Biological Cybernetics*, 67:183-190.

[43] Sompolinsky H, Yoon H, Kang K, M. S (2001) Population coding in neuronal systems with correlated noise. *Physical Review E, Statistical, Nonlinear and Soft Matter Physics*, 64:051904.

[44] Stone LS, Thompson P (1992) Human speed perception is contrast dependent. *Vision Research*, 32:1535-1549.

[45] Thompson P (1982) Perceived rate of movement depends on contrast. *Vision Research*, 22:377-380.

[46] Tolhurst D, Movshon J, Dean A (1982) The statistical reliability of signals in single neurons in cat and monkey visual cortex. *Vision Research*, 23:775-785.

[47] Weiss Y, Fleet DJ (2002) Velocity likelihoods in biological and machine vision. In Rao R, Oshausen B, Lewicki MS, eds., *Statistical Theories of the Cortex*, Cambridge, MA: MIT Press.

[48] Wilke SD, Eurich CW (2002) Representational accuracy of stochastic neural populations. *Neural Computation*, 14:155-189.

[49] Yoon H, Sompolinsky H (1999) The effect of correlations on the Fisher information of population codes. In Kearns MS, Solla S, Cohn DA, eds., *Advances in Neural Information Processing Systems*, pages 167-173, Cambridge, MA: MIT Press.

[50] Zemel R, Dayan P, Pouget A (1998) Probabilistic interpretation of population code. *Neural Computation*, 10:403-430.

[51] Zemel RS, Huys Q, Natarajan R, Dayan P (2004) Probabilistic computation in spiking populations. *Advances in Neural Information Processing Systems*, 17:1609-1616.

[52] Zhang K, Ginzburg I, McNaughton B, Sejnowski T (1998) Interpreting neuronal population activity by reconstruction: unified framework with application to hippocampal place cells. *Journal of Neurophysiology*, 79:1017-1044.

7 Computing with Population Codes

Peter Latham and Alexandre Pouget

One of the few things in systems neuroscience we are fairly certain about is that information is encoded in population activity. For example, a population of neurons coding for the orientation of a bar, (θ), might have firing rates $r_i = f(\theta - \theta_i) + \text{noise}$. Here $f(\theta)$ is a smooth, bell-shaped function and θ_i is the preferred orientation of neuron i.

Representing variables in populations codes, however, is only one step – just as important is *computing* with population codes. Sensorimotor transformations are a natural example: the brain receives information about the outside world; that information is represented in population activity at the sensory level; and to perform an action, such as reaching for an object, population codes in motor cortex must be generated to drive the appropriate joint movements. The transformation from the activity in sensory cortex to the activity in motor cortex is a computation based on population codes. Here we discuss how networks of neurons might implement such computations.

7.1 Computing, Invariance, and Throwing Away Information

Before we start, it's worth saying a few words about computing in general. Many, if not most, of the computations carried out by the brain involve *throwing away* information. For example, when computing a function, say $z = \phi(x, y)$, information about x and y is thrown away: z tells us nothing about the individual values of of x and y. This is a simple kind of invariance: all values of x and y such that $z = \phi(x, y)$ are effectively identical. These values thus form a manifold (in this case a one-dimensional curve) in the full two-dimensional x-y space. One can easily think of much more complex invariants. For example, the same face viewed from different angles, at different distances, in different lightings, and with various hair length, degree of sunburn, style of glasses, etc. is always recognized as belonging to the same person. Or, in terms of invariant manifolds, there are many different combinations of angle, distance, lighting, etc. that lead to the same outcome ("Hi, Fred"). Invariances like this, of course, live in high dimensions, and it is an open question how the brain computes them.

A second, less obvious, kind of invariance has to do with population activity. Because of neuronal noise, many different patterns of activity code for the same thing (e.g., the same value of a variable), and networks should be invariant with respect to these differences. In particular, they should do as good a job as possible extracting the relevant part of the activity (e.g., the position of the peak of a tuning curve) and ignoring the irrelevant part (e.g., the overall amplitude). The goal of this chapter is to develop an understanding of how networks of neurons handle both kinds of invariance.

7.2 Computing Functions with Networks of Neurons: A General Algorithm

Networks of neurons implement input-output functions: they take as input population activity from one set of neurons and produce as output population activity on another. If the input and output populations code for a set of variables, then we can think of the networks as computing functions of those variables. In this section we describe how to construct networks that can compute essentially any smooth function.

For simplicity we will assume that on the input side there are two populations, each coding for one variable, and on the output side there is one population, also coding for one variable (figure 7.1). As discussed in the introduction, we will also assume that the activity of each neuron is described by one number, r (which we generally think of as firing rate). The value of r is set by both a tuning curve and noise. Letting x and y refer to the input variables, the activity of the i-th neuron in each population is thus given by

$$
\begin{aligned}
r_i^x &= f_x(x - x_i) + \eta_i^x \\
r_i^y &= f_y(y - y_i) + \eta_i^y .
\end{aligned}
\tag{7.1}
$$

Here r_i^x and r_i^y are the firing rates of neuron i of the x and y populations, f_x and f_y are tuning curves (often taken to be Gaussian), x_i and y_i are referred to as *preferred values*, and η^x and η^y represent noise, which is zero mean and typically correlated. The peaks of the tuning curves correspond approximately to the encoded variables (figure 7.1). Although the horizontal axis in figure 7.1 is index (which labels neuron), we can, and often do, also think of it as labeling the value of the encoded variable. Thus, the statement "the population peaks at x," is shorthand for "the preferred value of the neuron with the highest firing rate is x."

If the population activity given in equation (7.1) is fed into a network, the output is a new population which codes for the variable z,

$$
r_i^z = f_z(z - z_i) + \eta_i^z .
\tag{7.2}
$$

The noise, η^z, is partially inherited from the input and is partially generated from internal noise in the network (stochastic transmitter release, for example).

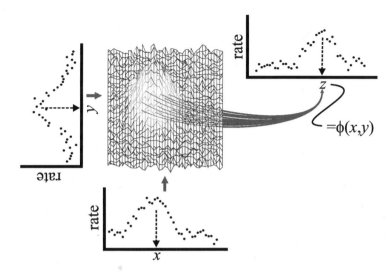

Figure 7.1 Feedforward network that computes $z = \phi(x, y)$. The input layers consist of populations that code for x and y, and thus peak near x and y. Feedforward connections to the intermediate layer, combined with recurrent connections in that layer, produced a bump at position (x, y). Connections from the position of that bump to $z = \phi(x, y)$ in the output layer complete the network.

The value of z in equation (7.2) (the approximate position of the peak of the population activity) depends on x and y (the approximate peaks of the two input populations). Thus, this network implements some function, which for definiteness we call ϕ: $z = \phi(x, y)$. Our goal is to understand how to design a network that can implement an arbitrary function.

The design we use is based on the algorithm described in [4], which takes advantage of the properties of basis function networks. The main idea, which is illustrated in figure 7.1, is the following: Consider two population codes peaking at x and y. Let these two populations project onto an intermediate network consisting of a two-dimensional array of neurons. With the appropriate connectivity (which we discuss below), the intermediate network can be made to peak at (x, y). If the neurons associated with that peak project to the output layer such that they most strongly activate the neurons whose preferred value is $\phi(x, y)$, then the network will compute the function $z = \phi(x, y)$.

To understand this architecture in more detail, we construct this network step by step, starting with simplified connectivity and working up to the complete connectivity that will allow the network to compute the function ϕ. Denoting the firing rates of the neurons in the intermediate layer r_{ij}, where i and j label position in a two-dimensional array, we first consider a network with only feedforward connections,

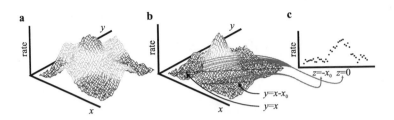

Figure 7.2 Intermediate layer in response to inputs like the ones shown in figure 7.1 (a). Pattern of activity when there are only feedforward connections from the input. (b). Pattern of activity when Mexican hat recurrent connectivity is introduced. Short-range excitation enhances the peak; long-range inhibition suppresses the ridges. (c). Connectivity that implements the function $z = y - x$: neurons in diagonal strips in the intermediate layer connect preferentially to the appropriate neurons in the output layer. Two strips are shown, one corresponding to $y - x = 0$ and the other to $y - x = -x_0$.

$$r_{ij} = \psi \left(\sum_k J_{ik} r_k^x + \sum_l J_{jl} r_l^y \right),$$

where the feedforward connection matrix, J_{ij}, is (relatively sharply) peaked at $i = j$ and ψ is a sigmoidal function of its argument (e.g., $\psi(u) = \nu_0(1 + \exp(u_0 - u))^{-1}$). As illustrated in figure 7.2a, this feedforward connectivity produces perpendicular ridges of activity in the intermediate layer, with a peak where the ridges cross.

The second step is to get rid of the ridges so that we have only a bump of activity at position (x, y). One way to do this is to add "Mexican hat" recurrent connectivity, which has the property that nearby neurons excite each other and distant neurons inhibit each other. Letting $W_{ij,kl}$ be the connection strength from neuron kl to neuron ij, a standard implementation of Mexican hat connectivity is

$$
\begin{aligned}
W_{ij,kl} &= W_E \exp\left(-[(i - k)^2 + (j - l)^2]/2\sigma_E^2 \right) \\
&- W_I \exp\left(-[(i - k)^2 + (j - l)^2]/2\sigma_I^2 \right)
\end{aligned}
$$

The parameters W_E, W_I, σ_E, and σ_I control the shape of the connectivity matrix; if we impose the conditions $W_E > W_I$ and $\sigma_E < \sigma_I$, then it will have the shape given in figure 7.3.

Introducing recurrent connectivity means that the network can no longer be characterized by a simple static nonlinearity, but instead must evolve in time. For this we use simple first-order kinetics,

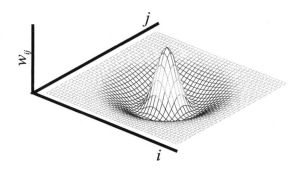

Figure 7.3 Weight matrix corresponding to Mexican hat connectivity.

$$\frac{dr_{ij}}{dt} = \psi \left(\sum_{kl} W_{ij,kl} r_{kl} + \sum_{k} J_{ik} r_k^x + \sum_{l} J_{jl} r_l^y \right) - r_{ij}. \tag{7.3}$$

The effect of these recurrent connections is to enhance regions of highest firing rates – the intersection of the two grids in figure 7.2a – and suppress lower firing rates. This results in a bump of activity at position (x, y). More accurately, the firing rate, r_{ij}, is highest for indices such that $x_i \approx x$ and $y_i \approx y$ where, recall, x and y correspond to the peaks of the input populations. A plot of the activity in the intermediate layer is shown in figure 7.2b.

The third step is to add the connectivity from the intermediate layer to the output layer. Conceptually, this is relatively straightforward: neurons in the intermediate layer whose preferred value is near (x_i, y_j) should excite neurons in the output layer whose preferred value is near $\phi(x_i, y_j)$. Formally, we write

$$r_i^z = \sum_{jk} G\left(z_i - \phi(x_j, y_k) \right) r_{jk}, \tag{7.4}$$

where $G(x)$ is a unimodal function with a peak at zero (e.g, a Gaussian) and the firing rates in the intermediate layer, r_{jk}, are taken to be the equilibrium rates ($t \to \infty$ in equation (7.3)). This connectivity, along with the pattern of activity it produces in the output layer, is shown in figure 7.2c for the function $\phi(x, y) = y - x$. For this function, neurons along diagonal strips in the intermediate layer connect preferentially to the appropriate neurons in the output layer. Specifically, neurons in the strip $y = x + a$ connect preferentially to the neurons in the output layer that code for a.

Manipulating the feedforward connectivity – adjusting $\phi(x, y)$ in equation (7.4) – allows any sufficiently smooth function ϕ to be computed. Moreover, networks of this type are not restricted to computations of only two variables; by increasing the dimension of the intermediate layer, functions of multiple variables can be computed. Thus, this network architecture provides us with a general algorithm for computing smooth functions of multiple variables.

7.3   Efficient Computing; Qualitative Analysis

In spite of the power and flexibility of these kinds of networks, there is room for improvement in at least two ways. First, the network architecture was purely feedforward, so information flowed only from the input to the output. In many situations, however, the distinction between input and output is not so clear. For example, when computing the location of an object relative to your head based on visual cues, the inputs are the location of the object on your retina and the location of your eyes in your head, and the output is the location of the object relative to your head. If the object makes noise, however, neurons in auditory cortex code directly for the location of the object, and so act as input. Second, the networks were not necessarily optimal; there was nothing preventing them from throwing away large amounts of information (an issue we will return to below). Both of these considerations are related to *efficient* computation – computation that makes use of all the available information. In this section we discuss how to build networks that compute efficiently.

Our starting point is the class of networks described above, augmented in two ways. First, we add feedback connections from the output layers to the intermediate layer and from the intermediate layer to the input layers, and we add recurrent connections within the input layers. This puts the input and output layers on equal footing, so we call all layers except the intermediate layer "input layers." Second, we construct the networks so that they exhibit multidimensional attractors; that is, so that the input and intermediate layers can display bumps of activity in the absence of input.

Replacing the largely feedforward network analyzed in the previous section with an attractor network is a key step, and the reason we do it was alluded to in the section 7.1: we want to construct networks that pay attention only to the relevant activity. To see why an attractor network might do this, consider for a moment just a single population that codes for one variable, say x. In this case there is a unique mapping from the population activity, $\mathbf{r}^x$, to an estimate of the encoded variable, denoted $\hat{x}$. In other words, there is some function h such that $\hat{x} = h(\mathbf{r}^x)$. This is a rather extreme kind of invariance: assuming there are n neurons, then there is an $(n-1)$-dimensional manifold that maps to the same value of $\hat{x}$. A very natural way to implement this in a network of neurons is to ensure that the dynamics collapses onto a one-dimensional manifold; that is, ensure that the network implements a one-dimensional attractor. Such an attractor has the property that all the points on an $(n-1)$-dimensional manifold are attracted to the same point on the attractor. That point can thus code directly for $\hat{x}$, and if the network is designed optimally it will provide an optimal estimate of $\hat{x}$. This idea is illustrated in figure 7.4, and in the remainder of the chapter we expand on it from a quantitative (and fairly high-level) perspective.

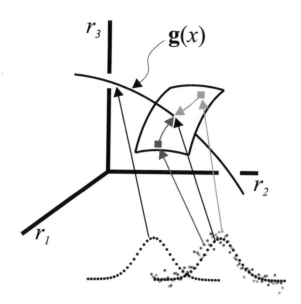

Figure 7.4   Cartoon of an attractor network; the three dimensions represent the full *n*-dimensional space. The line labeled $\mathbf{g}(x)$ represents a line attractor; each point on it corresponds to a smooth bump. The plane perpendicular to this line is invariant under network dynamics. Shown are two initial conditions (red and green squares) that correspond to two different realizations of noisy populations codes (red and green populations). Under the network dynamics, both initial conditions evolve to the same point on the line attractor (red and green arrows on the invariant manifold), and thus provide the same estimate, $\hat{x}$, for the encoded variable (see color insert).

7.4   Efficient Computing; Quantitative Analysis

To see how an attractor network can be used to estimate variables encoded in population activity, consider the following scenario. At time $t = 0$, the network is initialized, typically by transient input. This initialization, which provides all the information about the encoded variables that the network will receive, results in a noisy pattern of activity like the one shown in figure 7.5a. After that the network evolves deterministically[1] until it settles into a state with smooth hills of activity in both the input and intermediate layers, as shown in figure 7.5b. The peaks of these hills act as network estimates of the variables encoded in the initial conditions. The question we are interested in is: how accurate are those estimates? Or, more specifically, what is the variance of the estimates?

This question was first considered in [2], and discussed in gory detail in [3]. Here we give a simplified answer for the case of a single variable encoded in

---

1. The deterministic evolution is an approximation, but it is useful in that it allows detailed analysis of the network. See [3] for a further discussion of this point.

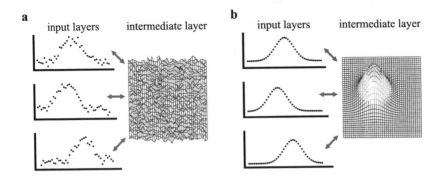

Figure 7.5 Evolution from noisy to smooth hills. (a). Initial conditions: noisy populations activities. Note that information has not yet propagated into the intermediate layer, so the neurons in that layer fire at the background rate. (b). After a long time the network has evolved to a set of smooth hills, including a smooth bump in the intermediate layer. The peaks act as network estimates of the encoded variables.

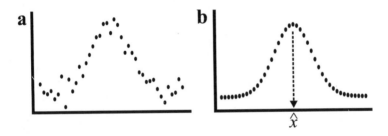

Figure 7.6 Same as figure 7.5 but for a single hill of activity. (a). Initial conditions: a noisy hill of activity. (b). After a long time the network has evolved to a smooth hill. The position of the peak is the network estimator, $\hat{x}$, of the encoded variable.

population activity (although our analysis applies to multiple variables). This corresponds to the situation shown in figure 7.6: a noisy hill of activity encoding a single variable, x, relaxes under the intrinsic network dynamics to a smooth hill whose peak is an estimate of the encoded variable. Because of trial-trial variability, the smooth peak is never in the same place twice. What we do now is compute the variance of the position of the peak; that is, the variance of the network estimate of the encoded variable.

This analysis requires more advanced math than we have been using so far. For a somewhat expanded (but also more general, and thus more difficult) exposition see [3]. A quick review of all that linear algebra that used to put you to sleep would also be useful.

Our starting point is network dynamics of the form

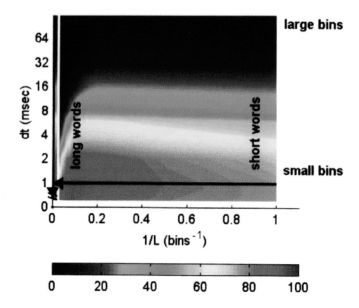

Figure 2.4 Information rate in spikes per second as a function of parameters of the spike-train representation, the bin width Δt, and the inverse total word length $1/L$. Reproduced with permission from Reinagel and Reid, [55].

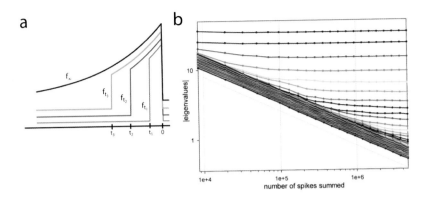

Figure 2.11 Apparent high dimensionality in the integrate-and-fire model due to spike interaction. (a). Family of filters labeled by the time to the last spike. (b). Spectrum eigenvalues, plotted as a function of the number of spikes N. The noise floor goes down as $1/N$. Many modes emerge as significant with large enough N.

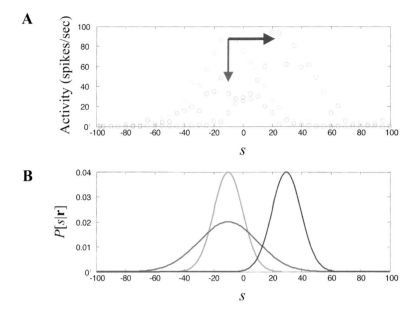

Figure 6.2 A. Population patterns of activity from a population of neurons with tuning curves as in figure 6.1, corrupted by Poisson noise. B. Posterior probability distributions obtained with a Bayesian decoder (equation 6.2) applied to the patterns in A. When the pattern of activity is simply translated (*blue arrow*), the peak of the distribution translates by the same amount and the width remains the same (*green* versus *blue curve* in *lower* panel). When the gain of the population activity decreases (*red arrow*), the posterior distribution widens (*green* vs. *red curves* in *bottom* panel).

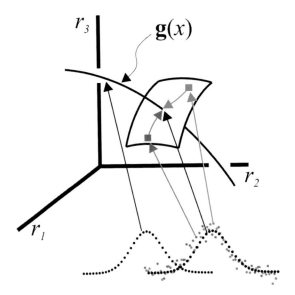

Figure 7.4 Cartoon of an attractor network; the three dimensions represent the full *n*-dimensional space. The line labeled g(x) represents a line attractor; each point on it corresponds to a smooth bump. The plane perpendicular to this line is invariant under network dynamics. Shown are two initial conditions (red and green squares) that correspond to two different realizations of noisy populations codes (red and green populations). Under the network dynamics, both initial conditions evolve to the same point on the line attractor (red and green arrows on the invariant manifold), and thus provide the same estimate, $\hat{x}$, for the encoded variable.

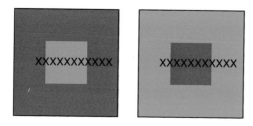

Figure 8.15 The static presentation paradigm: the receptive field sampling positions in the red square and the green square are labeled here by crosses.

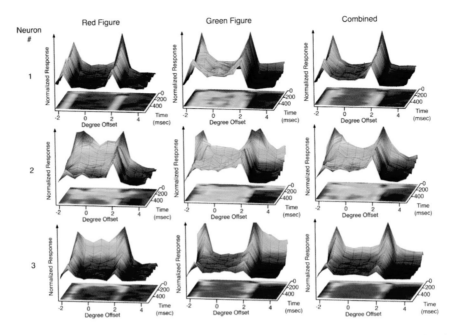

Figure 8.16 The temporal evolution of the responses of three different (typical) V1 neurons to different parts of the red figure in the green background (left column), and to different parts of the green figure in the red background (middle column). The right column sums the responses to the two stimuli at each spatial location to demonstrate the figure enhancement effect.

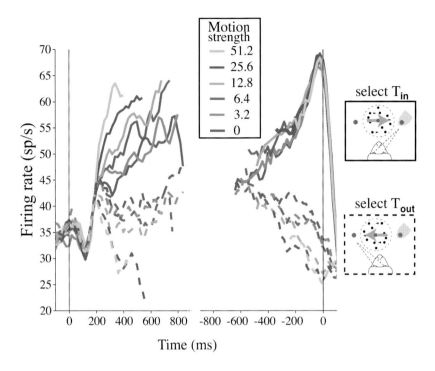

Figure 10.7 Time course of LIP activity during the reaction time version of the direction discrimination task. Average spike rates for 54 LIP neurons. Responses are grouped by choice and motion strength. Solid and dashed lines show responses for trials that were terminated with a T_{in} and T_{out} choice, respectively. The colors indicate the motion strength. The responses are aligned on the left to the onset of motion stimulus and drawn only up to the median RT for each motion strength, excluding any activity within 100 ms of the saccade. The responses on the right are aligned to the initiation of the saccadic eye movement response, and they are plotted backward in time to the median RT, excluding any activity occurring within 200 ms of motion onset. Only correct choices are included except for the 0% coherence case. Adapted with permission from J. D. Roitman and M. N. Shadlen, [27].

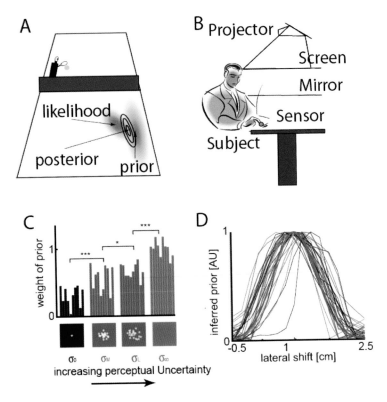

Figure 13.1 (A) Example: The other player is hitting the ball. Seeing the ball, we can estimate that it will land in the red region (with a likelihood proportional to the saturation). We have prior knowledge that the ball is likely to land in the green region (with a probability proportional to the saturation). The black ellipses denote the posterior, the region where the Bayesian estimate would predict the ball to land. (B) The experimental setup. (C) Human subjects' reliance on the prior as a function of increasing perceptual uncertainty. Replotted from Körding and Wolpert [33]). (D) The inferred prior for the different conditions and subjects. The real distribution is shown in red.

$$\frac{d\mathbf{r}}{dt} = \mathbf{H}(\mathbf{r}) - \mathbf{r}. \tag{7.5}$$

Here $\mathbf{r}$ represent the population activity encoding the variable x (since there is only one population, we drop the superscript that used to appear on $\mathbf{r}$) and $\mathbf{H}(\mathbf{r})$ contains all the information about the network dynamics. This function is in principle arbitrary, but in practice it typically has the form $H_i(\mathbf{r}) = \psi\left(\sum_j W_{i-j} r_j\right)$ where, as above, ψ is sigmoidal. A key aspect of this network is that it admits an attractor, and for the simple one-population model we are considering here it admits a line attractor. What this means is that there is some function $\mathbf{g}(x)$ that satisfies

$$\mathbf{g}(x) = \mathbf{H}\Big(\mathbf{g}(x)\Big).$$

For example, $\mathbf{g}(x)$ might satisfy the equation $g_i(x) = \psi\left(\sum_j W_{i-j} g_j(x)\right)$ where $g_i(x)$ vs. i is a smooth hill of activity.

As in equation (7.1), the activity is initialized according to a set of tuning curves, $r_i = f(x - x_i) + \eta_i$. It is convenient to write this in vector notation, and also to explicitly take into account the fact that the network is initialized with noisy activity,

$$\mathbf{r}(t = 0) = \mathbf{f}(x) + \mathbf{N}, \tag{7.6}$$

where $\mathbf{f}(x) \equiv (f(x - x_1), f(x - x_2), ...)$ is the set of tuning curves and $\mathbf{N} \equiv (\eta_1, \eta_2, ...)$ is the noise. The noise has zero mean, $\langle \mathbf{N} \rangle = 0$ (angle brackets represent an average over trials), and covariance matrix $\mathbf{R}$,

$$\langle \mathbf{NN} \rangle = \mathbf{R}. \tag{7.7}$$

We can now explicitly state the problem we are interested in: If a network that evolves according to equation (7.5) is initialized according to equation (7.6), it will evolve onto a point on the attractor; that is, in the limit $t \to \infty$, $\mathbf{r}(t)$ will approach $\mathbf{g}(\hat{x})$. Under this scenario, $\hat{x}$ is the network estimate of the encoded variable. Because of the noise, $\hat{x}$ will vary from trial to trial. However, we will assume the network is unbiased, so that when $\hat{x}$ is averaged over many trials it is equal to x: $\langle \hat{x} \rangle = x$. The first question we wish to answer is: what is the variance of $\hat{x}$? The second is: how does that variance compare to the variance of an optimal estimator?

To answer these questions we will assume that the noise is small, linearize the equations of motion around an equilibrium on the attractor, and solve explicitly for the variance. The only subtlety is deciding which point on the attractor to linearize around. It turns out to be convenient to linearize around $\hat{x}$, so we write

$$\mathbf{r}(t) = \mathbf{g}(\hat{x}) + \delta\mathbf{r}(t)\,. \tag{7.8}$$

The reason for this choice is that as $t \to \infty$ the network evolves to $\mathbf{g}(\hat{x})$ (i.e., $\mathbf{r}(t = \infty) = \mathbf{g}(\hat{x})$), which in turn means that $\delta\mathbf{r}(\infty) = 0$. This will greatly simplify our analysis.

To derive an expression for the time evolution of $\delta\mathbf{r}(t)$, we insert equation (7.8) into equation (7.5) and keep only terms up to first order in $\delta\mathbf{r}(t)$. This results in the evolution equation

$$\frac{d\delta\mathbf{r}}{dt} = \mathbf{J}(\hat{x}) \cdot \delta\mathbf{r}\,. \tag{7.9}$$

Here $\mathbf{J}(\hat{x})$ is the Jacobian,

$$J_{ij}(\hat{x}) \equiv \frac{\partial H_i(\mathbf{g}(\hat{x}))}{\partial g_j(\hat{x})} - \delta_{ij}\,,$$

where δ_{ij} is the Kronecker delta ($\delta_{ij} = 1$ if $i = j$ and 0 otherwise), and "$\cdot$" indicates a dot product ($\mathbf{A} \cdot \mathbf{u} \equiv \sum_j A_{ij} u_j$). Equation (7.9) has the solution

$$\delta\mathbf{r}(t) = \exp[\mathbf{J}(\hat{x})t] \cdot \delta\mathbf{r}(0)\,. \tag{7.10}$$

To simplify this equation we use the expansion

$$\mathbf{J}(\hat{x}) = \sum_k \lambda_k(\hat{x})\mathbf{v}_k(\hat{x})\mathbf{v}_k^{\dagger}(\hat{x})\,,$$

where $\mathbf{v}_k(\hat{x})$ and $\mathbf{v}_k^{\dagger}(\hat{x})$ are the eigenvectors and adjoint eigenvectors of $\mathbf{J}(\hat{x})$, respectively, with eigenvalue $\lambda_k(\hat{x})$. Using this expansion, equation (7.10) can be rewritten

$$\delta\mathbf{r}(t) = \sum_k \exp[\lambda_k(\hat{x})t]\mathbf{v}_k(\hat{x})\mathbf{v}_k^{\dagger}(\hat{x}) \cdot \delta\mathbf{r}(0)\,. \tag{7.11}$$

Since the network dynamics admits a line attractor, one eigenvalue is zero and the rest have negative real part. Thus, in the limit $t \to \infty$, only one term in equation (7.11) survives – the one corresponding to the zero eigenvalue. Letting $k = 0$ label this eigenvalue ($\lambda_0 = 0$; $\mathrm{Re}\{\lambda_{k \neq 0}\} < 0$), we have

$$\delta\mathbf{r}(\infty) = \mathbf{v}_0(\hat{x})\mathbf{v}_0^{\dagger}(\hat{x}) \cdot \delta\mathbf{r}(0)\,. \tag{7.12}$$

We now use the fact that $\mathbf{r}(\infty) = \mathbf{g}(\hat{x})$, which implies that $\delta\mathbf{r}(\infty) = 0$ (see discussion above). Combining this with equation (7.12) and using equations (7.6) and (7.8) to express $\delta\mathbf{r}(0)$ in terms of $\mathbf{f}$ and $\mathbf{g}$, we find that

$$\mathbf{v}_0^\dagger(\hat{x}) \cdot [\mathbf{f}(x) - \mathbf{g}(\hat{x}) + \mathbf{N}] = 0. \tag{7.13}$$

To solve this equation we assume that the noise is small, let $\hat{x} = x + \delta x$, and expand equation (7.13) to first order in both δx and the noise. This results in the expression

$$\mathbf{v}_0^\dagger(x) \cdot [\mathbf{f}(x) - \mathbf{g}(x)] + \mathbf{v}_0^\dagger(x) \cdot \mathbf{N} + \delta x \partial_{\hat{x}} \left\{ \mathbf{v}_0^\dagger(\hat{x}) \cdot [\mathbf{f}(x) - \mathbf{g}(\hat{x})] \right\}_{\hat{x} = x}. \tag{7.14}$$

For the network to be unbiased, δx must vanish in the limit $\mathbf{N} \to 0$. This happens only if $\mathbf{v}_0^\dagger(x) \cdot [\mathbf{f}(x) - \mathbf{g}(x)] = 0$, so we will assume that this holds (in practice it must be checked on a case-by-case basis). Using this condition, the second term in equation (7.14) reduces to $-\delta x \mathbf{v}_0^\dagger(x) \cdot \mathbf{f}'(x)$ where a prime denotes a derivative. Thus, equation (7.14) becomes

$$\delta x = \frac{\mathbf{v}_0^\dagger(x) \cdot \mathbf{N}}{\mathbf{v}_0^\dagger(x) \cdot \mathbf{f}'(x)}.$$

Since we are assuming zero mean noise, $\langle \delta x \rangle = 0$. The variance of δx is then given by

$$\langle \delta x^2 \rangle = \frac{\mathbf{v}_0^\dagger(x) \cdot \mathbf{R} \cdot \mathbf{v}_0^\dagger(x)}{[\mathbf{v}_0^\dagger(x) \cdot \mathbf{f}'(x)]^2}, \tag{7.15}$$

where $\mathbf{R}$, the noise covariance matrix, is defined in equation (7.7).

Equation (7.15) is important because it tells us that the efficiency of the network depends only on the adjoint eigenvector of the linearized dynamics whose eigenvalue is zero. Moreover, we can use this expression to find the adjoint eigenvector that minimizes the variance: differentiating equation (7.15) with respect to $\mathbf{v}_0^\dagger(x)$ and setting the resulting expression to zero, we find that the variance of the network is minimized when

$$\mathbf{v}_0^\dagger(x) \propto \mathbf{R}^{-1} \cdot \mathbf{f}'(x). \tag{7.16}$$

To satisfy equation (7.9) – and thus find the optimal network – we most modify network parameters, as it is those parameters that determine $\mathbf{v}_0^\dagger(x)$. Note that we can adjust parameters until the network is optimal *without running any simulations*, although in practice the line attractor, $\mathbf{g}(x)$ (which also depends on network parameters), must be found numerically.

How well does the network compare to an optimal estimator? To answer that, we need to find the variance of the optimal network, which we do by inserting equation (7.16) into (7.15). This yields

$$\langle \delta x^2 \rangle = \frac{1}{\mathbf{f}'(x) \cdot \mathbf{R}^{-1} \cdot \mathbf{f}'(x)} \, .$$

This expression should be compared to the Cramér-Rao bound, which is $\langle \delta x^2 \rangle \geq 1/I$ where I is the Fisher information. For a Gaussian distribution with covariance matrix $\mathbf{R}$, the Fisher information is given by [1]

$$I = \mathbf{f}'(x) \cdot \mathbf{R}^{-1} \cdot \mathbf{f}'(x) + \frac{1}{2}\text{Tr}\{\mathbf{R}^{-1} \cdot \partial_x \mathbf{R} \cdot \mathbf{R}^{-1} \cdot \partial_x \mathbf{R}\} \, .$$

If the second term is small, then the network comes close to the Cramér-Rao bound; otherwise it doesn't. Whether or not networks of the type discussed here are optimal, then, depends on the correlational structure. What the correlational structure actually is in realistic networks is an active area of research.

7.5   Summary

Our main thesis is that networks compute with population codes by taking as input one set of noisy population codes and producing as output another set. The art is figuring out how to build networks with interesting input/output relations and small information loss. Qualitatively, this means building networks such that the output population codes peak in the right places and the neurons in those populations aren't too noisy.

In this chapter we examined two related classes of networks. The first was a feedforward network that used basis functions; the second was an extension of the first, in which sufficient feedback and recurrent connections were added so that the network implemented a multidimensional attractor. The use of attractor networks allowed us to derive optimality conditions that told us when networks can compute with minimum information loss.

The networks discussed here work well in a few dimensions (when the input and output populations code for a few variables), but fail when the dimensionality becomes large, somewhere on the order of ten or so. This is because the number of neurons in the input layer increases with the dimension. Thus, networks of the type described here are not adequate to solve the really high-dimensional problems, such as those we encounter in vision or audition. Either new paradigms for computations will have to be invented, or we will have to figure out how to reduce high-dimensional problems to low-dimensional ones that can be solved using the network architecture described here.

References

[1] Abbott LF, Dayan P (1999) The effect of correlated variability on the accuracy of a population code. *Neural Computation* 11:91–101.

[2] Deneve S, Latham PE, Pouget A (2001) Efficient computation and cue integration with noisy population codes. *Nature Neuroscience* 4:826–831.

[3] Latham PE, Deneve S, Pouget A (2003) Optimal computation with attractor networks. *Journal of Physiology, Paris* 97:683–694.

[4] Pouget A, Sejnowski TJ (1997) Spatial transformations in the parietal cortex using basis functions. *Journal of Cognitive Neuroscience* 9:222–237.

8 Efficient Coding of Visual Scenes by Grouping and Segmentation

Tai Sing Lee and Alan L. Yuille

8.1 Introduction

The goal of this chapter is to present computational theories of scene coding by image segmentation and to suggest their relevance for understanding visual cortical function and mechanisms. We will first introduce computational theories of image and scene segmentation and show their relationship to efficient encoding. Then we discuss and evaluate the relevant physiological data in the context of these computational frameworks. It is hoped that this will stimulate quantitative neurophysiological investigations of scene segmentation guided by computational theories.

Our central conjecture is that areas V1 and V2, in addition to encoding fine details of images in terms of filter responses, compute a segmentation of images which allows a more compact and parsimonious encoding of images in terms of the properties of regions and surfaces in the visual scene. This conjecture is based on the observation that neurons and their retinotopic arrangement in these visual areas can represent information precisely, thus furnishing an appropriate computational and representational infrastructure for this task. Segmentation detects and extracts coherent regions in an image and then encodes the image in terms of probabilistic models of surfaces and regions in it, in the spirit of Shannon's theory of information. This representation facilitates visual reasoning at the level of regions and their boundaries, without worrying too much about all the small details in the image.

Figure 8.1 gives three examples which illustrate the meaning of higher-level efficient encoding of scenes. Firstly, consider Kanizsa's famous illusory triangle (figure 8.1a) [28]. It is simpler to explain it as a white triangle in front of, and partially occluding, three black circular disks rather than as three Pac-Men who are accidentally aligned to each other. Indeed, this simple explanation is what humans perceive and, in fact, the perception of a triangle is so strong that we hallucinate the surface of the triangle as being brighter than the background and perceive sharp boundaries to the triangle even at places where there are no direct visual cues. Secondly, when confronted with the image shown in figure

8.1b [58], we perceive it as a group of convex spheres mixed together with a group of concave indentations (e.g. an egg carton partly filled with eggs). This interpretation is more parsimonious than describing every detail of the intensity shading and other image features. Thirdly, at first glance, the image in figure 8.1c [18] appears to be a collection of random dots and hence would not have a simple encoding. But the encoding becomes greatly simplified once the viewer perceives the Dalmatian dog and can invoke a dog model. The viewer will latch on to this interpretation whenever he or she sees it again, underscoring the powerful interaction between memory and perception when generating an efficient perceptual description.

These three examples suggest that we can achieve a tremendous amount of data compression by interpreting images in terms of the structure of the scene. They suggest a succession of increasingly more compact and semantically more meaningful codes as we move up the visual hierarchy. These codes go beyond efficient coding of images based on Gabor wavelet responses [13, 37] or independent components [56, 6, 43].

In this chapter, we will concentrate on image segmentation, which is the process that partitions an image into regions, producing a clear delineation of the boundaries between regions and the labeling of properties of the regions. The definition of "regions" is a flexible one. In this chapter, we focus on early visual processing and so a region is defined to be part of an image that is characterized by a set of (approximately) homogeneous visual cues, such as color, luminance, or texture. These regions can correspond to 3D surfaces in the visual scene, or they can be parts of a 3D surface defined by (approximately) constant texture, albedo, or color (e.g. the red letters "No Parking" on a white stop sign). Based on a single image, however, it is often difficult to distinguish between these two interpretations. At a higher level of vision, the definition of region is more complex and can involve hierarchical structures involving objects and scene structures.

The approach we have taken stems from the following computational perspective about the function of the visual system. We hold it to be self-evident that the purpose of the visual system is to interpret input images in terms of objects and scene structures, so that we can reason about objects and act upon them. As thirty years of computer vision research has shown, interpreting natural images is extremely difficult. Tasks such as segmenting images into surfaces and objects appear effortlessly easy for the human visual system but, until recently, have proved very difficult for computer vision systems.

The principles of efficient coding and maximization of information transmission have been fruitful for obtaining quantitative theories to explain the behavior of neurons in the early stages of the visual system. These theories explain linear receptive field development, and various adaptation and normalization phenomena observed in these early areas [3, 12, 56, 68]. Moreover, the behaviors of the neurons in the early stages of the visual systems, such as the retina, lateral geniculate nucleus (LGN), and simple cells in V1, are reasonably well characterized and successfully modeled in terms of linear filtering, adaptation, and normalization [10]. But there is a disconnect between this quantitative research in early sensory coding and the more qualitative, function-oriented research that has been directed to the extrastriate cortex.

How can these principles of efficient encoding be extended to hierarchical encoding of images in terms of regions, surfaces, and objects? A more advanced way of encoding images is to organize the information in a hierarchy, in the form of a generative model [53]. In this hierarchical theory, a description at the higher level can synthesize and predict ('explain away') the representations at the lower level. For example, the theory would predict that when a face neuron fires, the eye neurons and the mouth neurons will need to fire less. This can lead to an efficient encoding of images, as illustrated in figure 8.1. Rao and Ballard's model [59], though limited in the type of visual interpretation it can perform, is a good illustrative example of this idea of predictive coding.

In reasoning about the functions of V1, it is natural to propose that this first visual area in the neocortex, which contains orders of magnitude more neurons than the retina, should participate in interpreting visual images rather than simply encoding and representing them. Decades of computer vision research on scene segmentation, surface inference, and object recognition can potentially provide theoretical guidelines for the study of brain function. This is where interaction between neurophysiological investigation and computer vision research could prove to be valuable: computer vision can provide knowledge of natural images, and the design of mathematical theories and computational algorithms that work, while biology can provide insights as to how these functions are being solved in the brain.

We will now describe an important class of theories that perform image segmentation in terms of efficient encoding of regions [16, 54, 7, 35]. Next, we will briefly discuss a second generation of theories which represent the current state of the art in computer vision. The first class of models has been instrumental for motivating physiological experiments discussed in the second part of this chapter, while the second-generation theories can provide insights for understanding some of the physiological observations not predicted by the first class of models.

These models are mathematically formulated in terms of probability models on graphs and, in particular, Markov random fields (MRFs) [80]. These graphs (see figure 8.2), consist of nodes whose activity represents image, or scene, properties (such as the presence or absence of a segmentation boundary). The connections between the nodes represent the likely probabilistic dependencies between the node activities. The graphical, or network, structure of these models makes it straightforward to implement them on networks reminiscent of the neural networks in the brain, as observed in Koch et al. [31] and Lee [36]. So these models can serve as useful guides for investigating the neural mechanisms which implement scene segmentation, as we will discuss later in this chapter.

An advantage of using computational theories of this type is that we can test their performance on natural images. If they fail to yield good segmentations, then we can design new theories which work better. This requirement, that these theories yield acceptable segmentation results when applied to real-

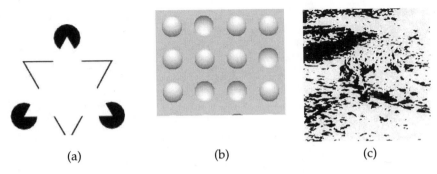

(a)   (b)   (c)

Figure 8.1 Examples that illustrate images are interpreted to make descriptions simpler and shorter. (a) Kanizsa's triangle. (b) Ramachandran's grouping by shape from shading. (c) Gregory's Dalmatian dog.

world images, ensures that they are not merely "toy models." Indeed, the first generation of theories will be adequate for the types of stimuli used in this chapter but the second generation will be needed to perform segmentation fairly reliably on natural images. There is a growing literature on more advanced theories which, for example, include Gestalt laws for perceptual grouping, and even object-specific knowledge.

We conjecture that the neural processes we describe in this chapter are representative of neural mechanisms that operate in other areas of the brain for performing other, higher-level, tasks such as categorization and analogical association. In other words, we propose that these mechanisms are not unique to the segmentation task nor to the visual areas V1 and V2. Certainly the types of theories described here for scene segmentation might have very close analogies, and mathematical underpinnings, to the theories underlying other cognitive abilities such as language, reasoning, categorization, and other aspects of thinking.

8.2   Computational Theories for Scene Segmentation

The earliest computational methods for scene segmentation were based on designing edge detectors to find the large changes in local intensity contrast which are associated with the boundaries of objects (e.g. [49]). These methods involve convolving the image with first-and second-order derivative operators which are smoothed by Gaussian filters and then thresholding the resulting images to extract the edges. This can be implemented by local filters which are similar to the properties of cells in V1. These methods can be extended to allow the filters to be influenced by local context. For example, the Canny edge detector [9] uses heuristics like hysteresis and nonmaximum suppression to facilitate the completion of contours and to thin out multiple responses to the same edge. But overall, these methods are often unable to yield a complete segmentation of the scene because they do not take into account the global structure.

Global approaches to image segmentation began with a class of models that were developed independently in the 1980s [16, 54, 7]. These were based on designing a global criterion for segmenting images into regions. The models assumed that regions have smoothly varying intensity patterns separated by boundaries where the intensity changes significantly. This corresponds to scenes containing smoothly varying spatial geometry separated by discontinuities (and with no texture or albedo patterns). We will describe later how these models can be extended to deal with more general images that include texture, albedo, and shading patterns.

We discuss these models using Leclerc's perspective which formulates scene segmentation as an inference problem in terms of efficient encoding [35]. This approach is based on the minimum description length (MDL) principle [60].

The computational goal is to choose the representation W of the regions, which best fits the image data D, or equivalently, which best encodes the data. In Bayesian terms, we seek to perform maximum a posteriori (MAP) estimation by maximizing the *a posteriori* distribution $P(W|D)$ of the representation conditioned on the data. By Bayes theorem, we can express this in terms of the likelihood function $P(D|W)$ and the prior $P(W)$ as follows:

$$P(W|D) = \frac{P(D|W)P(W)}{P(D)}.$$

The likelihood function $P(D|W)$ specifies the probability of observing data D if the true representation is W and $P(W)$ is the prior probability of the representation (before the data). In the weak-membrane model, the likelihood function is a simple noise distribution and the prior encodes assumptions that the image is piecewise smooth and the boundaries are spatially smooth (see next section for details).

In order to relate MAP estimation to efficient encoding, we take the logarithm of Bayes rule $\log P(W|D) = \log P(D|W) + \log P(W) - \log P(D)$. $P(D)$ is constant (independent of W), so MAP estimation corresponds to *minimizing* the encoding cost:

$$-\log P(D|W) - \log P(W)$$

We now interpret this in terms of minimal encoding. By information theory [65], the number of bits required to encode a variable X which has probability distribution $P(X)$ is $-\log P(X)$. The term $-\log P(W)$ is the cost of encoding the interpretation W. The term $-\log P(D|W)$ is the cost of encoding the data D conditioned on interpretation W. This cost will be 0 if the interpretation explains the data perfectly (i.e. $P(D|W) = 1$). But usually the interpretation will only partially explain the data and so $-\log P(D|W)$ is called the residual (see the detailed example below).

Observe that the encoding depends on our choice of models $P(W|D)$ and $P(W)$. Different models will lead to different encoding, as we will describe later.

The Weak-Membrane Model

The weak-membrane model deals with images where the intensity varies smoothly within regions, but can have sharp discontinuities at the boundaries of regions. We introduce it by the energy functional proposed by Mumford and Shah [54]. This model was defined on a continuous image space, rather than on a discrete lattice (hence the term "functional" rather than "function"). But, as we will show, it can be reformulated on a lattice. (There are differences between the Mumford and Shah model and closely related models by Geman and Geman [16] and by Blake and Zisserman [7]. The most important difference is that the Mumford and Shah model is guaranteed to segment the image into closed regions, while this is only strongly encouraged by the other models.)

The weak-membrane model represents the image by variables (u, B), where B is the set of boundaries between regions and u is a smoothed version of the input image d. More precisely, the image is described by intensity values $d(x, y)$ specified on the image space (x, y). The model assumes that the intensity values are corrupted versions of (unobserved) underlying intensity values $u(x, y)$. The underlying intensity values are assumed to be piecewise smooth, in a sense to be described below.

We formulate this problem by describing $-\log P(D|u, B) - \log P(u, B)$ directly. We write this as $E(u, B)$:

$$E(u, B) = \int \int_R \frac{(u(x, y) - d(x, y))^2}{\sigma_d^2} dx dy + \int \int_{R-B} \frac{1}{\sigma_u^2} \|\nabla u\|^2 dx dy + \alpha B,$$

where R is the image domain, B denotes the set of boundary locations, and $R - B$ indicates the entire image domain minus the boundary locations.

The first term in $E(u, B)$ is the data term, or $-\log P(D|u, B)$, where the distribution of the residues $P(D|u, B)$ is chosen to be Gaussian white noise with standard deviation σ_d. In other words, $P(D|u, B) = \prod_{x,y} P(d(x, y)|u(x, y))$, where $P(d(x, y)|u(x, y)) = \frac{1}{\sqrt{2\pi\sigma_d^2}} e^{-(u(x,y)-d(x,y))^2/(2\sigma_d^2)}$. The double integral over x and y is simply the continuous version of summing over all the pixels in the image domain R.

The second term is a smoothness prior, which assumes the variation on the estimated image intensity to be smooth within each region. Intuitively, the local variation following a Gaussian distribution, i.e. $P(\nabla u : (u, B)) = \frac{1}{\sqrt{2\pi\sigma_u^2}} e^{-(\frac{\nabla u}{2\sigma_u})^2}$, where σ_u is the standard deviation of this distribution, but this is an oversimplification (for a true interpretation, see [80]). Observe that when σ_u is very small, then the energy function enforces regions to have constant intensity. This smoothness term is deactivated (discounted) at the boundary B so the integral is over $R - B$. The intuition is that when the local image gradient is too steep, then it will be better to put in a boundary.

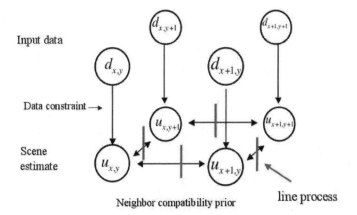

Input data

Data constraint →

Scene estimate

Neighbor compatibility prior   line process

Figure 8.2 A locally connected network for scene segmentation: A node (x, y) has value $u_{x,y}$. It receives direct input from the data $d(x, y)$. It is also connected to its immediate neighbors (or more generally, to nodes in a local neighborhood) by symmetric connections which embody the prior which enforces the estimated intensity to be piecewise smooth.

The third term is a penalty on the length of the boundaries. This is needed to prevent the image from breaking into too many regions or from creating regions with wildly zigzagging boundaries. The sum of the second and third term yields $-\log P(u, B)$ (technically this prior is improper, see [80], but this is not significant for this chapter).

To develop algorithms to minimize the energy function, it is convenient to reformulate it, in the style similar but not identical to that of Ambrosio and Tortorelli [1], so that the boundaries B are replaced by line process variables $l(x, y)$ which take on values in $[0, 1]$:

$$E_p[u, l|d] = \int\int_R \frac{(u(x, y) - d(x, y))^2}{\sigma_d^2} dxdy + \int\int_R (1 - l(x, y))^2 \frac{|\nabla u(x, y)|^2}{\sigma_u^2} dxdy$$
$$+ \alpha \int_R \{p|\nabla l(x, y)|^2 + p^{-1}l(x, y)^2/4\}dxdy. \tag{8.1}$$

The line process variables take value $l(x, y) \approx 1$ at the boundaries, thereby cutting the smoothness constraint. It can be shown that, in the limit as $p \mapsto 0$ the minimization of this corresponds to Mumford and Shah (and the line process variables take values either 0 or 1). The advantages of the second formulation equation (8.1) are: (i) that it is easier to find algorithms for it than for Mumford and Shah, and (ii) it can be directly discretized and implemented on a grid.

The weak-membrane model can be generalized to perform 3D surface inference [5] and to the coupled-membrane model [40] for texture segmentation. In natural images, many regions are defined by texture properties (e.g. stimuli in figure 8.12). The image intensities within each region are not smooth, but the texture properties are. To do this, we set the input $d(x, y)$ to be $WI(\sigma, \theta, x, y)$ which is a image of four continuous variables obtained by wavelet transform (which provides a simple local measure of texture). Each wavelet channel is fitted by a 2D weak-membrane but each of these membranes is coupled to its nearest neighboring membranes in the (σ, θ) domain. (The algorithm involves anisotropic diffusion which takes place in 4D but breaks are allowed in x and y only.) This model has been shown to be effective in segmenting some texture images, tolerating smooth texture gradients [40].

One justification for models like the Mumford-Shah formulation comes from the study of statistics of natural images. Zhu and Mumford [88] used a statistical learning approach to learn models for $P(d|u, B)$ and $P(u, B)$ from natural images, and their results are similar to the Mumford-Shah model (though with interesting differences). It is interesting to contrast how Zhu and Mumford use images statistics to learn the prior with how receptive fields can be learnt from similar statistics using efficient encoding principles [56].

8.3   A Computational Algorithm for the Weak-Membrane Model

When discretized on a grid, the weak-membrane model can be implemented in a network structure as shown in figure 8.2. Such a network contains a layer of input observation $d(x, y)$, a layer of hidden nodes $u(x, y)$, and a set of line processes (or boundary processes) $l(x, y)$. The u nodes can communicate (passing messages) to each other, but their communication can be broken when the line process between them becomes active. Thus, this is an interacting system of two concurrent processes.

For the weak-membrane implemented in a Markov network or Markov random field [16], the local connections between the nodes enforce the smoothness constraint, which make the states of the adjacent nodes vary as little as possible, subject to other constraints such as faithfulness to the data (the data term in the energy functional). More generally, Markov random fields can implement any form of compatibility constraint and do not have to be local connections [80].

We now describe algorithms that can find the solution of the weak-membrane model using such a network. Finding the solution that minimizes the energy functional of the weak-membrane model is not trivial, as there are many local minima due to the coupling of the two processes.

The simplest way of finding the scene estimate function u and partition boundary B that would minimize this class of energy functionals is to search through all possible sets of regions, calculating the cost for each set and choosing the set with the smallest cost. But the number of possible sets of regions is prohibitively large for images of any reasonable size, making an exhaustive search infeasible. Simple gradient descent algorithms will fail because the interaction with line processes makes the system highly nonconvex and gives it a lot of local minima to trap the algorithm into an inferior or incorrect solution.

The best algorithms that have emerged so far belong to a class of optimization techniques generally known as continuation methods [7, 1]. The basic idea of the continuation method is to embed the energy function in a family of functions $E_p(u, l)$ with the continuation parameter p. At large p, the energy function $E_p(u, l)$ is convex and will have only one single minimum. As p approaches zero, the energy function will transform gradually back to the original function which can have many local minima. The strategy is to minimize the energy at large p and then track the solution to small values of p. More precisely, we initialize p^0, select random initial conditions for (u, l), and perform steepest descent to find a minimum (u^0, l^0) of $E_{p^0}(u, l)$. Then we decrease p to p^1, and perform steepest descent on $E_{p^1}(u, l)$ using (u^0, l^0) as initial conditions, and so on. This approach is not guaranteed to find the global minumum of $E(u, B)$, but empirically it yields good results provided the initial value of p^0 is sufficiently large. The dynamics of the algorithm with the transformation of the energy landscape is shown in figure 8.3.

The steepest descent equations for the functional reformulation of the weak-membrane model, as in equation (8.1), are given by:

$$\frac{du(x, y, p, t)}{dt} = r_u\{-u(x, y, p, t) + d(x, y) + \nabla \cdot [\frac{\sigma_d^2}{\sigma_u^2}\nabla u(x, y, p, t)(1 - l(x, y, p, t))^2]\} \quad (8.2)$$

$$\frac{dl(x, y, p, t)}{dt} = r_l\{\alpha p \nabla^2 l(x, y, p, t) + \frac{1}{\sigma_u^2}(1 - l)\|\nabla u(x, y, p, t)\|^2 - \frac{\alpha l(x, y, p, t)}{2p}\}. \quad (8.3)$$

The parameters r_u and r_l are positive rate constants which control the rate of descent. At each stage with a particular p, which changes slowly from 1 to 0, the system relaxes to an equilibrium, i.e. $\frac{du}{dt}$ and $\frac{dl}{dt}$ are driven to 0.

In these equations, u follows a nonlinear diffusion process that is sensitive to the values of the line process. The line process at each location is a continuous variable, indicating that the boundaries are soft during the early stages of the algorithm and only become sharp at the end.

Figure 8.4 shows the outcome of such an algorithm given an input image (a). Minimizing $E(u, B)$ yields a map of boundary process B which, during the first stages of the algorithm, resembles an artist's sketch (b), and then develops into crisper boundaries (c) which partition the image into a set of piecewise smooth regions (d).

The gradual sharpening of the boundaries can be seen in the responses of a collection of line processes (over space) to a step edge at $x = 0$ (figure 8.5a). That is, the gradient along y is all zero, and the gradient along x is all zero except at $x = 0$, which is strong enough to activate $l(x = 0)$ fully, so that $l(x = 0) = 1$. Therefore the second term in equation (8.3) just vanishes, and at the equilibrium of each p relaxation stage (i.e. $\frac{dl}{dt} = 0$), the dynamical equation

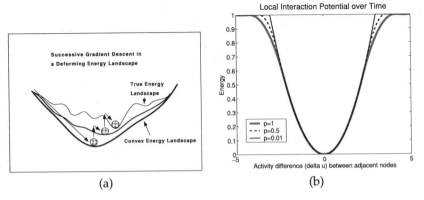

(a)   (b)

Figure 8.3 (a) The energy landscapes of a sequence of deforming energy functionals and the successive gradient descent of a 'ball' in this sequence of landscapes: the system first converges to the global minimum of the convex landscape, which is then used as the starting point for the next descent in the new energy landscape. This strategy of successive gradual relaxation will allow the system to converge to a state that is close to a global minimum of the original energy functional. This strategy can be considered a coarse-to-fine search strategy in the scale space of energy landscape. (b) The transformation of the approximating energy functional, from the convex one back to the original one, is achieved simply by modifying the local interaction potential as a function of p as shown here. The local interaction potential dictates the contribution of the second and third terms in the Mumford-Shah energy functional. At $p = 1$, the local interaction potential is a quadratic function $\lambda^2(\triangle u)$ smoothly saturates to 1 (in the unit of α). As p decreases, the transition becomes more and more abrupt, and converges to the local interaction potential prescribed by the original energy functional in the limit (see [7] for details).

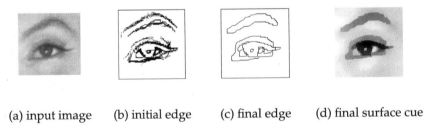

(a) input image   (b) initial edge   (c) final edge   (d) final surface cue

Figure 8.4 Segmentation of an image by the weak-membrane model. Results are encoded in two maps: the boundary map and the region map. (a) The input image. (b) The initial response of the edge (the line process $l(x, y)$) map resembles an artist's sketch of the scene, with uncertainty about the boundary. (c) The final response of the edge map B shows crisper boundaries. (d) The final estimate of the piecewise smooth intensity values $u(x, y)$ is like a smoothed and sharpened image, as if makeup had been applied. Adapted with permission from Lee [36].

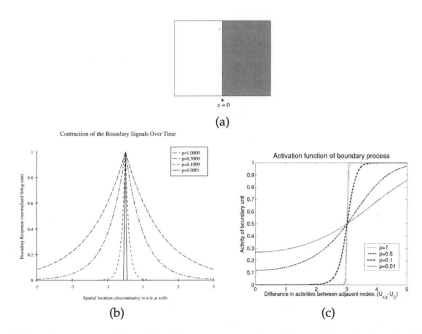

Figure 8.5   (a) An image with a luminance step edge. (b) In response to the step edge, initially, line processes near the edge will respond, resulting in a broader spatial response profile among these populations of nodes. Over time, as p decreases, the boundary responses start to contract spatially to the exact location of the step edge. The activity at each location represents the response of a line process at that location. The curve does represent the responses of a population of identical boundary processors distributed over space, or equivalently the spatial response profile of a boundary unit to different parts of the image with a step edge. As p decreases, the spatial response envelope becomes narrower and narrower [36]. (c) Another perspective on the continuation method is that the activation function of the line process becomes steeper as p decreases [15].

(8.3) yields

$$\alpha p \frac{\partial^2 l}{\partial x^2} = \frac{l\alpha}{4p} \implies l = e^{-\frac{|x|}{2p}}, \tag{8.4}$$

$\nabla^2 l$ controls the lateral interaction between the boundary signals l. As $p \to 0$, the boundary signal l in the surrounding is gradually suppressed, resulting in the contraction to a sharp boundary as shown in figure 8.5b.

Observing that a locally connected network is quite compatible with the known anatomical connections in the primary visual cortex (V1), Koch et al. [31] first proposed a neural circuit for implementing a variant of the weak-membrane model in V1 for the purpose of depth estimation (the same model was applied to segmenting images in [15]). Lee [36] explored the implemen-

tation of the coupled-membrane model [40] with V1 circuitry further based on
the energy functional stated in equation (8.1) and the descent equations described here. This circuit takes data input in the form of V1 complex cell responses, and might be considered more "neurally plausible." It was observed
that the two concurrent and interacting processes of region inference and boundary detection implicated by the descent equations are very similar in spirit to a
neural model proposed for V1 earlier in [21].

8.4   Generalizations of the Weak-Membrane Model

The main limitation of the weak-membrane model is that it uses very simple
assumptions about the intensity properties within regions. We have briefly described how this can be generalized to cases where the regions have smooth
texture patterns. But most natural images have richer properties. Some surface
regions are characterized by smooth texture properties, others have smooth
intensities, and yet others have shaded intensity properties which depend on
the tilt and slant of surfaces. The piecewise smooth intensities, assumed by
the weak-membrane model, are suitable for the 3D surfaces which are approximately flat but fail to accurately model images of more complicated surfaces,
such as spheres.

We now briefly describe some second-generation models of image segmentation. These are significantly more effective than the weak-membrane model
when evaluated on images with ground truth (as provided by the Berkeley
data set; see [48]). We will discuss three different aspects of these methods that
might be relevant to the interpretation of cortical mechanisms.

Firstly, we can generalize the weak-membrane model by observing that natural images are very complex. The images of object surfaces are characterized
by a combination of multiple factors such as textures, color, shapes, material
properties, and the lighting conditions. Each region is described by its own
model, for example shading or texture. The task of segmentation is now much
harder. We have to determine the segmentation boundaries while simultaneously determining the appropriate model for each region.

We can formulate this as a generalization [87, 89, 74] of the weak-membrane
model. We refer to these as region competition models.

$$E((R_r), n, (a_r), (\theta_r)) = \sum_{r=1}^{n} \int \int_{R_r} \{-\log P(d(x,y)|a_r, \theta_r)\} dx dy$$

$$-\sum_{r=1}^{n} \log P(a_r, \theta_r) + \frac{\alpha}{2} \sum_{r=1}^{n} |\partial R_r| + cn. \qquad (8.5)$$

This includes a set of generative models $P(d(x,y)|a_r, \theta_r)$ which are indexed by
model type index variable a_r (corresponding to texture, shading) and a variable θ_r, corresponding to the parameters of the model. This corresponds to encoding the image in terms of a richer language which allows different regions
to be encoded by different models (a texture model, or a shaded model, or an

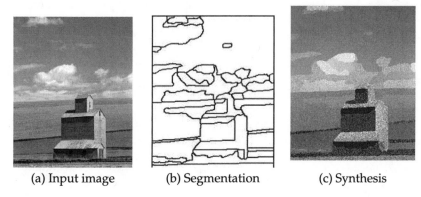

    (a) Input image   (b) Segmentation   (c) Synthesis

Figure 8.6 An illustration of how the region competition model can encode an image economically by encoding each region with a set of boundary elements and two numbers – the mean and the variance of the intensity values in each enclosed region. Different models of regions will compete to explain the image. (a) Input image. (b) Segmentation boundary. (c) Representation of image based on simple region models. Results produced by the data-driven Monte Carlo algorithm for the region competition class of models [74]. Figure courtesy of Z. Tu and S.C.Zhu.

alternative). Figure 8.6 illustrates coding regions of a segmented image with relatively simple models of regions. Regions can be encoded as one of three types: (i) a Gaussian model encoding the mean and variance of the intensity in the region, (ii) a shading model where the image intenesity follows a simple parameterized form, and (iii) a simple texture/clutter model. The segmentation thus encodes an image in terms of a set of boundaries as well as a set of region model codes (e.g. containing two values for each region the algorithm decides to encode as Gaussians). From such a representation, an approximation of the original image can be synthesized (figure 8.6c). More sophisticated generative models will give increasingly realistic synthesized images.

There is no limitation to the class of models that can be used. Recent work has generalized this approach to include models of objects, such as faces and text, so that segmentation and object recognition can be performed in the same unified framework [73].

This generalized model requires a significantly more complicated algorithm than the weak-membrane model. It needs processes to select the models and to "move" the boundaries. The movement of boundaries is dictated by a diffusion process on region properties similar to that for the weak-membrane model. We will discuss this further at the end of this section.

Secondly, there is a second class of models which are, in a sense, complementary to the region competition model. We will refer to these as affinity-based models.

This family of approaches uses affinity weights w_{ij} between different image pixels v_i and v_j. These affinity functions are based on properties measured from the image and are designed so that pixels in homogeneous image regions have high affinity ($w_{ij} \simeq 1$) with each other. For example, we can obtain a model with similar properties to the weak-membrane model, by setting $w_{ij} = e^{-\alpha|d_i - d_j|}$, where d_i is the intensity at lattice site v_i in the image. This construct is naturally regarded as a graph with the image pixels constituting the node set, and the weights between them as the edge set (here the boundaries occur when w_{ij} is small).

Given such a graph, a sensible goal is to label the nodes such that intraregion affinity is maximized (defined by the labels), while minimizing the interregion affinity. Given the label set $\{l_1, ..., l_k\}$, we assign a label to each image pixel so that pixels with the same labels define a region. Finding such a labeling can be formalized in the following minimization [83]:

$$E(m) = \min_{m \in \mathcal{P}(n,k)} \; : \; \frac{1}{k} \sum_{p=1}^{k} \frac{\sum_{i<j} w_{ij}(m_{ip} - m_{jp})^2}{\sum_{i<j} w_{ij}(m_{ip}^2 + m_{jp}^2)},$$

where n is the number of pixels, k the number of labels, and $\mathcal{P}(n,k)$ denotes the set of $n \times k$ indicator matrices. An indicator matrix m satisfies the following constraints, $m(i,p) \in \{0,1\}$ and $\sum_{p=1}^{k} m(i,p) = 1$. In this application the node indices i and j are taken as the indices of the image pixels. Accordingly, the indicator matrix takes the value $m_{ip} = 1$ when the ith pixel is assigned the pth label l_p, otherwise $m_{ip} = 0$.

The objective function falls into the class of NP-hard problems. Subsequently, a variety of algorithms have been developed to find nearly optimal solutions in polynomial time. One class of algorithms relaxes the discrete constraints on m to continuous values, transforming the minimization into a generalized eigenvalue problem [67]. The obtained continuous solutions are then rounded to discrete values producing the cut. Another interesting class uses hierarchical grouping and is fast and effective [64]. A third class of algorithm iteratively modifies the affinity matrix, using the eigenvectors as soft membership labels, until the graph eventually disconnects, producing reasonable segmentations [72].

This type of approach is appealing for several reasons. It simplifies the problem formulation as it does not require us to specify models. It enables a richer set of connections, defined by the affinities, than those implemented by the weak-membrane model (which is essentially a Markov random field with the nearest neighbors; see figure 8.2). These rich connection patterns are consistent with the known anatomy of V1. But these models are still being developed and detailed biological predictions have not yet been worked out. Finally, efficient computation of approximate solutions is possible.

Interestingly, there may be interesting connections between these types of theory and the algorithms used to implement the region competition models. In the data-driven Markov Chain Monte Carlo (MCMC) algorithm, Tu and Zhu [74] use "proposals" to activate the models. These proposals can be generated based on grouping pixels into regions based on affinity cues and then evaluating these groupings by accessing the models. From this perspective, the affinity-based methods can be used as sophisticated ways to generate proposals. In this way, it may be possible to combine these two approaches.

Thirdly, we have so far treated segmentation in terms of image intensity properties only. But the extended class of models, in principle, could enable us to integrate segmentation with the estimation of 3D shape properties such as 3D geometry or Marr's 2.5D sketch [49].

The inference of surface geometry, integrated into the segmentation framework, can be illustrated by a simple example where the image intensity corresponds to a shaded surface. This requires a model for how the image intensity has been generated from the surface of an object by light reflected from it. We assume the standard Lambertian model which is characterized by a reflectance function $R_{\vec{s}}(\vec{n}) = \vec{n}(x, y) \cdot \vec{s}$, with $\vec{n}(x, y)$ being the surface gradient at position (x, y) and $\vec{s}$ the light source (we assume a single light source here). We also assume that the light source $\vec{s}$ is known (there are techniques for estimating this). It is convenient to express the surface normal $\vec{n}(x, y)$ in terms of the surface slant (f, g) in the x and y directions respectively $(\vec{n}(x, y) = \frac{1}{\sqrt{1+f_x^2(x,y)+f_y^2(x,y)}}(-f_x(x, y), -f_y(x, y), 1))$.

We can use a classic shape-from-shading method due to Horn [22] as one of the models in region competition. There are more sophisticated models on shape from shading. But this is the simplest model that can illustrate the principle of surface inference. The cost function is of form:

$$E(f, g : x, y) = \int \int_{\Omega} \frac{(d(x, y) - R_s(f, g))^2}{\sigma_d^2} dxdy + \frac{1}{\sigma_s^2} \int \int_{\Omega} ((f_x^2 + f_y^2) + (g_x^2 + g_y^2)) dxdy,$$

where Ω is a subregion of the image, $d(x, y)$ is the intensity of the image at location (x, y). The first term is the standard Gaussian noise model. The second term is a smoothness prior on the surface orientation.

An additional constraint on the surface normal $\vec{n}(x, y)$ is available at the occlusion border $\partial\Omega$, where the surface normal is always perpendicular to the line of view. This provides boundaries conditions to start a surface interpolation process. Figure 8.7 illustrates how the surface orientation information, as represented by the needle map that indicates the direction of surface normals, can propagate in from the occlusion border to the surface interior during the process of surface interpolation. We would like to draw your attention to this propagation of signals from the border, as such propagation from the border to the interior has also been observed in neuronal activities in V1 as we shall discuss. This model provides one potential interpretation (among many) of such a signal being either a part of or at least a reflection of an ongoing surface inference process.

As in all the region competition theories (as well as the weak-membrane model), the boundary of the region Ω must be detected at the same time as inference of the regional properties – in this case, the 3D surface orientation

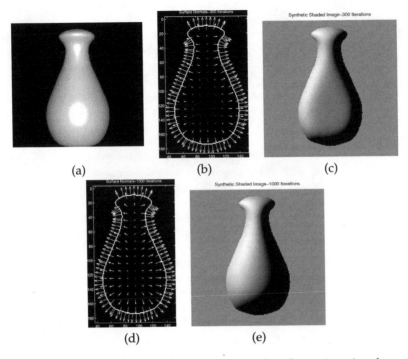

(a)   (b)   (c)

(d)   (e)

Figure 8.7 Surface interpolation by propagation of surface orientation from the boundary using locally connected network using Horn's algorithm. (a) Input image. (b) Initial estimate of surface as represented by the needle map. The needle points in the direction of surface normal. (c) A rendering of the surface as represented by (b) assuming lighting from the left, to illustrate the initial estimate of the surface. (d) Final estimate of surface orientations at each location and (e) its shaded rendering. This illustrates the propagation of surface orientation information from the border to the interior of the surface over time.

represented by the functions f, g.

It is important to remember that many other models of regions and boundaries have also been developed for the region competition theory, from simple models that describe each region by the mean and the variance of its intensity values within that region, or by covariance of the first derivatives along different directions for encoding texture (e.g. [87, 89]), to more advanced models of textures [88] and even objects [73].

In summary, the second generation of theories requires richer modeling for the types of intensity patterns that occur in real images. This can be considered to be a richer class of description of the image which can involve 3D surface shape and even models of objects. Such theories require complex inference algorithms because the segmentation of the image into regions must be performed while simultaneously determining what type of regions they are, and what are their regional properties. Different models cooperate and compete to explain different regions in the image. These inference algorithms can be helped by the use of proposals, some of which may be provided by the output of the affinity-based models. For more details on these classes of models, see [74, 73]. For related theories, from a different perspective, see [8, 84].

Three aspects of the second generation of segmentation models may relate to the physiological experiments described in the biological section. Firstly, the algorithms for the region competition methods (with multiple models) have aspects which are similar to the diffusion methods used for the weak-membrane model. The difference is that diffusion is only one of several components of the algorithm. Secondly, these algorithms make a natural use of bottom-up and top-down processing where the models are accessed by recurrent connections to different visual areas. Thirdly, this approach might also fit naturally in a hierarchical coding scheme which can potentially compress the total coding length by using higher-level (more abstract) description to replace or explain away the redundant information in the low-level representations, as suggested by Mumford [53].

8.5   Biological Evidence

In this section, we will discuss some neurophysiological experiments which suggest that the primary visual cortex is involved in image segmentation. We start by enumerating the predictions of the computational models, particularly those of the weak-membrane model for segmentation, then compare them to the experimental results.

1. There exists a dual representation of region and boundary properties. This is possibly represented by two distinct groups of neurons, one set coding region properties, while the other set codes boundary location.

2. The processes for computing the region and the boundary representations are tightly coupled, with both processes interacting with and constraining each other.

3. During the iterative process, the regional properties diffuse within each region and tend to become constant. But these regional properties do not cross the regional boundaries. For the weak-membrane model, such spreading can be described as nonlinear diffusion, which propagates at roughly constant speed. For more advanced models, the diffusion process may be more complicated and involve top-down instantiation of generative models.

4. The interruption of the spreading of regional information by boundaries results in sharp discontinuities in the responses across two different regions. The development of abrupt changes in regional responses also results in a gradual sharpening of the boundary response, reflecting increased confidence in the precise location of the boundary.

5. In the continuation method, there is additional sharpening of the boundary response. This is modulated by a global parameter p, which increases the sensitivity of all boundary-sensitive neurons gradually within each computational cycle (figure 8.3).

The computational models say nothing about where the representations, and the processes required to compute them, occur in the visual cortex. To relate these models to cell recordings requires making additional conjectures that we will now state.

We conjecture that segmentation computation is embodied in V1, with information about boundaries and regions explicitly represented there. However, not all the computations required for segmentation need take place in V1. For example, it is not clear, based on existing evidence, whether surfaces are represented in V1. There is evidence, however, on the sensitivity of V2 neurons to surface properties such as relative depth [70], border ownership [86], da Vinci stereo [4], and pop-out due to shape from shading [42]. Thus, it seems more likely that surface inference takes place in V2, but the process can be coupled to the segmentation process in V1 through recurrent connections.

This conjecture is related to the *high-resolution buffer* theory of V1 [39, 38] partially inspired by some of the experiments described in this section. In this theory, V1 acts as a high-resolution computational buffer which is involved in *all* visual computations that require high spatial precision and fine-scale detail, since V1 is the only visual area that contains small receptive fields AND with extensive recurrent connections with many areas of the extrastriate cortex. Some of these computations are performed in V1 directly, while others are performed by recurrent connections between V1 and the other visual areas in the extrastriate cortex. Processing in V1 detects salient regions which are enhanced by a recurrent feedback mechanism very much like the adaptive resonance or interactive activation mechanisms hypothesized by the neural modeling community [20, 51, 75]; see also [85] for a motion perception theory utilizing recurrent feedback and [14], for a model for integrateing what and where in the high-resolution buffer using on recurrent biased competition). In particular, Lee et al. [39] have argued that segmentation in V1 cannot be complete and robust without integrating with other higher-order computations, such as object recognition and shape inference. On the other hand, higher-order computations might not be robust without continuous consultation and interaction with the high-resolution buffer in V1. Thus, in their view, visual computations such as scene segmentation should involve the whole visual hierarchy utilizing the feedforward and recurrent feedback connections in the visual cortex. This relates to some of the second-generation computational models.

We now present neurophysiological findings that show experimental support for several of these computational predictions. In particular, we discuss evidence for (1) the gradual sharpening of the response to boundaries, (2) the simultaneous spreading of regional properties, and (3) the development of abrupt discontinuities in surface representations across surfaces.

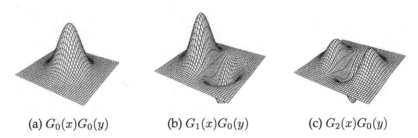

(a) $G_0(x)G_0(y)$ (b) $G_1(x)G_0(y)$ (c) $G_2(x)G_0(y)$

Figure 8.8 Graphs of (a) a 2D Gaussian, (b) the first x derivative of a 2D Gaussian which resembles the odd-symmetric Gabor filter/wavelet, (c) the second x derivative of a 2D Gaussian which resembles the even-symmetric Gabor filter/wavelet. Adapted from Young [82].

Edge and Boundary Representations and Their Spatial Temporal Evolution

We first review evidence that V1 neurons represent edge and boundary locations. The early experiments by Hubel and Wiesel [24] showed that neurons in V1 are sensitive to oriented intensity edges. Indeed Hubel and Wiesel conjectured that the neurons were edge detectors because of their orientation selectivity.

Detailed analysis of the receptive fields of simple cells, using the reverse correlation method, showed that they could be modeled by linear Gabor filters [13, 27]. The receptive fields at different scales resemble scaled and rotated versions of each other, which means they can be considered to be 2D Gabor wavelets [13, 37]. In the theoretical neuroscience community, the Gabor filter interpretation has been popular because Gabor filters achieve the limit of representing information with maximum resolution in the conjoint space of spacetime and frequency. Recently, it has been shown that they can be derived from the statistics of natural images as efficient codes for natural images based on independent component analysis [56]. Although such rationalization about efficient representation is interesting intellectually, we should not lose sight of the potential functional purposes of simple and complex cells as edge detectors, as proposed by Hubel and Wiesel [24]. Young [82] has long championed that simple cells can be described equally well in terms of the first-and second-order 2D Gaussian derivative operators (see figure 8.8). The odd-symmetric Gabors are sensitive to intensity edges and the even-symmetric Gabors to bars (such as peaks and valleys). In fact, Bell and Sejnowski [6] have aptly argued that the independent components likely arise from the structures of edges in natural images.

In summary, simple cells can serve as edge and bar detectors [24], with their maximum responses used to signal the location of the boundary [9]. But, considered as derivatives of Gaussian filters, they can also perform some of the other mathematical operations required by the computational models. The complex cells, which are not sensitive to the polarity of the luminance contrast at edges, would be particularly suitable for representing borders or boundaries of regions. The hypercomplex cells could serve as derivative operators which act on complex cells' responses to detect texture boundaries (see [36]).

We now turn to evidence of nonlocal interactions associated with computational models of edge detection. Studies by Kapadia et al. [29] showed that the activity of a V1 neuron to a bar within its receptive field can be enhanced by the presence of other bars outside the receptive field of the neuron, provided these bars are aligned to form a contour (longitudinal facilitation). Conversely, the neuron's response is suppressed if these bars are parallel to the bar within the receptive field (lateral inhibition). One manifestation of longitudinal facilitation is that V1 neurons looking at the short gaps in boundaries of the Kanizsa figures (see figure 8.1a) have been found to respond after a certain delay (100 ms after stimulus onset vs. the 40 ms required for the response to a real edge), as shown in the study by Lee and Nguyen [41]; (see [19, 66] for other subjective contour effects in V1, and [76] for classic results in V2). Lee and Nguyen [41] also found that V2 neurons responded earlier to the same stimuli. This raises the possibility that the illusory contour response found in V1 is in part due to feedback influence from V2, and in part carried out by the horizontal collaterals within V1.

Longitudinal facilitation and lateral inhibition are consistent with the mechanisms in basic edge detection models [9] and contour completion models [55, 79]). These mechanisms are also embodied in the weak-membrane model as described. The continuation method for the weak-membrane model further gives a quantitative prediction on the temporal evolution of the boundary process. Specifically, in response to a simple luminance border (as shown in figure 8.5), the neural response to boundaries gets sharper over time as the continuation parameter p decreases (predictions 4 and 5).

Analysis of data obtained from the experiment described by Lee and Nguyen [41] provides some evidence in support of the boundary contraction prediction. In that experiment, they used used a sampling paradigm to examine the spatiotemporal responses of neurons to a visual stimulus consisting of a square region whose boundaries were defined by a variety of cues (this sampling paradigm is used for many of the experiments reported in this chapter). In this paradigm, the monkey fixated on a dot on the computer monitor while the visual stimulus was presented for a short period of time (typically 400 ms for each trial). In different trials, the image was shifted spatially to a different location so that the receptive field of the neuron overlapped with different parts of the stimulus. This finely sampled the spatial response of the neuron at an interval of 0.25 degrees, as illustrated in figure 8.9. During each presentation, the stimulus remained stationary on the screen so that the temporal evolution of the neural responsess at each location could be monitored and studied.

Figure 8.10 shows the response of a cell to the different locations around the borders of two types of stimuli. The normalized responses at three different time windows reveal that the half-height width of the spatial response profile around the boundary decreases over time, which is consistent with the

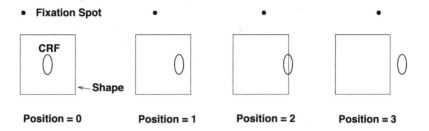

Figure 8.9 The spatial sampling scheme. The monkey fixates on the solid dot on the upper left. In successive trials, the image on the monitor is displaced relative to the fixation point of the monkey, or equivalently, relative to the recorded neuron's classical receptive field (CRF). This gives a spatial sampling of the neural response to different parts of the stimulus.

boundary-sharpening prediction. However, the absolute response of the neuron also decayed over time. This raises the possibility that this sharpening could potentially be simply be an "iceberg effect" where the response profile stays the same but simply sinks over time uniformly across space. The iceberg tip that remains visible, when normalized, might appear to be sharper. This seems unlikely, however, firstly because firing rate adaptation tends to be proportional to the firing rate (i.e. higher firing rates will adapt by a larger amount), so pure adaptation would flatten out the response profile; and secondly because the reduction of the half-height width of the response profile can be observed even when the absolute response of the neurons remains the same. Figure 8.11 shows the distribution of the half-height widths of the spatial response profiles of a population of neurons at three different time windows post-stimulus onset, which demonstrates a statistically significant effect of boundary contraction. Further experiments are needed to confirm this contraction of the boundary response, for example, by testing the neurons' responses to noisy and ambiguous figures which, we conjecture, should exaggerate and prolong the sharpening process.

It is evident from these data that a neuron's response often decays over time. This is traditionally considered to be an adaptation effect (the initial burst can partly be attributed to the neuron's temporal receptive field responding to the sudden onset of the stimulus). This adaptation is not a property of the weak-membrane model considered. Adaptation is not necessarily due to the neurons losing steam metabolically, since "habituating" neurons are capable of increasing their firing if a new and different stimulus suddenly appears [52]. For example, when the global orientation of the contour is more consistent to the neurons' orientation preference than the local texture, the later responses of the neurons are found to be stronger than the initial responses (figure 10 in [39]). The adaptation effect can potentially be understood as a "predictive coding" or "explaining away" effect proposed by Mumford [53] and Rao and Ballard [59].

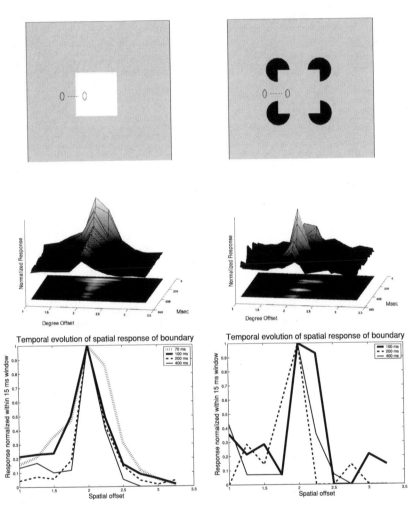

Figure 8.10   First row: two of the stimuli tested. Second row: A V1 neuron's spatiotemporal response to boundaries sampled at 1.5 degrees for a luminance boundary (left panel) and a subjective boundary (right panel). A gradual contraction of the spatial responses of the neurons to the boundary (at 2 degrees) can be observed for the line and the luminance border. Third row: When the peaks of the spatial response profiles were normalized to the same heights at different time windows, this reduction of the half-height width of the spatial response profile, a measure of sharpness of the boundary representation, becomes more evident.

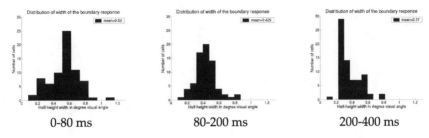

0-80 ms   80-200 ms   200-400 ms

Figure 8.11   The distributions of half-height widths in the spatial response profiles of a population of V1 neurons in response to the boundary of the luminance square at different time periods after stimulus onset. A successive reduction in the average boundary widths of the spatial response profile can be observed over time. The mean widths of boundary at three different time periods are 0.53, 0.42, and 0.37 degree visual angles, with standard error equal to 0.022, 0.016, and 0.016 respectively. The reduction of the boundary widths is statistically significant. Note that these boundary widths are necessarily overestimated as the sampling resolution was 0.25 degree visual angles, and the eye movement fixation window was about 0.5 degree window. Both factors would have increased the spatial width of the boundary response.

According to that theory, when there is a good high-level interpretation of an image region, as represented in a higher visual area, V1's responses are attenuated because they are partially explained away or replaced by the higher-order, presumably simpler description. V1, as a high-resolution buffer, is still needed to represent the residual information between the high-level prediction and the image stimulus. This information will include the local texture and color and disparity, because only V1 can represent such fine details in high resolution. Furthermore, not all predictive coding requires a top-down feedback mechanism. Recurrent center-surround or lateral inhibition mechanisms within V1 can also perform "predictive coding", just as the center-surround structure of the retinal receptive field has been considered a form of predictive code.

Segmentation of Texture Figures

The first study that systematically explored the responses of V1 neurons to a figure against the background in a visual scene was performed by Lamme [32]. In his experiments, there is a square region containing one type of texture surrounded by a background region with a different texture (figure 8.12). This stimulus is ambiguous, however, in terms of physical interpretation: it could be seen as a square foreground figure in front of a textured background, or alternatively, a window (background) on a textured wall. The simplest interpretation might be that there is a single square region with an albedo (pattern) discontinuity relative to the rest of the stimuli (e.g. a patch of texture cloth sewn into a hole in a cloth with a different texture). Since the cues embodied in the test images literally cannot distinguish between these interpretations, caution

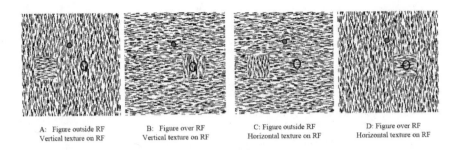

A: Figure outside RF   B: Figure over RF   C: Figure outside RF   D: Figure over RF
Vertical texture on RF   Vertical texture on RF   Horizontal texture on RF   Horizontal texture on RF

Figure 8.12   Lamme measured V1 neurons' responses to four conditions. In (A) and (B) the receptive field of the neuron is stimulated by vertical texture stimuli, but the receptive field is outside the figure in condition (A) and inside the figure in (B). Cases (C) and (D) are similar, except that now the receptive field of the neuron is now stimulated by horizontal texture. Lamme found that the neuron's activity is enhanced when its receptive field is inside the figure compared to when it is outside the figure. The solid dot indicates the fixation spot, while the ellipse indicates the receptive field of the neuron.

must therefore be taken not to overinterpret the results. With this caveat, we can agree that the common perceptual interpretation of this square is that of a foreground figure based on its many converging figure-ground organizational cues [57] such as smallness, convexity, and compactness.

Using a spatial sampling paradigm similar to the one we have described earlier for Lee and Nguyen's study [41], Lamme [32] examined neuronal responses at different spatial locations of the image relative to the texture square. In particular, he was interested in comparing the four conditions shown in figure 8.12. His findings are startling. First, he found that V1 neurons respond much more strongly (on the order of 40 % to 100 %) when their receptive fields are inside the figure than when they are in the background (i.e. responses to stimuli in figure 8.12 would be $B > A, D > C$). This occurred even though the size of the figure, (4 degrees $\times$ 4 degrees), was much larger than the classical receptive field of the neurons (which is typically 0.6 to 1 degrees for receptive fields from 2 to 4 degrees eccentricity). Second, this enhancement was uniform within the figure and terminated abruptly at the boundary.

It must be asked whether Lamme's results are significantly different from previous findings on surround suppression, which result from the well-known center-surround interactions in the primary visual cortex. It is well known that V1 neurons exhibit a phenomenon known as iso-orientation surround inhibition. That is, a neuron that prefers vertical orientation, in response to a vertical bar or vertical sinewave grating in its receptive field, will be inhibited by a surrounding vertical bar or grating (e.g. see, [47, 30, 44]. A cell inside a compact region of texture will receive less inhibition than a cell located in a large region of similar texture. But classical iso-orientation surround suppression theory has not anticipated a uniform enhancement within the figure, nor an abrupt discontinuity of enhancement response at the border.

Subsequent studies showed that the figure enhancement effect was weaker than Lamme described (about 15 % enhancement, [39]) or even less [61]) for a 4 × 4 degree texture square figure (see also, [45]). Lee et al. [39] nevertheless confirmed that the enhancement was indeed uniform within the figure, with an abrupt discontinuity at the boundary, as shown in figure 8.13a. This uniform enhancement response was obtained only when the cell's preferred orientation was *not* parallel to that of the border that it encountered along the spatial sampling line. When the cell's preferred orientation was parallel to that of the border, a significant response was observed at the border which can overshadow the small uniform enhancement observed within the texture figure (see figure 8.13b).

Figure 8.13c plotted the temporal evolution of combined responses at three different locations (inside the figure, in the background, and at the boundary) to compare the magnitude of the boundary effect to the figure enhancement effect. It shows that the enhancement effect (the difference between the response inside the figure and the response outside the figure) emerged at about 80 ms after the stimulus onset, after the initial burst of responses of the neurons, and that the boundary response, when the preferred orientation of the neurons is parallel to that of the texture boundary, is three to four times larger than the "figure enhancement" response [39].

Note that in the spatiotemporal response profiles shown in figure 8.13, the responses of each neuron to the two complementary cases (i.e. a vertically textured figure in a horizontally textured background vs. a horizontally textured figure in a vertically textured background) are summed together at each location for each point in time. For example, the combined response within the figure is obtained by summing the response for conditions B and D in figure 8.12, while the combined response in the background is the summation of the responses to A and C. By adjusting the position of the stimuli relative to the neurons, a spatiotemporal profile of the neuron's response to the images was obtained. If not summed, a vertical neuron will naturally respond more inside a vertically textured figure simply because of its orientation tuning. Summing the response helps to isolate the aspect of the response that is due to figure-ground context or compactness of the region, rather than the orientation tuning of the cell (see [39] for further details).

How do these experimental findings relate to the computational models described earlier? Clearly, several aspects of these results are consistent with the first class of computational segmentation models. There are uniform responses within each region with a sharp discontinuity at the border (prediction 3). There are responses to the boundaries (prediction 4). But there is a significant discrepancy, since none of the segmentation models predict the delayed enhancement within the figure. Some additional mechanisms not included in the weak-membrane model must also be involved.

Lamme [32] interpreted the enhancement effect as a signal for figure-ground segregation (i.e. a signal that can contrast a figure against the background). He argued that since figure-ground segregation is a high-order perceptual con-

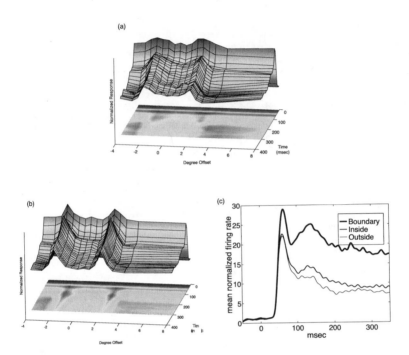

Figure 8.13   Population-averaged combined responses (30 cells recorded individually) to texture figures in a contrasting background. Panel (a): Spatiotemporal responses when the preferred orientation of the cells is orthogonal to the orientation of the border along the sampling line. The combined response inside the figure is uniform within the figure and greater than that in the background. Panel (b): Spatiotemporal responses when the preferred orientation of the cells is parallel to the border. In addition to the enhancement of response inside the figure relative to that in the background, a strong boundary response can be observed. The X-axis indicates the offset of the receptive field (RF) location relative to the center of the square, which is 4×4 degrees in size. The combined response in the figure in both cases was enhanced relative to the background at about 80 ms after stimulus onset. Panel (c) gives the population PSTHs (peristimulus time histograms) of the neurons at three locations (on the boundary, in the figure, and in the background) and shows that the elevation of the response at the boundary is over three times larger than the elevation of response inside the figure (both relative to the background). The enhancement inside the figure emerged at about 80 ms for texture figures.

struct, the delayed enhancement effect observed in V1 is likely a consequence of feedback from the extrastriate cortex. He has subsequently reported experiments showing that the enhancement effects disappeared when the extrastriate cortex was lesioned [34] or when the monkeys were under anesthesia [33] – see also [26]. The temporal delay in enhancement as evident in the PSTH (peristimulus-time histograms) is also consistent with the idea of feedback, as signals from even IT would be able to propagate back to V1 within 80 ms after stimulus onset (or 40 ms after the V1 initial response) [90]. However, it is still possible that the enhancement could be computed "bottom-up" with only feedforward and recurrent interaction within V1.

The Segmentation of Luminance and Color Figures

To demonstrate that the enhancement effect is more general, and not limited only to texture stimuli, Lee et al. [39] examined the responses of V1 neurons to luminance figure stimuli (a dark figure in a bright background, a bright figure in a dark background, or a gray figure in a texture background) and found similar but stronger enhancement effects (in terms of modulation ratio or percentage enhancement) for the luminance figures, even though the cells' absolute responses were much less because there were no oriented features inside their receptive fields. The enhancement was found to decrease as the size of the figure increased, but remained significant for figures as large as 7 degrees in diameter, far bigger than the size of the classical receptive field of the neurons.

Of particular interest were the responses to the gray figure in a texture background. In this test, the entire image was initially gray and then the background region was given a texture. Nevertheless, enhancement was observed even though there was no change in the stimulus within the receptive field of the neuron (only the surround was updated). Rossi et al. [61] repeated this experiment and found a progressive delay in the onset time of responses inside the gray figure as the size of the figure increased, as would be expected if the signal was propagated in from the border. They, however, did not believe the "enhancement" is necessarily related to figure-ground organization.

Similar observations have also been made for equiluminance color figures [81]. In this experiment, the entire screen was first set to a particular color, and then 300 ms later, a disk was made to appear centered at the receptive field of the neuron by changing the color of the background to the opponent color. This ensures, as for the gray figure case, that there was no change in the stimulus within or near the receptive field when the figure appears. Hence the transient response due to sudden color onset in the receptive field can be dissociated from the response due to the appearance of the figure due to background update. Figure 8.14 shows a typical neuron's temporal responses at the center of disks of four different diameters, ranging from 1 degree (border close to the receptive field) to 14 degrees (border far away from the receptive field). Even though the classical receptive field of the neuron (measured as the so-called minimum responsive area) was quite small, about 0.8 degrees in diameter, the neuron responded to the appearance of a color contrast border 7 degrees radius

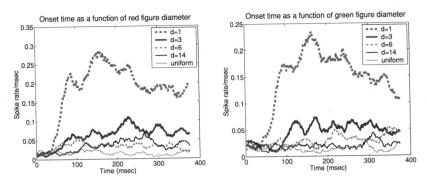

Figure 8.14   The PSTHs of a neuron in response to the onset of a color change in the disk surround that makes visible a disk figure of 1,2,3,4,6,14 degrees diameter centered at the receptive field of the neuron. The interior response was shown to be progressively delayed relative to the onset of response near the border (i.e. the RF is very close to the border when the figure is only 1 degree in diameter.

away! As the disk diameter became larger, the onset of the neural responses was progressively delayed, roughly in the order of 20 ms per degree. This result is consistent with the observation of Rossi et al. [61] on the luminance figure, and the hypothesis that signals are propagating (or diffusing) from the border to the interior surface of the figure. However, it is also possible the enhancement effect arises simultaneously in cells across the entire surface with a delay that is proportional to the size of the figure.

To resolve whether the progressive delay in onset of the enhancement is due to an increase in distance away from the border, or simply due to a larger figural size, the spatial sampling paradigm was applied to monitor the temporal emergence of the enhancement signals at different locations relative to the border for the chromatic stimuli. A red figure in a green background or vice versa, as shown in figure 8.16, were tested. The findings, as described below, were consistent with the border propagation hypothesis rather than the simultaneous emerging hypothesis (see [90] for the texture stimuli). In addition, the data showed that there were three major classes of neurons. One class of neurons responded primarily to the boundaries, while a second class responded well inside the figure, even though there are no oriented features within their receptive fields. The third class responded well at the boundaries, as well as inside the surface. Figure 8.16 shows three typical neurons which illustrate these three types of behavior.

Neuron 1 (row 1) was a cell that responded both to regions and boundaries. This cell responded much more strongly to the green figure than it did to the red background (middle column). Its response to the green background was weaker or about the same as the response to the red figure (left column). Therefore, the stronger response inside the green figure cannot be attributed to its

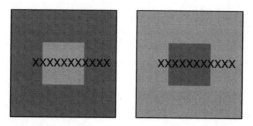

Figure 8.15   The static presentation paradigm: the receptive field sampling positions in the red square and the green square are labeled here by crosses (see color insert).

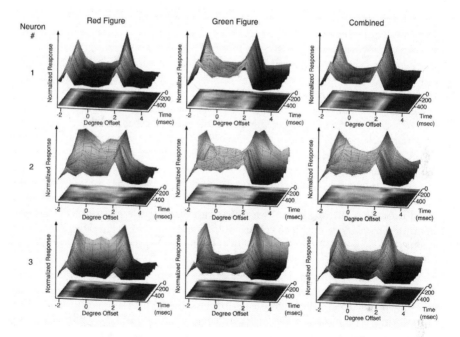

Figure 8.16   The temporal evolution of the responses of three different (typical) V1 neurons to different parts of the red figure in the green background (left column), and to different parts of the green figure in the red background (middle column). The right column sums the responses to the two stimuli at each spatial location to demonstrate the figure enhancement effect (see color insert).

preference to the green color alone. The combined response (to the red/green figure with the green/red background) shows a moderate enhancement in the figure relative to the background, as well as a robust boundary response. Many cells exhibited this kind of behavior.

Neurons 2 (row 2) and 3 (row 3) preferred the red color initially, as shown by their robust response to the onset of the red color in their receptive fields (left and middle columns). In fact, these neurons did not initially respond to the temporal onset of the green stimuli in their receptive fields. However, over time, the neurons started to respond more strongly inside the green figure to such an extent that the response to the green figure became stronger than the response to the red background (the color of which they initially preferred). In the case of the neuron 2, the later responses inside the figures were always stronger than the responses in the background, regardless of the color of the stimuli, with sharp discontinuities at the boundary. Its combined responses (the sum of the responses to the red and the green figures in contrast to the sum of the responses to the green and the red backgrounds) emphasized the enhancement responses inside the figure. Neuron 3 is similar to neuron 2 in exhibiting a dramatic reversal of the responses from initial preference for color to a later preference for figure (row 2, middle column). Its combined response emphasizes the boundary responses more than the enhancement of the figure.

These examples relate to prediction 1, since they show that some neurons responded more to the color region, others responded more to the boundaries, and a significant number of neurons, such as neuron 1, respond to both. In all these three neurons, the responses at the interior of the figure lag behind the responses at the figure border, particularly in the case of the green figure in a red background (middle column). This is manifested as a concave "wave front" in the responses to the green figure (middle column), which is consistent with the idea of information propagating inward from the border. This concave wavefront is not as obvious in the red figure case, perhaps because the initial chromatic change from gray (the initial screen color) to red within the receptive field provided a stronger bottom-up drive to the neurons as well. When this temporal transience in color is eliminated as in the experiment described in figure 8.14, a progressive delay in the onset time of the interior response relative to the boundary response is observed.

But perhaps the most striking aspects of these plots are the uniform responses within the figure and the abrupt discontinuity at the border of the figures. This is similar to the findings for texture, and is a clear indication of a mechanism similar to nonlinear diffusion as prescribed by the computational models. However, it is not entirely clear at this stage whether the propagated signals are related to color perception, surface representation, or perceptual saliency. Some neural models such as the BCFC model proposed in [21] suggest that color information in V1 is only carried by center-surround color-opponent cells, which means that both luminance and color information are available only at the contrast border. This necessitates the propagation of color and luminance signals from the boundary to the interior during the inference of color for each region. Evidence from von der Heydt et al. [77] seems to argue against this color-diffusion hypothesis. On the other hand, the propagation of neural activity from the border is also reminiscent of the border propagation of Horn's surface inference from shading algorithm. Further experiments are needed to clarify these issues.

The Nature of the Enhancement Signal

The evidence presented so far is broadly consistent with the nonlinear diffusion and boundary contraction predictions of the weak-membrane class of models. The main differences are the adaptation decay, and the enhancement within the figure that have been observed in neurophysiological studies.

Both of these two discrepancies can be understood in terms of the theory of the hierarchical generative model for predictive coding [53, 59]. The rapid decay in response after the initial outburst in response to stimulus onset can be understood mechanistically in terms of synaptic adaptation in the forward connection [11], as surround inhibition, or as feedback inhibition. Alternatively, it can be understood in terms of V1 neurons losing interest on the input because the input stimulus is being explained or "predicted" by the surrounding neurons or higher-level neurons [53, 59]. The delayed enhancement in responses could reflect the differential predictions that are offered by the contextual surround. The stimulus features in a small region or compact figure are not as well predicted by the surround stimuli; thus they are considered more surprising and appear to be more salient, which can elicit stronger attention. Features in a larger region of similar features are better predicted by the surrounding context, and hence are less salient. The delay in the enhancement response simply reflects the amount of time required to integrate the signals over each region: the larger a region, the longer the delay. From this predictive coding perspective, the enhancement response can be viewed as a measure of surprise or saliency.

An alternative perspective, however, is also possible. The enhancement could be signaling a fitness measure (informally a "happiness factor"), which is proportional to the probability of how well a higher-level description or model is fitting the input data in V1. A compact figure fits the model of an object better because its smooth and compact boundary might fit the spatial and shape prior better. This explanation is more consistent with the model of Tu et al.[73] in the second generation of segmentation theories in which a match of a model to the data can produce resonating "happiness". This view is also compatible with the classical ideas of interactive activation and adaptive resonance [51, 20]. The delay in the enhancement is expected because matching data with top-down models would need to involve recurrent interaction with the extrastriate cortex, and this takes time. Such resonance could enhance the relevant part of the V1 representation (see also [14]).

These two views are difficult to resolve at this stage, as they share many features in common, and it is likely both contain aspects of the truth. Both views involve recurrent bottom-up and top-down interaction, although the predictive coding theory includes both feedback and surround inhibition. Both views

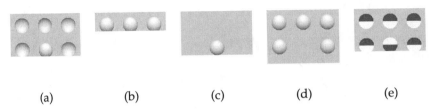

(a)   (b)   (c)   (d)   (e)

Figure 8.17   The basic stimuli conditions with LA (sphere with lighting from above) as the stimulus element presented to the receptive field of the neuron. The actual display contains many more stimulus elements repeated in the surround. (a) Oddball condition: RF stimulus is different from the surrounding stimulus elements. (b) Uniform condition: RF stimulus is the same as the surrounding stimulus elements. (c) Singleton condition. (d) Hole condition: RF not simulated, only the RF surround was stimulated. (e) An example of the 2D control. Oddball condition of the WA (white above) stimulus.

suggest that the response enhancement associated with a stimulus would be correlated to the perceptual saliency of that stimulus.

It is possible that the computation of the "saliency" of the texture and color figures can potentially be computed bottom-up using lateral inhibition. Lee et al. [42] performed another experiment to establish that this enhancement does involve top-down processes and is quantitatively related to perceptual saliency of a region. They tested V1 and V2 neurons with a set of stimuli with different degrees of bottom-up contrast saliency and perceptual "pop-out" saliency. Among them, a white-above (WA) stimulus (figure 8.17e) has a high contrast and thus strong bottom-up saliency. Yet when surrounded by a set of white-below (WB) stimuli, the WA oddball is difficult to detect, thus with low perceptual pop-out saliency. On the other hand, a light-from-above (LA) stimulus (figure 8.17a) has a lower stimulus contrast, but when surrounded by a set of light-from-below (LB) stimuli, the LA oddball easily pops out from the distractors.

In this experiment, the receptive field stimulus (the center of each display in figure 8.17) was presented to the center of the classical receptive field of the neuron, while the monkey performed a simple fixation task. Note that there were six types of stimuli tested in the actual experiment. Each of the stimulus elements (the target and distractors) was 1 degree in diameter while the receptive field ranged in size from 0.4 to 0.7 degrees. The center-to-center distance between the stimulus elements is 1.5 degree visual angles. The receptive field stimulus could be surrounded by identical stimulus elements (uniform condition) or the opposite stimulus elements (oddball condition). Can V1 neurons distinguish the difference in the surround stimuli between the oddball condition (figure 8.17a) and the uniform condition (figure 8.17b)?

We would expect that because of iso-orientation surround suppression, a vertically oriented neuron will respond more strongly to a vertical bar in the receptive field when the surround is populated by horizontal bars (oddball) than when the surround is populated by vertical bars (uniform). This has been observed by Knierim and Van Essen [30] as well as by other center-surround experiments based on sinewave gratings. However, the WA and WB stimuli, and likewise the LA and LB stimuli, would stimulate neurons of the same orientation. Since the iso-orientation suppression is not sensitive to the phase of the stimuli in V1, the amount of iso-orientation suppression from the surround will be the same for both the oddball and the uniform conditions. This is indeed the case for the WA and WB stimuli.

Lee et al. [42] found that, indeed, before the monkeys had learned to utilize the stimuli in some way (e.g. making a saccade to the oddball in the stimulus), V1 neurons were not sensitive to the difference in the surround stimuli between those two conditions, for both LA/LB and WA/WB stimuli. V2 neurons, on the other hand, responded more in the oddball condition than in the uniform condition for the LA/LB stimuli, but this is not observed for the WA/WB stimuli. Ramachandran [58] pointed out that the LA/LB stimuli were more salient pop-out targets because they afford opposite 3D interpretation when a single lighting direction is assumed. For example, when the LA stimuli are considered convex, the LB stimuli in the same image will be considered concave (although it is also possible to perceive all the stimulus elements as convex spheres but with lighting coming from different directions). The WA/WB stimuli have stronger bottom-up contrast, and thus can drive V1 and V2 neurons more rigorously. Yet the WA oddball does not jump out from the distractors because neither the WA nor the WB stimuli offer 3D interpretations. The initial negative finding by Lee et al. [42] of oddball enhancement effect in V1 but positive result in V2 might suggest that the "predictive inhibition" mechanisms for such shape from shading stimuli may be based in V2.

Interestingly, after they trained the monkeys to make a saccade to the oddball in each stimulus (for both LA/LB and WA/WB), they found the V1 neurons started to respond better to the oddball condition than the uniform condition for the LA/LB stimuli, but still not for the WA/WB stimuli, even when the monkeys were performing the same fixation task. Figure 8.18(a) shows that the singleton condition (i.e. no distractors) elicited the biggest response. The responses to the oddball and the uniform conditions are initially smaller than that for the singleton, perhaps due to surround suppression (if it is possible that lateral inhibition works within 3D representation as well). But at 100 ms, the response to the oddball condition became stronger than the response to the uniform condition, showing that the neuron was now sensitive to the difference in the surrounding stimuli between the two conditions. Observe that the latency of 100 ms is longer than the latency for the enhancement signals for the luminance/color figures (60 ms), and for the texture figures (80 ms) (see earlier figures). This longer delay probably reflects the greater complexity of the images being processed. In addition, the oddball (e.g. LA or LB) that is perceptually easier to detect is found to elicit a stronger enhancement response than the oddball that is more difficult to detect (e.g. WA or WB). This suggests that the enhancement may reflect how salient a stimulus element is.

To establish this observation, Lee et al. [42] compared the neural enhance-

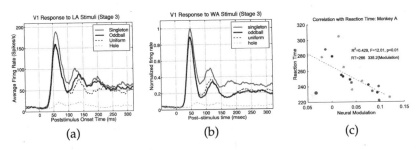

(a)   (b)   (c)

Figure 8.18   (a) The responses (PSTHs) of a neuron to the LA stimulus element in various contextual conditions. (b) The responses (PSTHs) of a neuron to the WA stimulus element in various contextual conditions. (c) The enhancement modulation ratio is found to be inversely correlated to the reaction time of the monkey in detecting the various stimuli with different degrees of saliency. The enhancement ratio is defined to be (A-B)/(A+B), where A is the response to the oddball condition and B is the response to the uniform condition. See Lee et al. [42] for details.

ment ratio against the speed and accuracy of the monkeys in detecting the oddball. They found that the enhancement ratio was inversely correlated to the reaction time of the monkeys (figure 8.18(c)), and positively correlated with the accuracy (not shown) in the monkeys' ability to correctly locate the oddball. This finding confirms that the enhancement signal is correlated with the perceptual saliency of the target stimuli.

A simple interpretation is that the responses to the oddball were enhanced in the extrastriate cortex because the monkeys started to pay more attention to it. This attentional signal was then fed back to enhance the responses of the V1 neurons. Could this enhancement in V1 be a simple passive reflection of activities higher up, an epiphenomenon that does not serve any functional purpose? First, the enhancement itself is not completely dependent on top-down attention because WA and WB stimuli fail to elicit the response even though the monkeys have been trained to detect them and should be paying as much attention to them as to the LA and LB stimuli. The interaction between attention and the underlying processing of these stimuli is important. Second, Lee et al. [42] argued from the high-resolution buffer perspective that V1 must provide the necessary segmentation boundary to constrain and contain the enhancement signals precisely. The participation of V1 is thus essential to produce a precise "coloring" of the figure to highlight it for further processing. To prove this point, they showed that the enhancement response is limited to the oddball stimuli but not to the distractor stimuli [42].

A recent pilot study in Lee's laboratory applied the spatial sampling paradigm to examine the precise spatiotemporal responses of neurons to these stimuli. Ten positions were sampled in the LA oddball condition, including a position centered on the LA oddball and another centered on one of its immediate neighboring distractors (figure 8.19(a)). Additionally, six positions were sam-

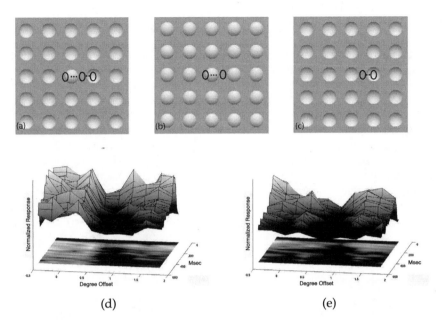

Figure 8.19 Spatial sampling of the shape from shading stimuli in oddball and uniform condition. (a) LA oddball condition: ten positions sampled covering the entire oddball and part of the distractor. (b) LA uniform condition: six positions sampled covering the pattern of the oddball when it is surrounded by identical elements, for comparison with the response to the oddball in (a). (c) LB uniform condition: four positions sampled covering the pattern of the distractor when it is surrounded by identical elements, for comparison with the response to the distractor in (a). Second row shows a neuron's response to the (a) (left column) and (b) and (c) (right column). (d) The spatiotemporal response to the oddball condition (a) shows that the response was strong and the enhancement was localized inside the figure, while (e) the response to the distractor vanished over time with only a weak boundary effect.

pled over the LA stimulus in the uniform condition (there is no need to sample centered on a distractor, since it is the same as the target) (figure 8.19(b)), and four positions were sampled over the shape of the distractor, also in the uniform condition (figure 8.19(c)). The idea is to compare the response to the oddball image against the uniform images while keeping the receptive field stimulus in each comparison constant. Figure 8.19(d) and (e) show the spatial activity profile of a cell in response to the oddball condition as well as the uniform conditions.

Several interesting phenomena can be observed. First, the neurons' responses inside the oddball were enhanced over time, with a sharp discontinuity at the boundary. By contrast, the responses to the distractors were initially strong, but decayed rapidly to very low levels. The later differential response between the oddball and the distractors presumably arose because the oddball was selected as the figure or target.

In addition, the discontinuity in response at the boundary of the distractors was weak and poorly localized. Similar weak discontinuity responses at the boundaries occur for both types of stimuli in the uniform condition. This suggests that the process of target selection and the process of segmentation might be tightly coupled: segmentation constrains the target enhancement, but segmentation itself also depends on target selection.

These oddball enhancement effects require several mechanisms. There is an initial stage where all the objects (the target and distractors) are detected. Next is a selection stage where the target is selected. In the case of the oddball, this can be mediated by surround competition. Finally, there is an enhancement of the response within the target and a strengthening of the discontinuity at its boundary. The oddball enhancement might arise from the same principle of the "figure enhancement" observed in texture, luminance, and color figures. When there is only one figure in the scene, the figure is salient and will be selected almost automatically as a target. When there are multiple figures in the scene, the less predicted one (i.e. the oddball) will pop out as the preferred target. As with the figure enhancement phenomena, this oddball enhancement or target selection phenomenon goes beyond the scope of the first class of segmentation models. It is partially consistent with theories where the recognition of objects and their segmentation are integrated [73]. In this theory, bottom-up processing activates higher-level object models, which feed back to explain the early representation. As before, such ideas can be understood either in terms of the predictive coding theory or in terms of interactive activation or resonance theory. Whether the excitement in the neurons is a sign of surprise or "happiness" remains to be elucidated.

8.6   Summary and Discussion

In this chapter, we have described how image segmentation can be formulated in terms of obtaining an efficient encoding of the image. We introduced a class of computational models consistent with this viewpoint and made predictions from these models. We described several experiments consistent with these conjectures which strongly suggest that neurons in V1 are involved in image segmentation. At the very least, we showed that activity in V1 is significantly more complex than the standard models of V1 as a filter bank, or as a way to efficiently encode intensity. Here is a summary of the evidence that has been discussed.

1. Evidence of region and boundary representations: Neurons in V1 responded to the interior and the boundaries of regions, even when there were no image features (oriented or otherwise) inside their classical receptive fields (figure 8.14). While some cells responded solely to boundaries and others responded strongly inside regions, many cells responded to both. This

suggests that the boundary and surface representations might be more distributed than the simple dual representations in boundary cells and region cells that some earlier computational models envisioned.

2. Evidence of interaction between the region and boundary processes: While the initial spatial response profile of a neuron tends to be smooth across boundaries, the later spatial response profile of the neuron always exhibited a sharp discontinuity between regions (figure 8.16). The gradual sharpening of the boundary responses coincides with the development of abrupt discontinuity in responses across regions, which suggests that the two effects might be coupled (figure 8.10). However, the boundary sharpening seems to continue to progress (200 to 300 ms) even after the response discontinuity has developed (100 ms) (figure 8.11).

3. Evidence of nonlinear diffusion in regional representation: There was a delay between the responses at the center of the figure vs. the response close to the boundary (figure 8.16). The delay is progressively larger as the size of the figure or the distance away from the border increases, suggesting that the signal is propagated (diffused) from the border to the interior surface of the figure (figure 8.14). The abrupt discontinuity in response between regions suggests diffusion is blocked by the region boundary (hence making it nonlinear).

4. Evidence of gradual sharpening of the boundary representation: Gradual sharpening of the boundary response was observed for both impulse edges (i.e. boundaries defined by lines) as well as for step edges (figure 8.10). This boundary sharpening may result from the continuation mechanism as p decreases.

5. Evidence of model selection or predictive coding between different visual areas: The enhancement of responses inside the figure is not predicted by most of the segmentation models. The experimental evidence from the odd-ball detection experiment (figure 8.19) suggested that feedback from other cortical areas is likely involved, and that top-down feedback in turn can facilitate segmentation, while segmentation helps to confine the enhancement process to precise spatial locations. Empirical evidence suggests the enhancement is proportional to perceptual saliency of the target. However, there are multiple interpretations on the nature of the enhancement effect. The predictive coding perspective suggests the enhancement is a measure of surprise, while the model selection perspective suggests the enhancement is a measure of happiness (or fitness or resonance) which emerges from the match between the selected top-down model and the V1 representation.

We propose that, in addition to furnishing a wavelet/filter bank for efficient detection and representation of image details, V1 performs image segmentation, and represents boundary locations and region properties in the activity of its neurons. This is consistent with Lee and Mumford's earlier proposal [39, 38] that V1 can serve as a high-resolution buffer to support *all* visual reasoning and interpretations which require high spatial precision and fine details available explicitly only in V1. We are not arguing that V1 by itself is sufficient for robust scene segmentation. In our view, early visual inference such as segmentation cannot be robust or complete without the interaction with global context and higher-order visual reasoning (e.g. object recognition). Such interaction can be mediated by the feedforward/feedback loops in the visual hierarchy [38]. Recent work in computer vision makes it clear that segmentation can be enhanced by object recognition [8, 84, 73]. Processing required to perform segmentation may be partially performed in higher-level areas using top-down feedback to V1. In this scenario, V1 performs an initial processing of the image and excites higher-level models and processing in other visual areas, which then in turn feed back to V1 to refine the representation.

Direct evidence in support of V1 performing higher-order processes such as figure-ground segregation (border ownership) and 3D surface encoding are either weak or unconvincing at this stage [90, 46]. Current compelling evidence seem to suggest that the representation of border ownership [86] and the representation of surface [4, 70] might start at V2. Many color and brightness illusions that are tied to surface perception have also been mainly observed in V2 [25, 23]. V1's sensitivity to shape from shading information, as demonstrated in Lee et al. [42], probably originated from V2 feedback. It is possible that the granularity of surface geometry representation is much coarser than the granularity for representing region and image properties, hence it is logical to factorize the functional representations into two separate areas. If surface inference and segmentation are to be integrated together, V1 and V2 have to work closely together.

How regions, boundaries, and their models can be encoded flexibly as a whole in V1 or in the extrastriate areas remains an open question. An interesting but controversial hypothesis is that cells belonging to the same region or same contour can synchronize, exhibiting a higher degree of functional connectivity. This is related to von der Malsburg's [78] binding-by-synchrony theory. The experimental evidence in support of this idea is mixed [63, 69]. Emerging evidence suggests that synchrony due to similarity in bottom-up input could potentially serve as a mechanism for Gestalt grouping [62], which might be related to the mechanisms for the affinity-based model [67, 83, 64, 71] and the compositional system of Geman et al. [17] . Further experiments are needed to clarify the connection between the phenomena of neuronal synchrony and figure enhancement, and their role in the encoding of the regions.

The computational models described in this chapter have provided important insights into the computational constraints and algorithms of segmentation. The biological predictions based on the weak-membrane class of models [31, 36] have motivated much of the experimental research discussed in this chapter. These first-generation theories are, at best, first-order approximations to true theories of segmentation since their performance on segmenting natural images is still limited. But the increasing successes of the next generation of theories, when evaluated on data sets with ground truth, suggest that the computational vision models for scene segmentation might be on the right track, and should be taken seriously in our investigation of visual systems. Insights from computer vision might prove to be instrumental in guiding our study on how V1 interprets images, extracting and representing abstract information rather than merely coding the raw input images. Theoretical framework will guide us where to look, and what to analyze. However, extra caution must be taken to guard against overinterpreting results to fit the theory in any theory-driven neurophysiological research.

The experimental results described in this chapter support some of the predictions derived from the computational models developed from computer vision. It is reassuring that the discovery of new phenomena such as region enhancement was parallel to the development of new computational algorithms in the computer vision community such as integration of top-down object recognition and bottom-up segmentation in various probabilistic inference frameworks. While current evidence, based on relatively simple image stimuli and experimental paradigms, cannot distinguish whether the enhancement within the figure is a sign of surprise (predictive coding) or happiness (model fitting and resonance), its correlation with perceptual saliency, and its various image-dependent properties provide credence to the hypothesis that image segmentation is a major computational task being performed in V1. Segmentation of the scene is a process of inference that produces a simpler and more compact description of the scene based on regions and boundaries, and their associated models. It can thus be considered as a form of efficient coding that goes beyond raw image coding.

Acknowledgments

This chapter benefits from the helpful discussions with David Mumford, David Tolliver, Gary Miller, Dan Kersten, Zili Liu, Jason Samonds, Tom Stepleton, Matthew Smith, and HongJing Lu. We thank Cindy Yang, Ryan Kelly, Lei Lu, My Nguyen, Xiaogang Yan, and Brian Potetz for technical assistance in the described experiments. Tai Sing Lee is supported by NSF IIS-0413211 and NIMH MH 64445, Penn State tobacco settlement grant and Alan L. Yuille is supported by NSF 0413214.

References

[1] Ambrosio L, Tortorelli VM (1990) On the approximation of free discontinuity problems. *Preprints di Matermatica, 86,* Pisa, Italy: Scuola Normale Superiore.

[2] Angelucci A, Levitt JB, Walton EJ, Hupe JM, Bullier J, Lund JS (2002) Circuits for local and global signal integration in primary visual cortex. *Journal of Neuroscience,* 22:8633-8646.

[3] Atick JJ, Redlich AN (1992) What does the retina know about natural scenes? *Neural Computation,* 4:196-210.

[4] Bakin JS, Nakayama K, Gilbert CD (2000) Visual responses in monkey areas V1 and V2 to three-dimensional surface configurations. *Journal of Neuroscience,* 20:8188-8198.

[5] Belhumeur, P (1996) A Bayesian approach to binocular stereopsis. *International Journal of Computer Vision*, 19(3): 237-260.

[6] Bell AJ, Sejnowski TJ (1997) The "independent components" of natural scenes are edge filters. *Vision Research*, 37(23):3327-38.

[7] Blake A, Zisserman A (1987) *Visual Reconstruction.* Cambridge, MA: MIT Press.

[8] Borenstein E, Ullman S (2001) Class specific top-down segmentation. *Proceedings of the European Conference on Computer Vision*, 110-122.

[9] Canny J (1986) A computational approach to edge detection. *IEEE Transactions on Pattern Analysis and Machine Intelligence*, B 207:187-217.

[10] Carandini M, Demb JB, Mante V, Tolhurst DJ, Dan Y, Olshausen BA, Gallant JL, Rust NC (2005) Do we know what the early visual system does? *Journal of Neuroscience*, 25(46):10577-97.

[11] Chance FS, Nelson SB, Abbott LF (1998) Synaptic depression and the temporal response characteristics of V1 cells. *Journal of Neuroscience*, 18(12):4785-99.

[12] Dan Y, Atick JJ, Reid RC (1996) Efficient coding of natural scenes in the lateral geniculate nucleus: experimental test of a computational theory. *Journal of Neuroscience*, 16: 3351-3362.

[13] Daugman JG (1985) Uncertainty relation for resolution in space, spatial frequency, and orientation optimized by two-dimensional visual cortical filters. *Journal of the Optical Society of America*, 2(7):1160-1169.

[14] Deco G, Lee TS (2004) The role of early visual cortex in visual integration: a neural model of recurrent interaction. *European Journal of Neuroscience*, 20:1089-1100.

[15] Geiger D, Yuille AL (1991) A common framework for image segmentation, *International Journal of Computer Vision*, 6(3):227-243.

[16] Geman S, Geman D (1984) Stochastic relaxation, Gibbs distribution, and the Bayesian restoration of images. *IEEE Transactions on Pattern Analysis and Machine Intelligence*, 6:721-741.

[17] Geman S, Potter D, Chi Z (2002) Composition systems. *Quarterly of Applied Mathematics*, 40: 707-736.

[18] Gregory, RL. (1970) *The Intelligent Eye.* London: Weidenfeld & Nicolson.

[19] Grosof DH, Shapley RM, Hawken MJ. (1993) Macaque V1 neurons can signal "illusory" contours. *Nature*, 365:550-552.

[20] Grossberg S (1987). Competitive learning: from interactive activation to adaptive resonance. *Cognitive Science*, 11:23-63.

[21] Grossberg S, Mingolla E (1985) Neural dynamics of perceptual grouping: textures, boundaries, and emergent segmentations. *Perception & Psychophysics*, 38:141-171.

[22] Horn BKP. (1986) *Robot Vision.* Cambridge, MA: MIT Press.

[23] Huang X, MacEvoy SP, Paradiso MA (2002) Perception of brightness and brightness illusions in the macaque monkey. *Journal of Neuroscience*, 22:9618-25.

[24] Hubel DH, Wiesel TN (1978) Functional architecture of macaque monkey visual cortex. *Proceedings of the Royal Society B (London)*, 198:1-59.

[25] Hung CP, Ramsden BM, Chen LM, Roe AW (2001) Building surfaces from borders in Areas 17 and 18 of the cat. *Vision Research*, 41:1389-1407.

[26] Hupe JM, James AC, Payne BR, Lomber SG, Girard P, Bullier J (1998) Cortical feedback improves discrimination between figure and background by V1, V2 and V3 neurons. *Nature*, 394:784-787.

[27] Jones JP, Palmer LA (1987). An evaluation of the two-dimensional Gabor filter model of simple receptive fields in the cat striate cortex. *Journal of Neurophysiology*, 58:1233-1258.

[28] Kanizsa G (1979) *Organization in Vision*. New York: Praeger.

[29] Kapadia MK, Westheimer G, Gilbert CD (2000) Spatial distribution of contextual interactions in primary visual cortex and in visual perception. *Journal of Neurophysiology*, 84:2048-2062.

[30] Knierim JJ, Van Essen DC (1992) Neuronal responses to static texture patterns in area V1 of the alert macaque monkey. *Journal of Neurophysiology*, 67:961-980.

[31] Koch C, Marroquin J, Yuille AL (1986). Analog "neuronal" networks in early vision. *Proceedings of the National Academy of Sciences of the United States of America*, 83: 4263-4267.

[32] Lamme VAF. (1995) The neurophysiology of figure-ground segregation in primary visual cortex. *Journal of Neuroscience*, 15:1605-1615.

[33] Lamme, VAF; Zipser, K; Spekreijse, H (1998) Figure-ground activity in primary visual cortex is suppressed by anesthesia. *Proceedings of the National Academy of Sciences of the United States of America*, 95(6): 3263-3268.

[34] Lamme VAF, Zipser K, Spekreijse, H (1997) Figure-ground signals in V1 depend on extrastriate feedback. *Investigative Ophthalmology & Visual Science*, 38(4) (Part 2): 4490.

[35] Leclerc YG (1989) Constructing simple stable descriptions for image partitioning. *International Journal of Computer Vision*, 3(1):73-102.

[36] Lee TS (1995) A Bayesian framework for understanding texture segmentation in the primary visual cortex. *Vision Research*, 35:2643-2657.

[37] Lee TS (1996) Image representation using 2D Gabor wavelets. *IEEE Transactions on Pattern Analysis and Machine Intelligence*, 18:959-971.

[38] Lee TS, Mumford D (2003) Hierarchical Bayesian inference in the visual cortex. *Journal of the Optical Society of America A*, 20:1434-1448.

[39] Lee TS, Mumford D, Romero R, Lamme VAF (1998) The role of the primary visual cortex in higher level vision. *Vision Research*, 38:2429-2454.

[40] Lee TS, Mumford D, Yuille A (1992) Texture segmentation by minimizing vector-valued energy functionals: the coupled-membrane model. *Lecture Notes in Computer Science*, 588:165-173.

[41] Lee TS, Nguyen M (2001) Dynamics of subjective contour formation in the early visual cortex. *Proceedings of the National Academy of Sciences of the United States of America*, 98:1907-1911.

[42] Lee TS, Yang C, Romero R, Mumford D (2002) Neural activity in early visual cortex reflects perceptual saliency determined by stimulus attributes and experience. *Nature Neuroscience*, 5:589-597.

[43] Lewicki MS, Olshausen BA (1999) Probabilistic framework for the adaptation and comparison of image codes. *Journal of the Optical Society of America A*, 16(7):1587-1601.

[44] Li CY, Li W (1994) Extensive integration field beyond the classical receptive field of cat's striate cortical neuron–classification and tuning properties. *Vision Research*, 34:2577-2598.

[45] Marcus DS, Van Essen DC. (2002) Scene segmentation and attention in primate cortical areas V1 and V2. *Journal of Neurophysiology*, 88:2648-2658.

[46] MacEvoy SP, Kim W, Paradiso MA (1998) Integration of surface information in primary visual cortex. *Nature Neuroscience*, 1:616-620.

[47] Maffei L, Fiorentini A (1976) The unresponsive regions of visual cortical receptive fields. *Vision Research*, 16:1131-1139.

[48] Martin D, Fowlkes C, Tai D, Malik J (2001) A database of human segmented natural images and its application to evaluating segmentation algorithms and measuring ecological statistics. *Proceedings International Conference of Computer Vision*, vol 2, 416-424.

[49] Marr D (1982) *Vision*. New York: WH Freeman.

[50] Marr D, Hildreth E (1980) Computational theory of edge detection. *Proceedings of the Royal Society B (London)*, 207:187-217.

[51] McClelland JL, Rumelhart DE (1981). An interactive activation model of context effects in letter perception. Part I: An account of basic findings. *Psychological Review*, 88:375-407.

[52] Miller EK, Desimone R (1994) Parallel neuronal mechanisms for short-term memory. *Science*, 28:263(5146):520-522.

[53] Mumford D (1992) On the computational architecture of the neocortex: II. The role of cortico-cortical loops. *Biological Cybernetics*, 66:241-251.

[54] Mumford D, Shah J (1989) Optimal approximations by piecewise smooth functions and associated variational problems. *Communications on Pure and Applied Mathematics*, 42:577-685.

[55] Nitzberg M, Mumford D, Shiota T (1993) *Filtering, Segmentation and Depth*. New York: Springer-Verlag.

[56] Olshausen BA, Field DJ (1996) Emergence of simple-cell receptive field properties by learning a sparse code for natural images. *Nature*, 381:607-609.

[57] Palmer S (1999) *Vision Science: Photons to Phenomenology*. Cambridge, MA: MIT Press.

[58] Ramachandran VS (1988) Perception of shape from shading. *Nature*, 331:163-166.

[59] Rao RPN, Ballard DH (1997) Predictive coding in the visual cortex: a functional interpretation of some extra-classical receptive-field effects. *Nature Neuroscience*, 2:79-87.

[60] Rissanen J (1987) Minimum Description Length Principle. In Kotz S, Read C, Banks D, eds., *Encyclopedia of Statistical Sciences, Volume 5*, pages 523-527, New York: Wiley.

[61] Rossi AF, Desimone R, Ungerleider LG (2001) Contextual modulation in pimary visual cortex of nacaques. *Journal of Neuroscience*, 21:1698-1709.

[62] Samonds JM, Bonds AB (2005) Gamma oscillation maintains stimulus structure-dependent synchronization in cat visual cortex. *Journal of Neurophysiology*, 93:223-236.

[63] Shadlen MN, Movshon JA (1999) Synchrony unbound: a critical evaluation of the temporal binding hypothesis. *Neuron*, 24(1):67-77, 111-25.

[64] Sharon E, Brandt A, Basri R (2001) Segmentation and boundary detection using multiscale intensity measurements, *Proceedings IEEE Conference on Computer Vision and Pattern Recognition*, Kauai, Hawaii, 1:469-476.

[65] Shannon CE (1948) A mathematical theory of communication. *Bell System Technical Journal*, 27:379-423, 623-656, July, October.

[66] Sheth BR, Sharma J, Rao SC, Sur M. (1996) Orientation maps of subjective contours in visual cortex. *Science*, 274:2110-2115.

[67] Shi J, Malik J (2000) Normalized cuts and image segmentation. *IEEE Transactions on Pattern Analysis and Machine Intelligence*, 22:8, 888-905.

[68] Simoncelli EP (2003) Vision and the statistics of the visual environment. *Current Opinion in Neurobiology*, 13(2):144-149.

[69] Singer W, Gray CM (1995) Visual feature integration and the temporal correlation hypothesis. *Annual Review of Neuroscience*, 18:555-586.

[70] Thomas OM, Cumming BG, Parker AJ (2002) A specialization for relative disparity in V2. *Nature Neuroscience*, 5:472-478.

[71] Tolliver D, Miller GL (2006) Graph partitioning by spectral rounding: applications in image segmentation and clustering. *Proceedings IEEE Conference on Computer Vision and Pattern Recognition*, New York City, 1:1053-1060.

[72] Tso DY, Gilbert CD, Wiesel TN (1988) Relationships between horizontal interactions and functional architecture in cat striate cortex as revealed by cross correlation analysis. *Journal of Neuroscience*, 6:1160-1170.

[73] Tu ZW, Chen XR, Yuille AL, Zhu SC (2005) Image parsing: unifying segmentation, detection and recognition *International Journal of Computer Vision*, 63(2):113-140.

[74] Tu Z, Zhu SC (2002) Image segmentation by data-driven Markov chain Monte Carlo. *IEEE Transactions on Pattern Analysis and Machine Intelligence*, 24(5): 657-673.

[75] Ullman, S (1994) Sequence seeking and counterstreams: A model for bidirectional information flow in the cortex. In C Koch, J Davis, eds., *Large-Scale Theories of the Cortex*, pages 257-270, Cambridge, MA: MIT Press.

[76] von der Heydt R, Peterhans E, Baumgarthner G (1984) Illusory contours and cortical neuron responses. *Science*, 224:1260-1262.

[77] von der Heydt R, Friedman HS, Zhou H (2003) Searching for the neural mechanisms of color filling-in. In Pessoa L, De Weerd P, eds., *Filling-in: From Perceptual Completion to Cortical Reorganization*, pages 106-127, Oxford: Oxford University Press.

[78] von der Malsburg C (1981) The correlation theory of brain function. *Internal Report*, Göttingen, Germany: Max-Planck Institute for Biophysical Chemistry.

[79] Williams LR, Jacobs DW (1997) Stochastic completion fields: A neural model of illusory contour shape and salience. *Neural Computation*, 9(4):837-858.

[80] Winkler G (1995) *Image Analysis, Random Fields and Dynamic Monte Carlo Methods.* Berlin: Springer-Verlag.

[81] Yan XG, Lee TS (2000) Informatics of spike trains in neuronal ensemble. *Proceedings of the 22nd Annual International Conference of the IEEE Engineering in Medicine and Biology Society*, WC, 5978-65226, 1-6.

[82] Young RA (1985) The Gaussian derivative theory of spatial vision: analysis of cortical cell receptive field line-weighting profiles. *General Motors Research Technical Report*, GMR-4920.

[83] Yu SX, Shi J (2003) Multiclass Spectral Clustering. *Proceedings of the Ninth International Conference on Computer Vision*, 313-319.

[84] Yu SX, Shi J (2004) Segmentation given partial grouping constraints. *IEEE Transactions on Pattern Analysis and Machine Intelligence*, 26:173-183.

[85] Yuille AL, Grzywacz NM (1998) A theoretical framework for visual motion. In Watanabe T, eds., *High-Level Motion Processing-Computational, Neurbiological, and Psychophysical Perspectives*, pages 187-211, Cambridge, MA: MIT Press.

[86] Zhou H, Friedman HS, von der Heydt R (2000) Coding of border ownership in monkey visual cortex. *Journal of Neuroscience*, 20:6594-6611.

[87] Zhu SC, Lee TS, Yuille A (1995) Region competition: unifying snakes, region growing and MDL for image segmentation. *Proceedings of the Fifth International Conference in Computer Vision*, 416-425.

[88] Zhu S, Mumford D (1997) Prior learning and Gibbs reaction diffusion. *IEEE Transactions on Pattern Analysis and Machine Intelligence*, 19(11):1236–1250.

[89] Zhu SC, Yuille AL (1996) Region competition: unifying snake/ balloon, region growing and Bayes/MDL/energy for multi-band image segmentation. *IEEE Transactions on Pattern Analysis and Machine Intelligence*, 18(9): 884-900.

[90] Zipser K, Lamme VAF, Schiller PH. (1996) Contextual modulation in primary visual cortex. *Journal of Neuroscience*, 16:7376-7389.

9 Bayesian Models of Sensory Cue Integration

David C. Knill

9.1 Introduction

Our senses provide a number of independent cues to the three-dimensional layouts of objects and scenes. Vision, for example, contains cues from stereo, motion, texture, shading, etc.. Each of these cues provides uncertain information about a scene; however, this apparent ambiguity is mitigated by several factors. First, under normal conditions, multiple cues are available to an observer. By efficiently integrating information from all available cues, the brain can derive more accurate and robust estimates of three-dimensional geometry (i.e. positions, orientations, and shapes in three-dimensional space)[23]. Second, objects in our environment have strong statistical regularities that make cues more informative than would be the case in an unstructured environment. Prior knowledge of these regularities allows the brain to maximize its use of the information provided by sensory cues.

Bayesian probability theory provides a normative framework for modeling how an observer should combine information from multiple cues and from prior knowledge about objects in the world to make perceptual inferences [21]. It also provides a framework for developing predictive theories of how human sensory systems make perceptual inferences about the world from sensory data, predictions that can be tested psychophysically. The goal of this chapter is to introduce the basic conceptual elements of Bayesian theories of perception and to illustrate a number of ways that we can use psychophysics to test predictions of Bayesian theories.

9.1.1 Basics

To illustrate the basic structure of Bayesian computations, consider the problem of integrating multiple sensory cues about some property of a scene. Figure 9.1 illustrates the Bayesian formulation of one such problem — estimating the position of an object, X, from visual and auditory cues, V and A. The goal

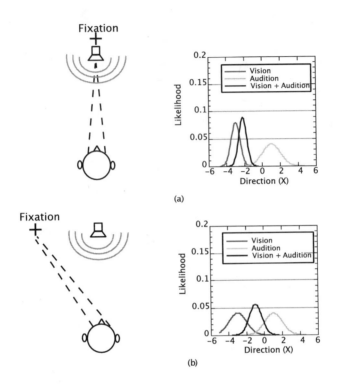

(a)

(b)

Figure 9.1 Two examples in which auditory and visual cues provide "conflicting" information about a target's direction. The conflict is apparent in the difference in means of the likelihood functions associated with each cue, though the functions overlap. Such conflicts are always present due to noise in the sensory systems. In order to optimally integrate visual and auditory information, a multimodal area in the brain must take into account the uncertainty associated with each cue. (a) When the vision cue is most reliable, the peak of the posterior distribution is shifted toward the direction suggested by the vision cue. (b) When the reliabilities of the cues is more similar, for example, when the stimulus is in the far periphery, the peak is shifted toward the direction suggested by the auditory cue. When both likelihood functions are Gaussian, the most likely direction of the target is given by a weighted sum of the most likely directions given the vision and auditory cues individually, $\hat{X}_{A,V} = w_V \hat{X}_A + w_A \hat{X}_V$. The weights are inversely proportional to the variances of the likelihood functions. (reprinted with permission from *Trends in Neuroscience*)

of an optimal, Bayesian observer would be to compute the conditional density function, p(X | V,A). Using Bayes' rule, this is given by

$$p(X \mid V, A) = \frac{p(V, A \mid X)p(X)}{p(V, A)}, \qquad (9.1)$$

where p(V, A | X) specifies the relative likelihood of sensing the given data for different values of X and p(X) is the prior probability of different values of X. Since the noise sources in auditory and visual mechanisms are statistically independent, we can decompose the likelihood function into the product of likelihood functions associated with the visual and auditory cues, respectively:

$$p(V, A \mid X) = p(V \mid X)p(A \mid X) \qquad (9.2)$$

p(V | X) and p(A | X) fully represent the information provided by the visual and auditory data about the target's position. The posterior density function is therefore proportional to the product of three functions, the likelihood functions associated with each cue and the prior density function representing the relative probability of the target being at any given position. An optimal estimator could pick the peak of the posterior density function, the mean of the function, or any of a number of other choices, depending on the cost associated with making different types of errors[34, 27]. For our purposes, the point of the example is that an optimal integrator must take into account the relative uncertainty of each cue when deriving an integrated estimate. When one cue is less certain than another, the integrated estimate should be biased toward the more reliable cue. Assuming that a system can accurately compute and represent likelihood functions, the calculation embodied in equations (9.1) and (9.2) implicitly enforces this behavior (see figure 9.1). While other estimation schemes can show the same performance as an optimal Bayesian observer (e.g. a weighted sum of estimates independently derived from each cue), computing with likelihood functions provides the most direct means available to "automatically" account for the large range of differences in cue uncertainty that an observer is likely to face.

9.2   Psychophysical Tests of Bayesian Cue Integration

9.2.1   The Linear Case

When several independent sensory cues are available to an observer for estimating some scene property like depth, we can write the average integrated percept as a function of the average value estimated from each cue individually, $z = f(z_1, z_2)$. Within a small neighborhood of one value of z, we approximate $f()$ as a linear function, so that we can write $z = w_1z_1 + w_2z_2 + k$. The weights w_1 and w_2 provide a measure of the relative contribution of the two cues to the integrated percept. A standard psychophysical procedure for measuring a set of cue weights is to find the point of subjective equality between

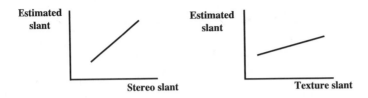

Figure 9.2 Perceived surface slant as a function of the slant suggested by one of the cues in a cue conflict stimulus. The example shown here illustrates a case in which a subject gives more weight to stereoscopic cues than to texture cues. (a) The slant suggested by texture information is fixed. (b) The slant suggested by stereo disparities is fixed. In practice, what we have labeled as perceived slant would be the value of a corresponding psychophysical measure, such as the point of subjective equality between a cue-conflict and a cue-consistent stimulus.

a cue-consistent stimulus with a stimulus in which the cues are made to conflict by a small amount. If we fix the value of one cue and vary the value of the other cue used to create the cue conflict stimulus, we can derive a set of functions like those in figure 9.2. The relative slopes of the two curves provide a measure of the relative weights, w_1/w_2. Were we to apply this method to an optimal integrator, we would find that the relative weights satisfy the relationship, $w_1/w_2. = \sigma_2^2/\sigma_1^2$, where σ_1^2 and σ_2^2 are the variances (uncertainty) in the estimates derived from each cue individually.

Discrimination thresholds, the difference in the value of z needed by an observer to correctly discriminate stimuli at some fiduciary level of performance (e.g. 75% of the time), provide the standard psychophysical measure of uncertainty. For a Gaussian model of uncertainty, thresholds are proportional to the standard deviation of internal perceptual representations. A psychophysical test of Bayes' optimality, then, would be :

Step 1: Measure discrimination thresholds T_i for stimuli containing only one or the other cue being investigated. These are approximately proportional to σ_i.

Step 2: Measure cue weights using the procedure described above.

Step 3: Test the predicted relationship, $w_1/w_2. = T_2^2/T_1^2$.

Knill and Saunders[22] applied this logic to the problem of integrating binocular depth cues with texture information for estimating planar surface slant. Figure 9.3 shows images of a number of textured, flat surfaces that are slanted away from the line of sight. The figure illustrates the fact that texture information is more unreliable at low slants than at high. The uncertainty in binocular cues (e.g. disparity), however, does not change as rapidly as a function of slant. This observation leads to the prediction that observers will give more weight to texture cues at high slants than low slants. Figure 9.4a shows a plot of the average discrimination thresholds for stimuli containing only one or the other

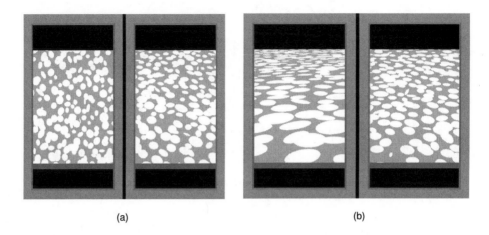

(a)   (b)

Figure 9.3 (a) Two textured surfaces rendered at slants of $0°$ and $40°$. The difference in slant is barely discernible. (b) Two textured surfaces rendered at slants of $70°$ and $60°$. The difference is clearly discernible. The example illustrates the fact that texture information is a much more reliable indicator of 3D surface slant for surfaces at high slants than for surfaces at low slants.

cue. Figure 9.4b shows a plot of the predicted texture cue weights derived from these thresholds (normalized so that the texture and binocular weights sum to 1) along with the average weights measured for all subjects. The measured weights closely follow those predicted from the thresholds. What appears as a slight underweighting of texture information may reflect the fact that the stimuli used to isolate binocular cues for estimating single-cue thresholds (random-dot patterns) were not equivalent to those used to measure cue weights (randomly tiled patterns). The disparity information in the latter may well have been more reliable than in the former, making the binocular cues more reliable in the combined cue stimuli used to measure cue weights.

Studies of human cue integration, both within modality (e.g., stereo and texture)[14, 22] and across modality (e.g., sight and touch or sight and sound)[32, 9, 5, 3] consistently find cue weights that vary in the manner predicted by Bayesian theory. While these results could be accounted for by a deterministic system that adjusts cue weights as a function of viewing parameters and stimulus properties that covary with cue uncertainty, representing and computing with probability distributions (as illustrated in figure 9.1) is considerably more flexible and can accommodate novel stimulus changes that alter cue uncertainty.

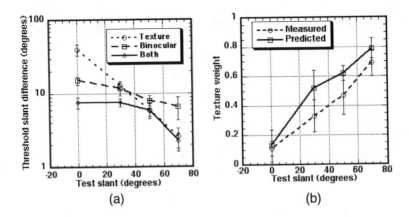

Figure 9.4   (a) Average slant discrimination thresholds when only texture information was available (monocular viewing of a texture similar to those in figure 9.3), when only stereo disparities were available (stimuli contained small random dots) or when both cues were available (binocular viewing of textures like those in figure 9.3. (b) Average texture cue weights measured using the cue perturbation technique described in the text. Stereo and texture cue weights were normalized to sum to 1, so that a texture weight of 0.5 would reflect equal weighting of the two cues.

9.2.2   A Nonlinear Case

When the likelihood functions associated with one or another cue are not Gaussian, simple linear mechanisms do not suffice to support optimal Bayesian calculations. Non-Gaussian likelihood functions arise even when the sensory noise is Gaussian as a result of the nonlinear mapping from sensory feature space to the parameter space being estimated. In these cases, computations on density functions (or likelihood functions) are necessary to achieve optimality.

Skew symmetry is an example of a 3D cue that has a highly non-Gaussian likelihood function[29]. Mirror-symmetric planar patterns project to approximately skew-symmetric figures in the image plane (under orthographic projection, the approximation is exact) (see figure 9.5). The information provided by skew can be parameterized by the angles of a figure's projected symmetry axes. When humans view images of symmetric figures slanted away in depth, even with correct stereoscopic viewing, they see the figures to have orientations that are slightly biased from the true orientation. These biases vary with the "spin" of a figure (its orientation around the normal to the surface). These spin-dependent biases are well accounted for by a Bayesian model that optimally combines skew symmetry information (represented by a highly non-Gaussian likelihood function in figure 9.6) with stereoscopic information about 3D surface orientation. Figure 9.7 shows subjects' data along with model pre-

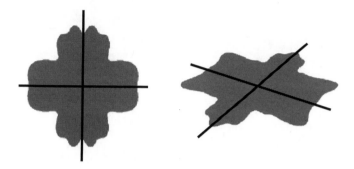

Figure 9.5 Skew symmetric figures appear as figures slanted in depth because the brain assumes that the figures are projected from bilaterally symmetric figures in the world. The information provided by skew symmetry is given by the angle between the projected symmetry axes of a figure, shown here as solid lines superimposed on the figure.

dictions.

A Bayesian integration model predicts that changing the 3D slant suggested by stereo disparities will lead to changes in the perceived tilt of a stereoscopically viewed symmetric figure (see figure 9.6). Subjects show exactly this behavior. The results would not be predicted by a deterministic scheme of weighting the estimates derived from each cue individually.

9.3 Psychophysical Tests of Bayesian Priors

Three-dimensional vision is well understood to be an ill-posed problem in the sense that multiple interpretations of a scene are generally consistent with a given set of image data. This is in part due to the inherent ambiguity of inverting the 3D to 2D perspective projection and in part due to noise in the image data. Despite this, our percepts of the 3D world are remarkably accurate and stable. The fact that our environment is highly structured makes this possible. Prior knowledge of statistical regularities in the environment allows the visual system to accurately estimate the 3D layout of surfaces in a scene, even in images with seemingly impoverished information. Specific models of this type of knowledge, in the form of a priori constraints, play a major role in computational theories of how the visual system estimates 3D surface shape from a variety of cues. Examples include motion (rigidity [31], elastic motion [2]), surface contours (isotropy [7], symmetry [15], lines of curvature [30], geodesics [16]), shape from shading (lambertian reflectance [13], linear reflectance [28], general reflectance [4], point light source [13], hemispheric light source [24]), and texture (homogeneity [10, 26], isotropy [33, 11]).

Building accurate Bayesian models of human perceptual performance re-

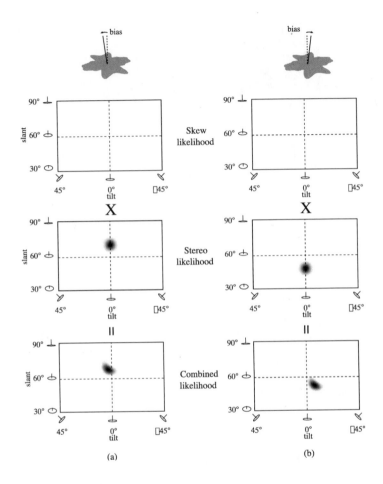

(a)   (b)

Figure 9.6 When viewed stereoscopically, slanted, symmetric figures appear tilted away from their true orientation. The bias is determined by the spin of the figure within its 3D plane. Assuming that visual measurements of the orientations of the skew symmetry axes in the image are corrupted by Gaussian noise, one can compute a likelihood function for 3D surface orientation from skew. The result, as shown here is highly non-Gaussian. When combined with stereoscopic information from binocular disparities, an optimal estimator multiplies the likelihood functions associated with skew and stereo to produce a posterior distribution for surface orientation, given both cues (assuming the prior on surface orientation is flat). (a) When binocular disparities suggest a slant greater than that from which a figure was projected, the posterior distribution is shifted away from the orientation suggested by the disparities in both slant and tilt, creating a biased percept of the figure's tilt. (b) The same figure, when binocular disparities suggest a smaller slant, gives rise to a tilt bias in the opposite direction. This is exactly the pattern of behavior shown by subjects. (Reprinted with permission from *Trends in Neuroscience*)

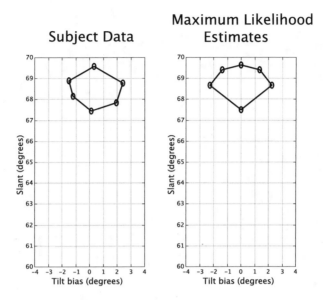

Figure 9.7 When viewed stereoscopically, slanted, symmetric figures appear tilted away from their true orientation. The bias is determined by the spin of the figure within its 3D plane. Shown here are average 3D orientation estimates from subjects viewing symmetric figures slanted away from the line of sight by 60 degrees. Also shown are predictions of an optimal Bayesian integrator that assumes subjects overestimate slant-from-stereo (explaining the overall positive bias in slant judgments).

quires that we formulate psychophysically testable predictions from models of the possible prior constraints that subjects might incorporate into their perceptual inferences. I will illustrate this using the example of texture isotropy. Texture patterns like those shown in figure 9.3 clearly provide information about 3D surface orientation; however, this can only be true if one has prior knowledge of the statistical structure of natural textures. Previous studies have shown that foreshortening information is a dominant cue for judgments of surface orientation and shape [8, 19, 20]. Since this cue relies on prior assumptions about the "shape" statistics of surface textures, knowing what assumptions human observers use is key to understanding how humans estimate surface orientation from texture.

A particularly strong constraint would be that surface textures are isotropic - that their statistical properties are invariant to orientation on a surface (they have no global orientation). Because isotropic textures have a specific average shape (circular), images of isotropic textures support much stronger inferences about surface geometry from the foreshortening cue than do images of anisotropic, homogeneous textures. In effect, when using an isotropic constraint, observers can use the local statistics of texture element shape (texture

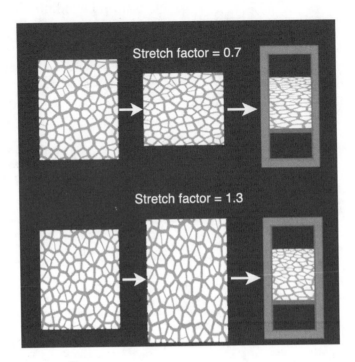

Figure 9.8 Stimuli for the experiments were created in three stages. First, a random, isotropic texture pattern was generated. This was then stretched by some amount in the vertical direction (here shown stretch factors of 0.7 and 1.3). The resulting texture was projected into the image at a slant of 65° and a vertical tilt. A subject that assumes surface textures are isotropic would overestimate the slant of the top stimulus and underestimate the slant of the bottom one. (Reprinted with permission from *Vision Research*)

shape statistics) to make inferences about local surface orientation.

We tested whether humans assume that surface textures are isotropic by measuring the perceived 3D orientations of planar textures that were compressed or stretched by small amounts away from being isotropic (see figure 9.8)[18]. Were subjects to assume that image textures were projected from isotropic surface textures, these manipulations would lead to predictably biased estimates of surface orientation. Figure 9.9 shows the results of an experiment performed to test these predictions. Subjects' judgments were biased in the manner predicted by the hypothesis that their visual systems assume surface textures are isotropic.

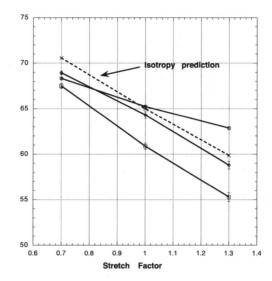

Figure 9.9   Plots of subjects' estimates of 3D surface slant as a function of the stretch factor used to create the surface textures prior to projecting them into the image. The dashed line shows the results predicted by the hypothesis that subjects assumed the surface textures were isotropic.

9.4   Mixture models, Priors, and Cue Integration

Notable in the list of prior constraints given in the previous section is that most cues can be interpreted using any one of several constraints. Common to all of these cues is that one or another qualitatively different prior may apply. This gives rise to a model selection problem that the brain apparently solves when interpreting 3D cues [18]. Solutions to the model selection problem can come in two forms. First, a single cue can, of itself, provide the information necessary to determine when a particular prior should be applied. For example, in a noiseless image, three video frames of four points is sufficient to determine if the points are moving rigidly relative to one another[6]; that is, whether the rigidity constraint should be applied to estimating their relative 3D positions from the motion sequence. Second, other cues may effectively resolve ambiguities as to which prior to use for cue interpretation. This is a form of cue interaction that is clearly highly nonlinear, but which can easily be shown to occur commonly in our visual experience. I will consider each of these in turn.

9.4.1   Model Self-Selection

A notable feature of the prior constraints that make depth cues informative is that they are not constraints on the scene property being estimated (e.g. shape)

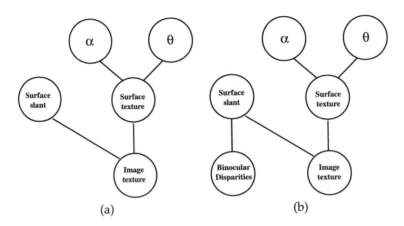

Figure 9.10   (a) A simple Bayes' net describing the principle variables that determine the texture appearing in an image. The surface texture is determined by the parameters of the stochastic process that generated it. here we have simplified these to parameters describing how much a texture is stretched away from being isotropic (α) and the direction in which it has been stretched (θ). The image texture depends both on the surface texture and the orientation of the surface in depth. The informativeness of the image texture about surface slant depends critically on the prior distribution on the "hidden" parameters, α and θ. (b). Another cue like stereo disparities depends on the slant of the surface and can disambiguate α and θ.

but on another variable that is often not of interest to an observer (e.g. light source direction). Statisticians refer to such variables as nuisance parameters and they may be represented using a simple Bayes' net, as in figure 9.10a (here applied to the problem of estimating surface orientation from texture). The key observation is that a cue like image texture is only as good as the prior constraints that apply to these nuisance parameters. In this case, the figure shows two such parameters, α and θ, the amount by which a texture is stretched away from being isotropic and the direction in which it is stretched. An assumption that surface textures are isotropic amounts to assuming that $\alpha = 1$ (θ is undefined in this case).

At a minimum, surface textures come in two broadly different classes, textures that are statistically isotropic and textures that are not. The values of α and θ that characterize a particular surface texture for the anisotropic textures are clearly less constrained than for isotropic textures. Estimating surface orientation from texture implicitly requires choosing which of the two models to use to interpret the texture. To see how the information provided by a cue like texture by itself can support this choice, note that the likelihood for surface orientation, given observed texture data, can be expressed as an integral over all possible values of α and θ:

$$p(\vec{T}\,|\,\sigma,\tau) = \int_0^\pi \int_0^1 p(\vec{T}\,|\,\sigma,\tau,\alpha,\theta)p(\alpha,\theta)d\alpha d\theta, \tag{9.3}$$

where $\vec{T}$ is a vector of image texture measurements, σ is the slant of the surface, and τ is the tilt of the surface. $p(\alpha,\theta)$ is the prior density function on the texture generating parameters. Since we have assumed that textures come in two categories, isotropic and anisotropic, the prior on the hidden variables, $p(\alpha,\theta)$ can be written as a mixture of priors for isotropic textures and for anisotropic textures,

$$p(\alpha,\theta) = \pi_{\text{isotropic}}p_{\text{isotropic}}(\alpha,\theta) + \pi_{\text{anisotropic}}p_{\text{anisotropic}}(\alpha,\theta), \tag{9.4}$$

where $\pi_{\text{isotropic}}$ and $\pi_{\text{anisotropic}}$ are the prior probabilities of a texture being isotropic and anisotropic, respectively. Since the isotropic prior on α and θ is a delta function at $\alpha = 1$, we can simplify the likelihood function to a mixture of two likelihood functions,

$$p(\vec{T}\,|\,\sigma,\tau) = \pi_{\text{isotropic}}p(\vec{T}\,|\,\sigma,\tau,\alpha=1) +$$

$$\pi_{\text{anisotropic}} \int_0^\pi \int_0^1 p(\vec{T}\,|\,\sigma,\tau,\alpha,\theta)p_{\text{anisotropic}}(\alpha,\theta)d\alpha d\theta \tag{9.5}$$

The isotropic likelihood function is a slice through the likelihood function expressed over slant, tilt, and the two texture parameters. When the likelihood function is peaked near $\alpha = 1$, this will have a large peak value. When it is peaked far away from $\alpha = 1$, it will have a much smaller peak value. The anisotropic likelihood function, on the other hand, is an integral over the space of possible values of α and θ. This integration has the effect of shrinking the magnitude of the likelihood function, but keeps it relatively constant regardless of the position of the peak. The integration causes an an Occam's razor effect - likelihood functions that depend on priors that leave a number of hidden variables free to vary are shrunk more and more as the number of unconstrained hidden variables increases [18, 25]. Consider what will happen when viewing an image of an isotropic texture. The peak value of the isotropic likelihood function will be quite high, while the peak value of the anisotropic likelihood function will be low. This will remain true as long as α stays near 1. When it deviates too far from 1 (that is, one is viewing the image of a highly anisotropic texture like a wood grain), the misfit of the isotropic model will overcome the Occam's razor effect of the integration in the anisotropic model and the peak value of the isotropic likelihood function will shrink below that of the anisotropic model and the latter will begin to dominate.

This leads to the prediction that for surface textures that were anisotropic, but close to isotropic (e.g. the textures used in the experiment described in the previous section), observers would be biased by the isotropy assumption. For images of textures that were highly anisotropic, however, observers would be

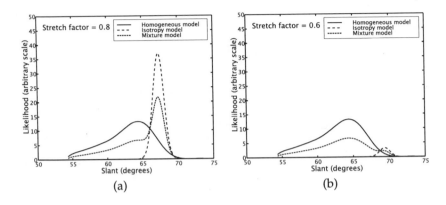

Figure 9.11   Likelihood functions derived for surface slant for stimuli like the ones shown in figure 9.8. The surface textures used to generate the stimuli were stretched before projection into the image. (a) Surface textures stretched by a factor of 0.8 (compressed in the direction of surface tilt), (b) surface textures stretched by a factor of 0.6. The peak of the isotropic likelihood function shifts with the stretch factor because it is derived with the assumption that the stretch factor = 1 (isotropic textures); that is, an "isotropic" observer is biased to interpret the texture compression in the image as entirely due to perspective effects and would over-estimate the slant of the surface. As the surface texture projected into the image becomes more compressed, the homogeneous likelihood function begins to dominate the mixture (as in b). (Reprinted with permission from *Vision Research*)

unbiased, or at least less biased. Figure 9.11 illustrates the effect for a texture like the one shown in figure 9.8, where we have calculated the likelihood functions using a reasonable model of the surface texture generator [17] and the uncertainty in surface slant arises from random variations in the surface texture itself. Note that the peak of the anisotropic likelihood function remains constant near the true slant of 65 degrees.

Figure 9.12 shows the results of an experiment designed to test whether and how subjects switch between isotropic and anisotropic models when estimating surface orientation from texture. The experiment was almost equivalent to the one initially described to test the isotropy assumption in the previous section, but we stretched textures by much larger amounts before projecting them into a stimulus image. As can be seen in the figure, subjects were strongly biased by the isotropy assumption for intermediate values of the stretch factor, but that this effect disappeared at large stretch factors.

One of the quantitative predictions of the statistical formulation is that the range over which subjects show an isotropic bias depends on the reliability of the information in the image. In the case of texture, the visual angle subtended by a texture has the largest impact on how reliably the information determines whether or not the isotropy assumption should apply, since the information derives from perspective effects which grow with field of view size. Figure

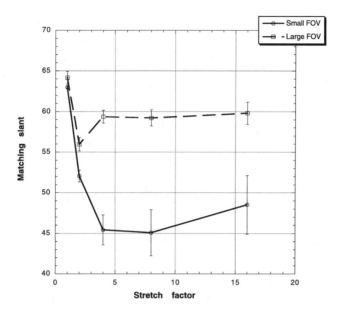

Figure 9.12   Plots of subjects' estimates of 3D surface slant as a function of the stretch factor used to create the surface textures prior to projecting them into the image. The stretch factors used here were considerably larger than in the previous experiment. Subjects show strong perceptual biases for images of surface textures stretched by a factor of 2 away from being isotropic, but the bias disappears for surface textures stretched by very large amounts. Note that the effect is stronger for the small field of view stimuli, in which the image data does not as reliably indicate whether or not the isotropy model should apply.(Reprinted with permission from *Vision Research*)

9.12 shows that, as predicted, the magnitude and range of the isotropy biases were larger for small field of view stimuli than for large.

9.4.2   Model Selection and Cue Integration

Figure 9.10b shows a Bayes' net for a stimulus containing both an image texture and binocular disparities. In this case, the binocular disparities provide information about the orientation of the surface, but not about the surface texture itself. Nevertheless, disparity information can disambiguate which model to use for interpreting the surface texture by selectively amplifying or squashing the likelihood functions associated with the isotropy and anisotropy models for surface textures. One can easily see this effect in stereoscopic computer displays of ellipses. When the ellipses have aspect ratios near one, they appear as circles slanted in depth, but when they have much smaller aspect ratios, they appear as slanted ellipses.

This type of cooperative cue integration provides one account for what Landy, Maloney, Johnston, and Young termed cue vetoing [23]. If one includes in the list of models that can be used to interpret a cue an uninformative prior (e.g. for texture, that would be a prior that assumes textures can be inhomogeneous; that is, surface textures can have statistics that vary over space), one can show that two cues appear to be combined by some form of average when one cue's interpretation is near the constrained interpretation of the other cue (e.g. the isotropic interpretation of textures), but that one cue will completely dominate when it suggests an interpretation very different from the constrained interpretation of the other cue. This can happen even when the reliability of the disambiguating cue is low. Thus, weak disparity information can "turn off" otherwise reliable texture information about surface orientation.

9.5   Conclusion

Bayesian probability provides a normative framework for combining sensory information from multiple cues and for combining sensory information with prior knowledge about the world. Experiments to date that have quantitatively tested the predictions of Bayesian models of cue integration have largely supported the hypothesis that human observers are "Bayes optimal" in their interpretation of image data. Perhaps more importantly, Bayesian accounts of these processes provide insights into the computational structure of perceptual problems that provide a deeper understanding of how perceptual computations work (e.g. cue reweighting, applying prior models, model selection). Work is only now beginning on how humans learn the statistics needed to support optimal perceptual inference [1] and how to extend these ideas to study temporal aspects of cue integration which more typically take place in dynamic settings [12].

References

[1] Adams WJ, Graf EW, Ernst MO (2004) Experience can change the "light-from-above" prior. *Nature Neuroscience,* 7:1057-1058.

[2] Aggarwal JK, Cai Q, Liao W, Sabata B (1998) Nonrigid motion analysis: articulated and elastic motion, *Computer Vision and Image Understanding,* 70:142-156.

[3] Alais D, Burr D (2004) The ventriloquist effect results from near-optimal bimodal integration. *Current Biology,* 14(3): 257-262.

[4] Bakshi S, Yang YH (1997) Towards developing a practical system to recover light, reflectance and shape, *International Journal of Pattern Recognition,* 11(6): 991-1022.

[5] Battaglia PW, Jacobs RA, Aslin RN (2003) Bayesian integration of visual and auditory signals for spatial localization. *Journal of the Optical Society of America A,* 20(7):1391-1397.

[6] Bennett BM, Hoffman DD, Nicola JE, Prakash C (1989) Structure from two orthographic views of rigid motion, *Journal of the Optical Society of America A,* 6:1052-1069.

[7] Brady M, Yuille AL (1984) An extremum principle for shape from contour, *IEEE Transactions on Pattern Analysis and Machine Intelligence*, PAMI-6, No. 3, 288-301.

[8] Buckley D, Frisby J, Blake A (1996) Does the human visual system implement an ideal observer theory of slant from texture? *Vision Research*, 36(8):1163-1176.

[9] Ernst MO, Banks MS (2002) Humans integrate visual and haptic information in a statistically optimal fashion, *Nature*, 415(6870):429-433.

[10] Garding J (1992) Shape from texture for smooth curved surfaces in pespective projection. *Journal of Mathematical Imaging and Vision*, 2(4):327-350.

[11] Garding J (1995) Surface orientation and curvature from differential texture distortion. In *Proceedings of 5th International Conference on Computer Vision*, Cambridge, MA, 733-739.

[12] Greenwald H, Knill DC, Saunders J (2005) Integrating depth cues for visuomotor control: a matter of time, *Vision Research*, 45(15): 1975-1989.

[13] Ikeuchi K, Horn BKP (1981) Numerical shape from shading and occluding boundaries, *Artificial Intelligence*, 17:141-184.

[14] Jacobs RA (1999) Optimal integration of texture and motion cues to depth, *Vision Research*, 39:3621-3629.

[15] Kanade T (1981) Recovery of the three-dimensional shape of an object from a single view. *Artificial Intelligence*, 17: 409-460.

[16] Knill DC (1992) Perception of surface contours and surface shape: from computation to psychophysics, *Journal of the Optical Society of America A*, 9(4): 1449 - 1464.

[17] Knill DC (1998) Surface orientation from texture: ideal observers, generic observers and the information content of texture cues. *Vision Research*, 38(17): 2635-56.

[18] Knill DC (2003) Mixture models and the probabilistic structure of depth cues, *Vision Research*, 43(7):831-854.

[19] Knill DC (in press) Discriminating surface slant from texture: Comparing human and ideal observers, *Vision Research*.

[20] Knill DC (1998) Ideal observer perturbation analysis reveals human strategies for inferring surface orientation from texture, *Vision Research*.

[21] Knill DC, Richards W, eds. (1996) *Perception as Bayesian Inference*, Cambridge, UK: Cambridge University Press.

[22] Knill DC, Saunders JA (2003) Do humans optimally integrate stereo and texture information for judgments of surface slant? *Vision Research*, 43(24):2539-58.

[23] Landy MS, Maloney LT, Johnston EB, Young M (1995) Measurement and modeling of depth cue combination: in defense of weak fusion. *Vision Research*, 35(3):389-412.

[24] Langer MS, Zucker SW (1994) Shape from shading on a cloudy day. *Journal of the Optical Society of America A*, 11: 467-478.

[25] Mackay DJC (1992) Bayesian interpolation, *Neural Computing*, 4:415-447.

[26] Malik J, Rosenholtz R (1995) Recovering surface curvature and orientation from texture distortion: A least squares algorithm and sensitivity analysis. In *Proceedings of 3rd European Conf. on Computer Vision*, Volume 800 of *Lecture Notes in Computer Science*, 353-364, Berlin, Springer-Verlag.

[27] Maloney LT (2002) Statistical theory and biological vision. In Heyer D, Mausfeld R, eds., *Perception and the Physical World: Psychological and Philosophical Issues in Perception*, 145-189, NY: Wiley.

[28] Pentland AP (1990) Linear shape from shading, *International Journal of Computer Vision*, 4:153-163.

[29] Saunders J, Knill DC (2001) Perception of 3D surface orientation from skew symmetry. *Vision Research*, 41(24):3163-3185.

[30] Stevens KA (1981) The visual interpretation of surface contours. *Artificial Intelligence*, 17: 47-73.

[31] Ullman S (1979) The interpretation of structure form motion. *Proceedings of the Royal Society of London. Series B., R.*, 203:405-426.

[32] van Beers RJ, Sittig AC, Denier van der Gon JJ, (1999) Integration of proprioceptive and visual position information: An experimentally supported model. *Journal of Neurophysiology*, 81:1355-1364.

[33] Witkin AP(1981). Recovering surface shape and orientation from texture. *Artificial Intelligence*, 17(1): 17-45.

[34] Yuille A, Bülthoff H (1996) In Knill DC, Richards W, eds., *Perception as Bayesian Inference*, 123 - 161, Cambridge, UK: Cambridge University Press.

PART IV

Making Decisions and Movements

10

The Speed and Accuracy of a Simple Perceptual Decision: A Mathematical Primer

Michael N. Shadlen, Timothy D. Hanks, Anne K. Churchland,
Roozbeh Kiani, and Tianming Yang

10.1 Introduction

A decision is a commitment to a proposition among multiple options. Often this commitment leads to a particular course of action. It might be said that the life of an organism consists of a series of decisions made in time [29]. Leaving aside the moral dimension of choices, it is reasonable to view even pedestrian decisions as a window on higher cognitive function, for they offer a glimpse of how the brain connects information to behavior in a contingent manner. Indeed, even simple visual decisions are based on a sophisticated confluence of available sensory information, prior knowledge, and the potential costs and benefits associated with the possible courses of action. Thus, understanding the neural basis of these decisions provides a model for the principles that govern higher brain function. An important step in making progress toward this goal is to develop frameworks for understanding simple decisions.

In this chapter, we describe one such framework, sequential sampling, which has been used to explain a variety of reaction-time decision tasks. This framework has a rich history in statistical decision theory and mathematical psychology. Our review is at best cursory, but we provide some key citations to the literature. Our main goal in this chapter is to provide an introductory tutorial on the mathematics that explains the psychometric and chronometric functions — that is, accuracy and speed of decisions as a function of difficulty. Then, to underscore our enthusiasm for this framework, we briefly summarize recent data from our laboratory that suggest a possible neural implementation of the computational principles in the parietal cortex of the monkey.

10.2   The Diffusion-to-Bound Framework

In this chapter, we consider simple binary decisions made upon the sequential analysis of evidence. In principle this evidence could arrive continuously in time or in discrete time steps. At each time step, the decision-maker either stops the decision process by committing to one of the alternatives or continues the process by waiting for the next piece of evidence. Thus, in a very general sense, the process involves tradeoffs between speed and accuracy and costs associated with obtaining more information. The framework is sufficiently rich to show up in a variety of problems, from quality control decisions (ship or reject a lot), to pricing bonds, and perception [15, 19]. Our interest is in perception and higher brain function. Perhaps it is worth saying at the outset that not all problems in perception involve the sequential arrival of information, and even when information is provided this way, there is no guarantee that it will be accumulated across time. However, in the particular case we study, it clearly is. Furthermore, we believe this gives us some insight into how the brain can solve more complex decisions that involve the accumulation of evidence obtained at different points in time.

For students of neuroscience and perception, the sequential analysis of information to some termination point lies at the heart of understanding measurements of reaction time and perceptual accuracy. Reaction-time tasks are important because they highlight the tradeoff in speed and accuracy of perception and because they permit identification of the time epoch in which a decision is forming but has not yet been completed. Simultaneous measurement of choices and reaction times provides multiple quantitative constraints that must be satisfied by any theory that aims to explain the neural mechanisms underlying the decision process.

For these reasons, we study decision-making in the context of a reaction-time motion discrimination task. In this task, fixating subjects are presented with a patch of moving dots. Some of these dots move together, or "coherently" in a given direction, while the remaining dots move randomly. At any time after motion onset, subjects can indicate their choice about the direction of motion of the stimulus by making a saccade to one of two targets. To make the task easier or more difficult, the percentage of coherently moving dots is increased or decreased. This task can be performed by both human and monkey subjects, allowing for both psychophysical and physiological investigation. Multiple studies have shown that accuracy depends on the coherence of the moving dot stimulus (figure 10.1 A) [6, 27]. Furthermore, both humans and monkeys reach their decisions faster when the motion coherence is larger, that is, when the task is easier (figure 10.1 B). Ultimately, we would like to understand the neural mechanisms that underlie both the choices and reaction times measured in this task.

The diffusion-to-bound framework, illustrated in figure 10.2, explains the pattern of behavior shown in figure 10.1. In this framework, noisy momentary evidence for one alternative or the other displaces a decision variable in the positive or negative direction. The expected size of the momentary evidence

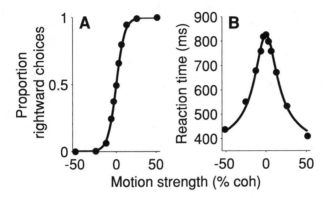

Figure 10.1   Behavioral data from one monkey performing reaction time (RT) version of the direction discrimination task. A. Psychometric function. The probability of a rightward direction judgment is plotted as a function of motion strength. Positive coherence refers to rightward motion and negative coherence to leftward motion. B. Effect of motion strength on RT. Mean RT for correct trials is plotted as a function of motion strength as in A. Error bars are smaller than the symbols. The solid lines show a combined diffusion model fit to the choice and RT data.

Diffusion to bound model

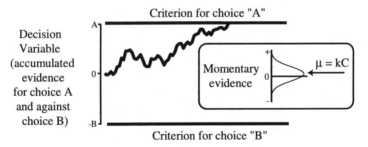

Figure 10.2   Diffusion-to-bound model of the decision process. Momentary evidence in favor of the " A " choice and against the " B " choice is accumulated as a function of time. The process terminates with an " A " or " B " choice when the accumulated evidence reaches the upper or lower bound, respectively, at $+A$ or $-B$. The momentary evidence is distributed as a unit-variance Gaussian whose mean, μ, is proportional to motion strength. The decision variable on a single trial follows a random " diffusion " path, like the one shown. The average of many of these paths would appear as a ramp with slope μ and variance proportional to time. Both decision time and the proportion of " A " and " B " choices are governed by A, B, and μ.

is related to the direction and strength of the motion stimulus, but in any one moment, the evidence is a random number. Over time, these random momentary evidence values are accumulated, giving rise to a random trajectory. The decision process terminates when the trajectory encounters a bound at $\pm A$. The particular bound that is crossed determines the choice, and the time taken to reach that bound determines the decision time. The important idea is that a single mechanism explains both which choice is made and how long it takes to make it.

These predictions can be described by relatively simple analytical equations, which give rise to the fits in figure 10.1. The psychometric function describes the probability of choosing the positive direction as a function of the motion strength, C:

$$P_+ = \frac{1}{1 + e^{-2kCA}} \tag{10.1}$$

where k and A are fitted parameters. The direction of motion is indicated by the sign of C. The probability of choosing the positive motion direction is P_+. We assume that the subjects are unbiased. Therefore, when $C = 0$, $P_+ = 1 - P_+ = \frac{1}{2}$.

The chronometric function describes the reaction time as a sum of decision and nondecision times. The decision time function shares the same parameters as in the psychometric function:

$$E[t] = \frac{A}{kC} \tanh(kCA) \tag{10.2}$$

When C=0, this equation is interpreted as a limit

$$\lim_{C \to 0} \frac{A}{kC} \tanh(kCA) = A^2 \tag{10.3}$$

We will derive these equations in a later section, but for now, it suffices to say that they capture the data reasonably well. Indeed, this model explains the choices and reaction times of monkey and human subjects on a variety of simple, two-choice discrimination tasks under different speed-accuracy pressures [14, 24]. Before working through the derivations, let's acquaint ourselves with the fitted parameters in equations (10.1) and (10.2).

The simplest form of the diffusion model, as employed in this example, has three parameters. First, there is the bound height, A, which mainly controls the balance between speed and accuracy. We place these bounds equidistant from the starting point because at the beginning of the trial, before any evidence has arrived, the two alternatives are equally likely. We will restrict our analysis to this simple condition. The value of $\pm A$ represents the total amount of evidence that is required before a decision is made. Because random variations in the momentary evidence tend to average out with larger numbers of samples, a larger absolute value of A results in a greater level of accuracy. But the cost is time: a higher bound takes longer to reach, on average, resulting in a slower reaction time.

The second parameter, k, converts the stimulus strength into the drift rate of the diffusion process. The average drift rate is effectively the average value for the momentary evidence that accumulates per unit time. We will elaborate the concept of momentary evidence and its accumulation in later sections. For now, kC can be thought of as the mean of the momentary evidence normalized by its variance. For the random-dot motion experiments, it provides a very simple conversion from stimulus intensity and direction to the mean of the random number that accumulates sequentially. We are free to think about the momentary evidence or its accumulation. The momentary evidence is described by a distribution of random numbers: at each time step there is a draw. The accumulation has an expected drift rate equal to this mean per time step.

A third parameter is required to fit the reaction time data. The average non-decision time, $\bar{t}_{nd}$, accounts for the sensory and motor latencies outside the decision process per se. On any one trial, t_{nd} is a random number, but for present purposes, we are only concerned with its mean value. The mean reaction time is the sum of the mean decision time and the mean nondecision time.

The three parameters, k, A, $\bar{t}_{nd}$, are chosen to fit the choice and reaction time data in figure 10.1. Clearly they do a reasonable job of capturing the shapes of both functions and their relative position on the motion strength axis. This is by no means guaranteed. It suggests that a single mechanism might underlie the choices and decision times on this task. We emphasize that we do not expect all perceptual decisions to obey this framework. But many probably do.

10.3   Derivation of Choice and Reaction Time Functions

We will now explain how the accumulation of noisy momentary evidence to a positive or negative bound leads to the equations above: a logistic choice function and a $\tanh(x)/x$ decision time function in terms of stimulus strength. The exercise explains the origins of these functions, exposes the key assumptions, and gives us some insight into how these expressions generalize in straightforward ways to other decisions. The mathematics was developed by Wald and summarized in several texts [9, 15]. Here, we attempt to provide a straightforward explanation of the essential steps, because these ideas can be challenging to students and they are not well known to most physiologists. We emphasize that this is a synthesis of well-established results; certainly many important extensions of the theory are omitted. For additional reading, we recommend Link's book [19] and several insightful and didactic papers by Philip Smith [32, 33]. Other key references are cited below.

10.3.1   Overview

Boiled down to its essence, the problem before us is to compute the probability that an accumulation of random numbers will reach an upper bound at $+A$ before it reaches a lower bound at $-A$. This has an intuitive relationship with accuracy in the following sense. If the evidence should favor the decision instantiated by reaching the upper bound, what we will call a positive response, then the expectation of the momentary evidence is a positive number. Obviously, the accumulation of random numbers that tend to be positive, on average, will end at $+A$ more often that at $-A$. We desire an expression that returns the probability of such an accurate "positive" choice based on a description of the random numbers that constitute the momentary evidence. Our primary goal is to develop this formulation. Our second goal is to develop an expression for the number of samples of momentary evidence that it takes, on average, to reach one or the other bound. This is the decision time. Along the way, we will provide some background on the essential probability theory.

10.3.2   Statement of the Problem

Consider a series of random numbers, $X_1, X_2, \ldots, X_n$, each drawn from the same distribution. We are interested in the stochastic process that unfolds sequentially from the sum of these random numbers

$$Y_n = \sum_{i=1}^{n} X_i \tag{10.4}$$

We assume that each value of X is drawn from the same distribution and each draw is independent of the values that preceded it. In other words, the X_i are independent and identically distributed (*i.i.d.*). Like the X_i, the Y_i are also a sequence of random numbers. In fact there is a one-to-one correspondence between the two series. However, unlike the X_i, the Y_i are neither independent nor identically distributed. They are the accumulation of the X_i. Each subsequent value in the sequence of Y depends on the value that had been attained at the previous step. So there is clearly some correlation between Y_n and Y_{n-1}, and we certainly would not say that the distribution of Y on the nth step is the same as it was on the step before. On the other hand, the distribution of Y_n is easy to describe if Y_{n-1} is known. It is just $Y_{n-1} + X_n$. Since it is unnecessary to know how Y_{n-1} attained its particular value, we say that the sequence, Y_i, is a Markov process.

$Y_1, Y_2, \ldots, Y_n$ represents a random path from the origin, the accumulation of random numbers, $X_1, X_2, \ldots, X_n$. The path, Y, can be written as a function of t or as a function of the number of time steps, $n = t/\Delta t$. If the time steps are discrete the stochastic process is termed a random walk, and if t is continuous, Y is a termed a diffusion process. We tend to gloss over these distinctions (but see Appendix 10.1). We can do this because we are always considering time steps that are small enough (with respect to the bounds) so that it takes a large number to reach the bounds. This means that even if time steps come at irregular intervals, the number of steps multiplied by the average time step is a good approximation to the time to reach the bound, and the increments are small enough that we can treat the last step as if it reached the bound at $\pm A$ exactly, without overshoot.

According to our formulation, the process stops when Y_n reaches $+A$ or $-A$.

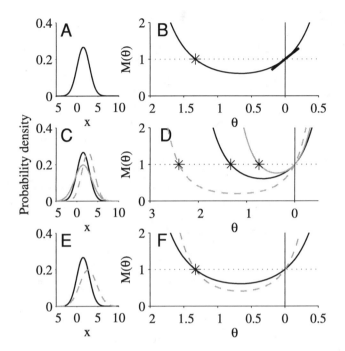

Figure 10.3   Effect of changes in mean and variance of a distribution on its moment-generating functions (MGFs). A. Probability density function (PDF) for a Gaussian distribution with a mean of 1.5 and a variance of 2.25 and standard deviation of 1.5. B. MGF associated with the PDF in A. Tangent line at $\theta = 0$ indicates the first derivative at 0. This is $E[X]$ (the mean), which equals 1.5 (note scaling of ordinate and abscissa). Asterisk indicates the θ_1 zero crossing. C. Same PDF as in A (black trace), alongside a normal PDF with a larger mean and the same variance (gray dashed trace), and a normal PDF with the same mean and a larger variance (gray solid trace). D. MGFs associated with each PDF in C. Line styles are the same as in C. Asterisk indicates the θ_1 zero crossing. E. Same PDF as in A (black trace), alongside a normal PDF with a larger mean and larger variance (gray dashed trace). F. MGFs associated with each PDF in E. Line styles are the same as in E. Asterisk indicates the θ_1 zero crossing.

Our goal is to derive expressions for the probability of reaching these bounds and the average stopping times. We want these expressions to be functions of the stimulus strength (sign and magnitude of the evidence). Because the distribution of the values to be accumulated, X_i, depends on the stimulus intensity, our goal is to derive these expressions in terms of the distribution of X_i.

10.3.3   Background: Moment Generating Functions

A concept that will be useful in this endeavor is that of the moment-generating function (MGF) of a probability distribution. The MGF (when it exists) is simply an alternative description of a probability distribution, and it can be thought of as a transformation that is convenient for certain calculations (much like a Laplace or Fourier transform). The MGF of a random variable X is the expectation of $e^{\theta X}$ over all possible values of X:

$$M_X(\theta) \equiv E\left[e^{\theta X}\right] = \int_{-\infty}^{\infty} f(x)e^{\theta x}dx, \tag{10.5}$$

where $f(x)$ is the probability density function for X, and θ can be any arbitrary value. If you are familiar with Fourier analysis or the Laplace transform, think of θ as the frequency variable. If this is a foreign concept, just think of θ as a number; and the MGF is a function of this number.

Figure 10.3B shows the MGF for the normal distribution with mean = 1.5 and standard deviation = 1.5 as shown in figure 10.3a. Interestingly, the slope of the function at $\theta = 0$ is the mean (or first moment) of X. We can see this by taking the derivative of equation (10.5), with respect to θ:

$$M_X'(\theta) = \frac{d}{d\theta}E\left[e^{\theta X}\right] = \frac{d}{d\theta}\int_{-\infty}^{\infty} f(x)e^{\theta x}dx = \int_{-\infty}^{\infty} xf(x)e^{\theta x}dx \tag{10.6}$$

At the point $\theta = 0$,

$$M_X'(0) = \int_{-\infty}^{\infty} xf(x)dx = E[x], \tag{10.7}$$

(Some students may need to be reminded that an expectation of a function of x is nothing more than a weighted sum of all possible values of that function; the weights are defined by the probability of observing each of the possible random values of x. The simplest case is the weighted sum of the x values themselves, that is, the expectation of x, which is termed the mean or first moment.)

It is also worth mentioning that the second derivative of the function shown in figure 10.3B evaluated at zero is the expectation of the squared values of the random variable, also known as the second moment. Just differentiate the expression in equation (10.7) again. Now an x^2 appears in the integral. This provides a little insight into the shape of the function shown in figure 10.3B. Since the expectation of a squared random number must be positive, we know that the convexity of the MGF at 0 is positive. It also explains the term "moment-generating": when evaluated at $\theta = 0$, the $1^{st}, 2^{nd}, \ldots, n^{th}$ derivatives of $M(\theta)$ return the expectations of $x, x^2, \ldots, x^n$.

Figure 10.3D and F show examples of MGFs associated with the normal distributions shown in figure 3C and E, each having a different mean and variance. You can see that higher means steepen the slope of the function at $\theta = 0$, whereas higher variance exaggerates the convexity. The figure also highlights a feature of the MGF that will be important to us in a moment. Notice that the $M(0) = 1$ (because e^{0X} is 1 for all X). The MGF then returns to 1 at another point. These are marked in the figure with an asterisk. We refer to this special root of the MGF as θ_1; so

$$M_X(\theta_1) = M_X(0) = 1 \tag{10.8}$$

θ_1 is going to play an important role in the argument we are about to share. You'll want to return to this figure later. For now, notice that θ_1 moves further from 0 when the mean is a larger positive number (figure 10.3C,D, dashed gray trace), it moves toward 0 when the variance is larger (figure 10.3C,D, solid gray trace), and it is unchanged when the ratio of the mean to variance remains the same (figure 10.3E,F).

MGFs are useful for analyzing the sums of random numbers. For example, suppose we add two random numbers to produce a new one:

$$S = X_1 + X_2 \tag{10.9}$$

The distribution of S can be written as a convolution of the distributions for X_1 and X_2:

$$f_S(s) = \int_{-\infty}^{\infty} f_{X_1}(r) f_{X_2}(s - r)\, dr, \tag{10.10}$$

where f_{X_1} and f_{X_2} are the probability density functions for the X_1 and X_2. An intuition for this is that the probability of making a particular sum, $S = s$, is the probability that $X_1 = r$ and $X_2 = s - r$ for all possible values of r. Effectively, the distribution of the new variable, S, is achieved by shifting and blurring the distribution for one of the added variables by the other.

Now suppose X_1 and X_2 have MGFs $M_{X_1}(\theta)$ and $M_{X_2}(\theta)$. The MGF for S is simply the product of these:

$$M_S(\theta) = M_{X_1}(\theta) M_{X_2}(\theta) \tag{10.11}$$

Thus convolution of the probability functions is replaced by multiplication of these transformed functions, which is often a more convenient operation. This general idea is a concept that should be familiar to readers acquainted with Fourier and Laplace transforms. It turns out to play a key role in the derivation of the psychometric function.

Thus, the MGF associated with Y_n, as defined in equation (10.4), is the MGF associated with the momentary evidence, X, multiplied by itself n times.

$$M_{Y_n}(\theta) = M_X^n(\theta) \tag{10.12}$$

This is the MGF associated with the height of the trajectory after n steps, ignoring the bounds.

10.3.4   A Moment Generating Function for the Terminated Accumulation

The decision process ends when the accumulation of evidence reaches one of the bounds, that is, when $\tilde{Y} = \pm A$. The tilde above the Y is there to indicate that we are considering the accumulation at its termination. There is no subscript, because the number of steps is a random number: the distribution of decision times.

Using the concept introduced above, we can also express this distribution in terms of its MGF,

$$M_{\tilde{Y}}(\theta) = E[e^{\theta\tilde{Y}}] = P_+e^{\theta A} + (1 - P_+)e^{-\theta A}, \qquad (10.13)$$

where P_+ is the probability of stopping at the positive bound. Notice the brute force expansion of the expectation as the weighted sum $e^{\theta A}$ and $e^{\theta(-A)}$. Our plan is to use this equation to obtain an expression for P_+. As it is, the equation is not practical because it contains an MGF and the variable θ. We would like instead to have terms that we can relate to stimulus intensity (e.g., motion coherence). To achieve this, we seek another way to represent the MGF for the terminated accumulation.

10.3.5   Wald's Martingale

This can be done in the following way. First, we create a new stochastic process, $Z_1, Z_2, \ldots, Z_n$ that parallels the sequence $Y_1, Y_2, \ldots, Y_n$:

$$Z_n = M_x^{-n}(\theta)e^{\theta Y_n} \qquad (10.14)$$

For any particular choice of θ, the MGF part becomes a number raised to the negative n^{th} power. In that case (and if $\theta \neq 0$) the Z_i form a sequence of random numbers in one-to-one correspondence with the Y_i. In fact, we could say that before the process begins, the accumulation starts at $Y_0 = 0$ and $Z_0 = 1$.

This newly created sequence has the following important property. If at the nth step, the process happens to have attained the value Z_n, then the expectation of the random value that it will attain on the next step is also Z_n

$$E[Z_{n+1} | Z_n] = Z_n : \qquad (10.15)$$

Think about what this means. Z_n is a random number—the nth value in a sequence of random numbers. Imagine observing this sequence as it plays out, one step at a time. Suppose we have just seen the nth step and we are now waiting for the next random number in the sequence. At this point, the value of Z_n is known. Now, we know that the next step will produce a random number. But the expectation of this random number (i.e., the average if only we could repeat this next step many times) is the number we have in hand. That is the meaning of equation (10.15). It says that on average, we do not expect the next step in the sequence to change from the value that it happened to attain on the pervious step. Of course, this is only true on average. Any given sequence of

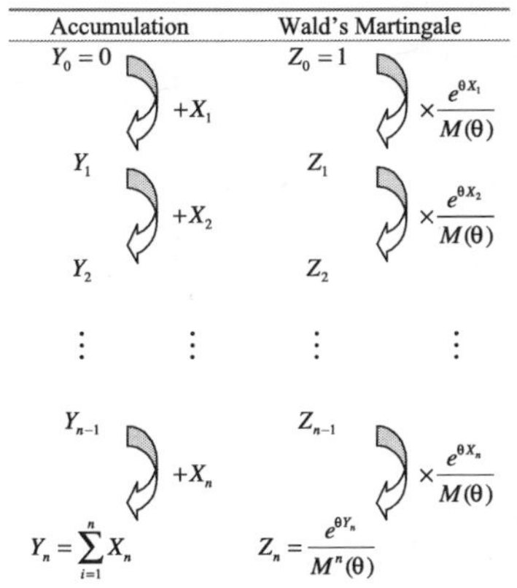

Accumulation	Wald's Martingale
$Y_0 = 0$	$Z_0 = 1$

$+X_1$ $\quad\times\dfrac{e^{\theta X_1}}{M(\theta)}$

Y_1 $\qquad Z_1$

$+X_2$ $\quad\times\dfrac{e^{\theta X_2}}{M(\theta)}$

Y_2 $\qquad Z_2$

$\vdots \qquad \vdots \qquad \vdots \qquad \vdots$

Y_{n-1} $\qquad Z_{n-1}$

$+X_n$ $\quad\times\dfrac{e^{\theta X_n}}{M(\theta)}$

$Y_n = \sum_{i=1}^{n} X_n$ $\qquad Z_n = \dfrac{e^{\theta Y_n}}{M^n(\theta)}$

Figure 10.4   Two stochastic processes. The two lists of random numbers are created by updating the previous value in the list using a random draw, X_n. Each, $X_1, X_2, X_3, ...,$ is drawn from the same distribution, and each draw is independent from the others. The formulas show how to use the current draw to update the previous value of Y or Z using the previous value attained and the new draw of X.

Z_i will wander about because the next number is unlikely to actually be the last number that was attained—that's just the expectation.

We can appreciate this in another way by considering an alternative recipe for generating the Z_i, illustrated in figure 10.4. To make any Z_{n+1}, begin with Z_n, draw a random value, X_{n+1}; multiply Z_n by $e^{\theta X_{n+1}}$ and divide by $M_X(\theta)$. Since $M_X(\theta)$ is $E\left[e^{\theta X_{n+1}}\right]$, the expectation of Z_{n+1} is Z_n.

A random variable sequence that has such properties is called a *martingale*. In fact, the stochastic process $Z_0, Z_1, \ldots, Z_n$ is a martingale with respect to the Y_n because $E\left[Z_{n+1} | Y_0, Y_1, Y_2, \ldots, Y_n\right] = Z_n$. This property can also be worked out directly from the definition of Y and Z, as follows:

$$E\left[Z_{n+1} | Y_0, Y_1, Y_2, \ldots, Y_n\right] = E\left[M_X^{-(n+1)}(\theta)e^{\theta Y_{n+1}} | Y_0, Y_1, Y_2, \ldots, Y_n\right]$$
$$= E\left[M_X^{-(n+1)}(\theta)e^{\theta(Y_n + X_{n+1})}\right] \text{ (by the rule for generating } Y_{n+1})$$
$$= E[M_X^{-1}(\theta)M_X^{-n}(\theta)e^{\theta Y_n}e^{\theta X_{n+1}}]$$
$$= E[M_X^{-1}Z_n(\theta)e^{\theta X_{n+1}}](\text{using the definition of } Z_n)$$
$$= M_X^{-1}(\theta)Z_n E\left[e^{\theta X_{n+1}}\right] \text{ (because } Z_n \text{ and } M_X(\theta) \text{ are known)}$$
$$= Z_n$$

$$(10.16)$$

Any particular instantiation of Z is a random process that is one to one with a particular instantiation of a random walk, Y. Yet, the expectation of any Z_n is always the same. In fact it is always 1.

$$E\left[Z_n\right] = E\left[M_X^{-n}(\theta)e^{\theta Y_n}\right] = M_X^{-n}(\theta)E\left[e^{\theta Y_n}\right] = M_X^{-n}(\theta)M_{Y_n}(\theta) = 1 \quad (10.17)$$

Notice that the MGF is a function of θ — at any particular value of θ, it is just a number — so it can be removed from the expectation in the first line of equation (10.17). The last equality follows from equation (10.12).

The stochastic process, Z, is known as Wald's martingale and the identity in equation (10.17) is known as Wald's identity, usually written

$$E\left[M_X^{-n}(\theta)e^{\theta Y_n}\right] = 1 \qquad (10.18)$$

The usefulness of creating Z is not yet apparent, but in a moment, we will exploit an important property it possesses.

10.3.6   Another Moment Generating Function for the Terminated Accumulation

Equation (10.14) gives us an expression that relates each Z_n to its associated Y_n and therefore to the distribution of each X_i, but remember that our goal is to relate the stopped variable $\tilde{Y}$ to that distribution. Fortunately, an important property of martingales, the optional stopping theorem, will enable us to do so. Suppose the sequence Z is forced to stop when the accumulation Y reaches one of the bounds. Let $\tilde{Z}$ represent the "stopped" value of Z.

$$\tilde{Z} = M_X^{-\tilde{n}}(\theta)e^{\theta\tilde{Y}} \qquad (10.19)$$

We placed a tilde over the n in this expression to indicate that we do not know the number of steps it takes to terminate. In fact n is a random number that we will relate to decision time. Because n is a random number, we cannot simply take the stopped accumulation and convert it to a stopped value for Wald's martingale. We do not know how many times we need to divide by $M_X(\theta)$. Fortunately, we can work with the expectation of $\tilde{Z}$.

The optional stopping theorem for martingales states that $E\left[\tilde{Z}\right] = E\left[Z_n\right]$ even though the number of steps, n, is a random number. We will not prove this theorem, but it ought to come as no surprise that this would hold, because the expectation of Z is always the same, in this case 1. Thus,

$$E\left[M_X^{-\tilde{n}}(\theta)e^{\theta\tilde{Y}}\right] = 1 \qquad (10.20)$$

The left side of this expression almost looks like the definition of an MGF for $\tilde{Y}$, which is what we desire. But alas, there is the $M_X^{-\tilde{n}}(\theta)$ bit inside the expectation. This expression is especially problematic because it introduces a random variable, $\tilde{n}$. If only we could make this bit disappear.

Here is how. Equation (10.20) holds for any value of θ that we choose. So let's choose θ such that $M_X(\theta) = 1$. Then it no longer matters that $\tilde{n}$ is a random

number, because 1 raised to any power is always 1. Recall from the discussion
of MGFs above that there are two values for θ that satisfy this identity: 0 and
the point marked θ_1 (the asterisk in figure 10.3B). For all MGFs, $M(0) = 1$, but
this is not useful (Z is not a stochastic process — it is always 1). However,
this other value away from the origin is profoundly interesting. It is guaranteed to exist if (*i*) X has a MGF, (*ii*) X has finite variance, (*iii*) $E[X] \neq 0$, and
(*iv*) the range of X includes positive and negative values. The first two conditions are formalities. The third omits a special case when the slope of the
MGF is zero at 0 (effectively, $\theta_1 = 0$). The last condition implies that the random increments can take on positive and negative values — in other words,
the conditions leading to a random walk or diffusion process. Suffice it to say
that for the conditions that interest us, θ_1 exists. At this special value, $\theta = \theta_1$,
equation (10.20) simplifies to

$$E\left[e^{\theta_1 \tilde{Y}}\right] = 1 \tag{10.21}$$

Equation (10.21) is not an MGF for the stopped random value $\tilde{Y}$, but it is a
point on that MGF.

10.3.7   The Psychometric Function

We have now found a value of θ for which the expression $E[e^{\theta \tilde{Y}}]$ is known, and
we can plug this back into equation (10.13), yielding:

$$M_{\tilde{Y}}(\theta_1) = E[e^{\theta_1 \tilde{Y}}] = P_+ e^{\theta_1 A} + (1 - P_+)e^{-\theta_1 A} = 1 \tag{10.22}$$

Solving for P_+

$$P_+ = \frac{1 - e^{-\theta_1 A}}{e^{\theta_1 A} - e^{-\theta_1 A}} = \frac{1 - e^{-\theta_1 A}}{e^{-\theta_1 A}\left(e^{\theta_1 A} + 1\right)\left(e^{\theta_1 A} - 1\right)} = \frac{1}{1 + e^{\theta_1 A}} \tag{10.23}$$

The probability of terminating a decision in the upper vs. lower bound is a
logistic function of the argument $\theta_1 A$.

We have very nearly achieved an expression for the psychometric function.
All that remains is to relate θ_1 to the stimulus intensity variable (e.g., motion
coherence). We know that θ_1 is a root of the MGF associated with the distri-
bution of X, the momentary evidence that accumulates toward the bounds.
Suppose X obeys a normal distribution with mean μ and standard deviation
σ. The MGF associated with the normal distribution is

$$M_X(\theta) = e^{\theta \mu + \frac{1}{2}\theta^2 \sigma^2}, \tag{10.24}$$

which is 1 when

$$\theta_1 = -\frac{2\mu}{\sigma^2} \tag{10.25}$$

Suppose that stimulus intensity leads to a proportional change in the mean of the momentary evidence but no change in the variance. Then, we can write

$$\theta_1 = -2kC/\sigma^2 \qquad (k > 0), \tag{10.26}$$

which gives us a logistic function resembling equation (10.1). The only difference is the σ^2 term here. This term, which we set to 1, provides a scaling for A and μ. We will justify these assumptions (at least partially) in a later section and consider the meaning of the fitted parameters, k and A, in terms that connect to noisy neurons in the visual cortex.

The form of the equation will depend ultimately on whatever particular assumptions we make about the relationship between motion coherence and the distribution of momentary evidence. The important point of the exercise is not to justify these assumptions but to recognize what it is about the distribution of momentary evidence that will lead to a prediction for the psychometric function (PMF). We prefer to leave this section with the PMF in its most general form prescribed by equation (10.23). This is a remarkable insight with many fascinating implications [19], some of which we will describe in detail later.

10.3.8   Decision Time

Now that we have computed the probability of terminating a decision in the upper vs. lower bound, we will derive an expression for the average time to reach the bound. This is the length of a time step multiplied by the number of steps taken to reach the bound, what we called $\tilde{n}$. We will derive an expression for the mean of this quantity, $E[\tilde{n}]$. The first step is to take the derivative of both sides of equation (10.20) with respect to θ:

$$E\left[e^{\theta \tilde{Y}} \tilde{Y} M_X^{-\tilde{n}}(\theta) - e^{\theta \tilde{Y}} \tilde{n} M_X^{-1-\tilde{n}}(\theta) M_X'(\theta)\right] = 0 \tag{10.27}$$

Evaluating this expression at $\theta = 0$ greatly simplifies matters. Recall that an MGF is always 1 at $\theta = 0$ and the first derivative is the first moment (i.e., the mean). Therefore

$$E\left[\tilde{Y} - \tilde{n}\mu\right] = 0, \tag{10.28}$$

which can be rearranged

$$E[\tilde{n}] = \frac{E[\tilde{Y}]}{\mu} \qquad (\text{for } \mu \neq 0) \tag{10.29}$$

This is a deceptively simple expression. It tells us that the mean number of steps to reach one of the bounds is the average accumulation at the time of the decision divided by the average increment in the evidence. Now $\tilde{Y}$ is either $+A$ or $-A$, but it is more often $+A$ when $\mu > 0$, and it is more often $-A$ when $\mu < 0$. The expectation is just a weighted sum of these two values. Therefore

$$E[\tilde{Y}] = P_+A + (1 - P_+)(-A) = (2P_+ - 1)A \tag{10.30}$$

and

$$E[\tilde{n}] = \frac{(2P_+ - 1) A}{\mu} \tag{10.31}$$

Substituting the expression for P_+ from equation (10.23), yields

$$E[\tilde{n}] = \frac{A}{\mu} \left(\frac{2}{1 + e^{\theta_1 A}} - 1 \right) = \frac{A}{\mu} \left(\frac{1 - e^{\theta_1 A}}{1 + e^{\theta_1 A}} \right) \tag{10.32}$$

Multiplying numerator and denominator by $e^{-\frac{\theta_1 A}{2}}$ yields a simple expression based on the hyperbolic tangent function:

$$E[\tilde{n}] = \frac{A}{\mu} \left(\frac{e^{-\frac{\theta_1 A}{2}} - e^{\frac{\theta_1 A}{2}}}{e^{-\frac{\theta_1 A}{2}} + e^{\frac{\theta_1 A}{2}}} \right) = \frac{A}{\mu} \tanh\left(-\frac{\theta_1 A}{2} \right) \tag{10.33}$$

This general expression tells us that the number of steps is related to the bound height, the mean of the momentary evidence, and θ_1. The value for θ_1 depends on the distribution that gives rise to the values of momentary evidence that are accumulated. We offer some helpful intuition on this below, but it is a number that tends to scale directly with the mean and inversely with the variance of that distribution. For the normal distribution, this tendency holds exactly. If we assume that the X_i are drawn from a normal distribution with mean μ and variance σ^2, then

$$E[\tilde{n}] = \frac{A}{\mu} \tanh\left(\frac{\mu A}{\sigma^2} \right) \tag{10.34}$$

In the special case where the momentary evidence favors the two decision outcomes equally, $\mu = 0$ and

$$E[\tilde{n}] = \lim_{\mu \to 0} \frac{A}{\mu} \tanh\left(\frac{\mu A}{\sigma^2} \right) = \frac{A^2}{\sigma^2} \tag{10.35}$$

Again, suppose a change in the motion strength, C, leads to a proportional change in the mean of the momentary evidence, but no change in the variance. Then substituting $-2kC/\sigma^2$ for θ_1 into equation (10.33) yields

$$E[\tilde{n}] = \frac{A}{\mu} \tanh\left(\frac{kCA}{\sigma^2} \right) \tag{10.36}$$

Equation (10.36) resembles equation (10.2), which we fit to the reaction time data in figure 10.1. The only difference is the σ^2 term here. This term, which we set to 1, provides a scaling for A and μ. The average decision time at $C = 0$ is therefore $E[\tilde{n}] = A^2$. This implies that the variance associated with the momentary evidence at each time step is 1. This implies that the variance associated with the momentary evidence at each time step is 1, and the coefficient, k, should be interpreted as follows: $\mu = kC$ is the mean of a normal distribution whose variance is 1 in a single time step. The momentary evidence is drawn from this distribution in each time step. This gives us a way to reconcile the fitted parameters, k and A, with measurements from neurons. We will resume this thread below.

Before leaving this section, we should point out one other aspect of the equations for decision time: they apply to both choices. In the equations above, $E[\tilde{n}]$ is the expected number of steps to reach *either* bound. It is the expected number of steps to finish, regardless of which bound is reached. However, when the upper and lower bounds are equidistant from the starting point, it is often the case that the expected number of steps to one or the other bound is exactly the same. This holds when the momentary samples (X_i) are drawn from the normal distribution. This is obvious when the mean of the momentary evidence is 0 — the case of a purely random walk. For any path of steps that ends in the upper bound, there is an equally probable path to the lower bound. It may be less obvious when there is a tendency to drift in the positive or negative direction. In that case, the claim is that the average number of steps to reach the "correct" bound (e.g., the positive bound when the evidence is positive, on average) is the same as the average number of steps to reach the "incorrect" bound. In fact, the entire distribution of stopping times should be identical and merely scaled by P_+ and its complement.

Consider a "path" that ends in the upper bound after n steps. The likelihood of observing this path is a product of likelihoods of obtaining the n values, $X_1, X_2, \ldots, X_n$ from $N\{\mu, \sigma\}$. Any such path has a mirror image that ends in the lower bound. The likelihood of observing this path is the product of the likelihoods of drawing $-X_1, -X_2, \ldots, -X_n$ from the same normal distribution. The ratio of these likelihoods is

$$\frac{P(X_1, X_2, \ldots, X_n \,|\, \mu, \sigma)}{P(-X_1, -X_2, \ldots, -X_n \,|\, \mu, \sigma)} = \frac{\prod_i \frac{1}{\sqrt{2\pi}\sigma} e^{-\frac{(X_i-\mu)^2}{2\sigma^2}}}{\prod_i \frac{1}{\sqrt{2\pi}\sigma} e^{-\frac{(-X_i-\mu)^2}{2\sigma^2}}} = e^{\frac{2\mu \sum_i X_i}{\sigma^2}} = e^{\frac{2\mu A}{\sigma^2}},$$

(10.37)

where A is the sum of the increments, X_i. Since all paths sum to this same value, every path that ends in the upper bound (+A) has a corresponding path that ends at the lower bound. The probability of observing any path to the upper bound is the same as the one to the lower path multiplied by a constant, which happens to be the odds of hitting the upper bound. We can see this by computing the odds from equation (10.23);

$$\frac{P_+}{1-P_+} = \frac{\left(\frac{1}{1+e^{\theta_1 A}}\right)}{\left(1 - \frac{1}{1+e^{\theta_1 A}}\right)} = e^{-\theta_1 A} = e^{\frac{2\mu A}{\sigma^2}}$$

(10.38)

From the perspective of the present exercise, the equality of mean decision time regardless of which bound terminates the decision is convenient on the one hand and damaging on the other. It is convenient because our equation for fitting the reaction time is appropriate even when we fit just the correct choices, as in figure 10.1. It is damaging because it predicts that the mean reaction time for error trials ought to be the same as for correct choices. In our experiments, they are close, but the reaction time on error trials is typically slightly longer than on correct trials [27, 24]. A variety of solutions have been proposed to remedy this deficiency. The most obvious, but the least explored, is to use a non-Gaussian distribution for the momentary evidence [20]. It turns out that if the slopes of the MGF at θ_1 and at 0 are not equal and opposite, then $E[\tilde{n}]$ are not the same when the process terminates at the upper or lower bound. Link and Heath illustrate this for the Laplacian distribution. Other solutions include variability in E[X] and starting point [17, 26] and a nonstationary bound. For example, if an "urgency" signal lowers the bounds as a function of time (or an equivalent addition is made to the accumulation) then longer decisions will be less accurate [10]. Variants on the nonstationary bound idea include adding a cost of computing time.

   If the bounds are not equidistant from the starting point of the accumulation, then the decision times for the two choices are wildly different. Expressions for these conditionalized stopping times can be found in [24] and [31] for Gaussian increments, and in [20] for non-Gaussian increments based on θ_1.

10.3.9 Summary

We derived general forms of expressions for P_+, the probability that an accumulation of random numbers will reach a positive bound before it reaches a negative bound, and $E[\tilde{n}]$, the number of random numbers that are added, on average, to reach either bound. The most general forms of these expressions are functions of the absolute value of the criterion and a special root of the MGF associated with the random increments. To achieve our fitting functions, we assumed that the random increments were drawn from a normal distribution. The special root is proportional to the mean divided by the variance of the increments: $\theta_1 = -2\mu/\sigma^2$. To construct our psychometric and chronometric functions, we made the additional simplifying assumption that this term is proportional to our stimulus intensity variable, motion strength. Recall that motion strength is a signed quantity; the sign indicates the direction. Thus, positive motion strengths give rise to positive increments, on average, and negative values of θ_1.

   The real dividend of this argument, we hope, is in the general expression that revolves around θ_1. The random numbers that accumulate in the brain may not be normally distributed (see Appendix 10.1) and the mapping between strength of evidence and the parameterization of momentary evidence may not be as simple as a proportional relationship to the mean. The connection between quality of evidence (e.g., stimulus intensity) and behavior (i.e., choice and decision time) are mediated via θ_1. If we know how intensity affects θ_1, then we can predict the shape of the psychometric and chronometric functions. It is reasonable to consider this term proportional to the mean/variance ratio for increments drawn from a variety of distributions. And it is not too hard to

Preferred   Null

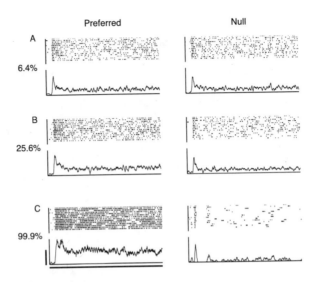

Figure 10.5   Response of MT neurons to stimuli with different motion strengths. A. Responses to motion at 6.4% coherence. Left column shows responses to motion in the preferred direction, and the right column shows responses to motion in the opposite direction. Top: Rasters of neural spike times. Solid line indicates onset of stimulus motion. Bottom: Average firing rate. The vertical bar at stimulus onset represents 100 sp/s, and the horizontal bar under the abscissa shows the 2-second duration of stimulus presentation. B. Same as A for 25.6% coherence. C. Same as A for 99.9% coherence. (Reproduced with permission from K. H. Britten, Shadlen, W. T. Newsome, J. A. Movshon, Response of neurons in macaque MT to stochastic motion signals. Vis. Neurosci. 10:1157-1169. ©1993 by the Cambridge University Press.)

appreciate how neurons could give rise to such a quantity.

10.4   Implementation of Diffusion-to-Bound Framework in the Brain

Our enthusiasm for the random walk to bound framework emanates from physiology experiments. For the random-dot motion task, there are neural correlates for both momentary evidence and its accumulation. Although there is much to learn about many of the most important details of the mechanism, we understand enough to believe that this mechanism, or something very close to it, actually underlies decisions on the random-dot motion task.

10.4.1   The Momentary Evidence for Direction is Represented by Neurons in area MT/V5

MT/V5 is an area of extrastriate visual cortex first identified by Zeki [12] and Allman and Kaas [2] and appears to be specialized for processing visual motion [1, 5, 23, 4]. The random-dot motion stimulus used in our task was tailored by Newsome, Britten, and Movshon [22] to match the receptive field preferences of neurons in the middle temporal area (MT). We know from a variety of stimulation and lesion experiments that area MT plays an essential role in allowing a monkey to perform the discrimination task. Indeed microstimulation of a cluster of rightward-preferring MT neurons causes the monkey to decide that motion is rightward more often [28] and to do so more quickly than when there is no stimulation [11]. Moreover, stimulating these same right-preferring neurons affects leftward decisions negatively. When the monkey decides that the motion is leftward, he does so more slowly when right-preferring neurons have been activated by microstimulation.

MT neurons respond to random-dot motion stimuli by elevating their firing rates. As shown in figure 10.5, the firing rate rises the most when highly coherent motion is in the neuron's preferred direction, and it is lowest when highly coherent motion is in the opposite (null) direction. Notice that the response is elevated relative to baseline when low coherence motion is shown in *either* direction, but the firing rate is slightly greater when the motion is in the neuron's preferred direction. After a brief transient associated with the onset of the random dots, the response reaches a fairly steady (but noisy) firing rate while the random-dot motion is displayed. It is the firing rate during this steady period that constitutes the momentary evidence. Notice that there is no sign of accumulation in these responses. They look nothing like the trajectories of a random walk. Rather, they provide the momentary evidence that is accumulated elsewhere in the brain.

10.4.2   A Crude Estimate of θ_1 from the Neural Recordings

The experiments suggest that the momentary evidence for rightward, say, is based on a difference in firing rates between right-preferring and left-preferring MT neurons [11]. There is good reason to believe that a decision is not based on a pair of neurons but on the activity from ensembles of neurons. For the random-dot displays used in our experiments, a typical MT neuron will change its average firing rate by ~40 spikes per second (sp/s) as motion strength increases from 0% to 100% in its preferred direction, and it will decrease its response by ~10 sp/s over this same range of motion strengths when the direction is opposite to its preferred direction [7]. If this difference in spike rates between ensembles of right- and left-preferring MT neurons constitutes the momentary evidence for rightward,

$$\mu_{MT} \equiv E\left[X_R - X_L\right] = 50C, \tag{10.39}$$

where once again C is motion coherence on a scale from -1 to 1.

What happens to the variance of this difference variable? For a single neuron, the variance of the number of spikes emitted by an MT neuron in a fixed epoch is typically a constant times the mean of this number, termed the Fano factor, ϕ. For a single MT neuron, $\phi_1 \approx 1.5$. Suppose the spike rate is 20 sp/s when C = 0. Then the expected number of spikes in 1 second is $E[s] = 20$ and the variance of the spike count in a 1 second epoch is $\phi_1 E[s] = 30$ sp². The average of N spike counts is the sum of N random numbers, $\frac{s_1}{N}, \frac{s_2}{N}, , \frac{s_N}{N}$. So the expected mean count is the same as the expectation of the count from a single neuron:

$$E[\bar{s}] = NE\left[\frac{s}{N}\right] = E[s] \tag{10.40}$$

However, the variance of the mean count is

$$Var[\bar{s}] = NVar\left[\frac{s}{N}\right] = N\frac{Var[s]}{N^2} = \frac{\phi_1 E[s]}{N} \tag{10.41}$$

This expression for the variance of a mean holds when the counts that are averaged are statistically independent. For sums of independent variables, the variance of the sum is the sum of the variances associated with each random variable.

Unfortunately, MT neurons are not independent in their responses. In that case, the variance of the sum is the sum of all the terms in the N by N covariance matrix depicted here,

$$\begin{pmatrix} \sigma_1^2 & \cdots & r_{1n}\sigma_1\sigma_n \\ \vdots & \ddots & \vdots \\ r_{n1}\sigma_n\sigma_1 & \cdots & \sigma_n^2 \end{pmatrix} \tag{10.42}$$

where r_{ij} is the correlation coefficient between the count from the ith and j^{th} neurons. In addition to N variance terms along the main diagonal, there are the other $N^2 - N$ covariance terms (when the correlation is nonzero). Assuming that all the variances are the same and all the coefficients are the same, we can specify these terms as follows. When we take the average spike count, each of the diagonal terms is

$$Var\left[\frac{s}{N}\right] = \frac{Var[s]}{N^2} = \frac{\phi_1 E[s]}{N^2} \tag{10.43}$$

and each off-diagonal term is

$$rVar\left[\frac{s}{N}\right] = \frac{rVar[s]}{N^2} = \frac{r\phi_1 E[s]}{N^2} \tag{10.44}$$

The variance of the mean is the sum of the N terms in equation (10.43) plus the $N^2 - N$ terms in equation (10.44)

$$Var[\bar{s}] = N\left(\frac{\phi_1 E[s]}{N^2}\right) + (N^2 - N)\left(\frac{r\phi_1 E[s]}{N^2}\right) \tag{10.45}$$

From this expression, it is easy to see that in the limit of large N,

$$\lim_{N\to\infty} Var[\bar{s}] = r\phi_1 E[s] \tag{10.46}$$

This limit is a reasonable approximation to the variance of the mean count from as few as $N = 100$ neurons in the ensemble.

Pairs of MT neurons with overlapping receptive fields exhibit correlation coefficients of $r \approx 0.15$ to 0.2. This implies that the average spike count from an ensemble of rightward motion sensors in MT is a random number whose expectation is the mean spike count from a neuron and whose variance is 0.225 to 0.3 times this expectation. We will use the top end of this range for our exercise below. We will also assume that the right-preferring MT neurons respond independently from left-preferring MT neurons. In other words, neurons with common response properties share some of their variability, but neurons with different preferences do not [38, 3, 16].

When $C = 0$, right- and left-preferring MT neurons both respond at about 20 sp/s. In 1 second, we expect the mean count from N right-preferring neurons to be 20 spikes per neuron with a variance of 6 spikes^2 per neuron^2. The same numbers apply for the left-preferring neurons. Thus, the expected difference is 0. The variance associated with this difference is 12 spikes^2 per neuron^2, assuming that the right- and left-preferring MT neurons are independent. For the strongest rightward motion condition shown in figure 10.5, $C = 0.51$. In that case, we expect the mean and variance of the average count from right-preferring neurons to be 40 spikes per neuron and 12 spikes^2 per neuron^2. For the left-preferring neurons, the mean and variance are 15 spikes per neuron and 4.5 spikes^2 per neuron^2. So the difference in the ensemble averages has expectation and variance of 25 and 16.5, respectively. The signal-to-noise ratio is $25/\sqrt{16.5} \approx 6.2$. For motion in the opposite direction, the expectation of the difference reverses sign, but the variance remains the same. If $C = 1$, then the expected difference is $60 - 10 = 50$ spikes per neuron with variance $(0.3)(60 + 10) = 21$. So the signal-to-noise ratio is $50/\sqrt{21} \approx 11$.

Based on these assumptions, we plotted in figure 10.6 the expected signal-to-noise ratio that right- and left-preferring MT neurons furnish in 1 second. We can see from this example that the signal-to-noise ratio is approximately linear over the range of motion strengths used in our experiments. The best line in this figure has a slope of 12.7. Now relate this to the equation for the psychometric and chronometric functions shown in figure 10.1. The fitting equation presumes that in each millisecond, a random number representing momentary evidence is drawn from a normal distribution with mean $\mu = kC$ and variance 1. What is the value of k that would provide the signal-to-noise ratios graphed in figure 10.6 after 1000 ms? After 1000 samples, the numerator must be 1000μ and the denominator must be the square root of the accumulated variance from 1000 samples. Therefore

$$\frac{1000kC}{\sqrt{1000}} = 12.7C$$
$$k = \frac{12.7}{\sqrt{1000}} \approx 0.4 \tag{10.47}$$

This value is remarkably close to the value for k estimated by fitting the behavioral data in figure 10.1 (0.43 ± 0.01). Of course, we can also express this number in terms of θ_1. Under the assumption that the momentary evidence

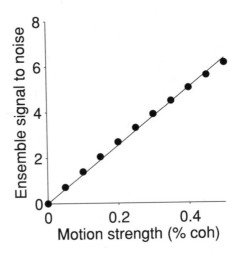

Figure 10.6   Estimated signal-to-noise ratio from an ensemble of MT neurons at different motion strengths. The calculations used to make these estimates are described in the text, and they are based on a stimulus duration of 1 second. The relationship is approximately linear over the range of motion strengths used in our experiments.

in each millisecond is a random draw from a normal distribution with unit variance and mean equal to kC, $\theta_1 = -2\mu/\sigma^2 \approx -0.8C$.

10.4.3   The Accumulated Evidence for Direction is Represented by Neurons in the Lateral Intraparietal Area (LIP)

Several observations argue that the LIP might be a suitable place to mediate decisions during the motion task. First, neurons in LIP receive a major input from direction selective neurons in area MT. Second, neurons in LIP project to the superior colliculus, an area that likely generates the choice response (an eye movement) [13, 25, 18]. Third, many neurons in LIP discharge in a sustained, spatially selective fashion when a monkey is instructed to make a delayed eye movement. This persistent activity can last for seconds before the eye movement is made, and it does not require the continued presence of a visual target. It is enough to flash a visual cue and to ask the monkey to make an eye movement to its remembered location some time later. Thus LIP neurons should be capable of representing the outcome of the decision about motion — a plan to make an eye movement to one of the targets. Indeed their capacity to emit persistent elevations in firing rate motivates the hypothesis that they can represent the integral of their inputs — the integral of a pulse is a step in activity. Thus, we suspected that these neurons might play a role in the conversion of momentary evidence to a binary decision (for review, see [30]).

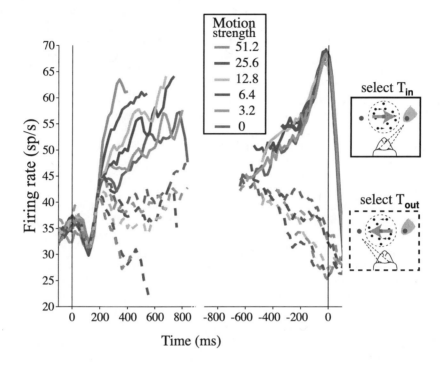

Figure 10.7   Time course of LIP activity during the reaction time version of the direction discrimination task. Average spike rates for 54 LIP neurons. Responses are grouped by choice and motion strength. Solid and dashed lines show responses for trials that were terminated with a T_{in} and T_{out} choice, respectively. The colors indicate the motion strength. The responses are aligned on the left to the onset of motion stimulus and drawn only up to the median RT for each motion strength, excluding any activity within 100 ms of the saccade. The responses on the right are aligned to the initiation of the saccadic eye movement response, and they are plotted backward in time to the median RT, excluding any activity occurring within 200 ms of motion onset. Only correct choices are included except for the 0% coherence case. Adapted with permission from J. D. Roitman and M. N. Shadlen, [27] (see color insert).

During decision-making in the reaction time motion task, neurons in area LIP undergo ramplike changes in spike rate (figure 10.7). These changes are evident from ~225 ms after onset of the random-dot motion until the monkey initiates its eye movement response. The neural activity represents the process leading to the monkey's choice, rising when the monkey chooses the target in the neuron's response field (T_{in}) and declining when the monkey chooses the target outside the neuron's response field (T_{out}). The graphs shown in figure 10.7 were obtained in the choice-reaction time experiments that produced the behavioral data shown earlier. The responses on the left side of the graph begin when the motion is turned on and stop at the median reaction time for each coherence. The responses on the right side of the graph are aligned to the end of the trial when the monkey initiates an eye movement response either to the choice target in the response field or to the other target.

During the epoch of decision formation, there is a clear effect of motion strength on the rate of change in activity. Strong (easy) stimuli cause a rapid and consistent increase or decrease in the spike rate. Weak (difficult) stimuli cause smaller increases and decreases that can change direction from moment to moment and thus meander like a particle in Brownian motion. For all stimuli, however, when the spike rate reaches a critical value, a decision for T_{in} is reached, and an eye movement ensues ~70 ms later [27]. LIP neurons represent which choice the monkey will make, the evolution of this decision in time, and the quality of the evidence upon which this decision is based.

With one important caveat, the responses in figure 10.7 can be related to the diffusion-to-bound model. The decision variable we focused on in this chapter is the accumulation of momentary evidence from MT, what we think of as a difference in spike rates from two ensembles of neurons selective for motion toward T_{in} and T_{out}, respectively. Suppose that beginning 225 ms after onset of motion, the firing rate of the LIP neuron represents the accumulation of this spike rate difference. Then its spike rate on any trial will meander like a sample trajectory shown in figure 10.2 until it reaches a bound. The solid curves in figure 10.7 are the expected averaged trajectories that end in the upper bound. They are averages conditionalized on choice. This is why even when the motion strength is 0%, the average response (solid cyan curve) seems to have a positive drift. This is true for error trials too (not shown).

The dashed curves force the caveat mentioned above. These are also conditionalized averages, but not to the response reaching a lower bound. For every LIP neuron with a right-choice target in its receptive fields, there is an LIP neuron with the left-choice target in its receptive fields. According to our ideas, these neurons also accumulate momentary evidence: a difference in spike rates from two ensembles of neurons selective for motion toward T_{in} and T_{out}. Of course these neurons tend to accumulate the evidence with an opposite sign. If T_{in} and T_{out} refer to right and left for the neuron we are recording, then T_{in} and T_{out} refer to left and right for these other LIP neurons. Suppose these neurons terminate the decision process with a left choice if their firing rates reach an upper bound. On these trials, the neurons we recorded (which signal right choices) will tend to decrease their responses because the evidence is against right. However, the end of the trial is highly variable relative to T_{in} neurons because the recorded neurons are not controlling the end of the trial when motion is in their null direction. This explains why the response averages shown by the dashed curves on the right side of figure 10.7 do not come to a stereotyped lower value before the saccade.

Rather than a single diffusion process (or random walk) that ends in two bounds, the physiology forces us to consider a process that is more like a race between two processes. One gathers evidence for right and against left, say. The other gathers evidence for left and against right. If these sources of momentary evidence were exactly the same and if they account for all of the variability in the LIP firing rates, then the two accumulations would be copies of one another, simply mirrored around the starting firing rate. If this inverse correlation were perfect, we could represent the two accumulations on a single graph with stopping bounds at $\pm A$. Of course, the two LIP neurons (or ensembles) are not perfectly anticorrelated. We see evidence for this in the conditionalized response averages in figure 10.7. But it turns out that so long as the race is between processes that are to a large extent anticorrelated, the equations we developed above hold. This is perfectly sensible because although we call this a race, there is no real competition. When one accumulator takes a positive step, the other takes a negative step. The correlation is not perfect, but this tendency renders moot any potential for the two mechanisms to actually compete to reach their respective upper bounds.

It is useful to think of a race between accumulators because this architecture is likely to extend to decisions among more than two options. It is hard to see how the model in figure 10.2 would extend to three, four, or more choices (see [17]). But a race among N accumulators is straightforward [35]. We are conducting experiments to test these ideas, and they look promising [8].

10.5   Conclusions

We have described a framework, diffusion to bound, for understanding how simple decisions are made in the brain. We have explained the mathematical tools that allow us to make predictions about the speed and accuracy of such decisions and have shown that these predictions match the behavior we observe. Lastly, we have provided evidence that the neural basis for the machinery we have described is in the parietal cortex.

We hope the mathematical tutorial will be useful to students interested in applying the equations. Indeed, the more general forms of the equations developed in terms of θ_1 may provide deeper insight into processes that are less straightforward than our motion experiments. Insights of fundamental importance to perception and decision-making can be found in [20, 19].

Decision-making in the random-dot motion task certainly takes place in a rarefied context: only two choices are present, they are equally probable *a priori*, there is only one source of relevant evidence, and all correct answers are of the same reward value. Yet, even these simplified conditions provide insights into the basic computations involved in decision-making. By suggesting the simple framework of accumulation of noisy momentary evidence to bound, we have a firm foundation from which we can begin to ask questions about more complicated decisions.

Are there certain kinds of decisions for which simply accumulating evidence over time is a poor strategy? Certainly. To integrate, the brain must know when the relevant information should be gathered. It would be detrimental to accumulate noise when the stimulus is not present. For example, many detection experiments in vision show little evidence for temporal integration beyond ~80 ms, the limits of Bloch's law [36, 37]. Even if there is no uncertainty about when to integrate, it may make little sense to do so if sufficient information can be acquired in a short epoch. We suspect that many discrimination problems in vision involve analyses of spatial correspondences (e.g., curvature, texture, elongation) that are best achieved on a stable representation of the image in the visual cortex. These analyses are typically performed in a snapshot, so to speak, before the pieces of the representation have time to shift about on the cortical map. While the fidelity of any decision variable could improve with further temporal integration, we suspect that often the benefit in accuracy is not sufficient to overcome natural tendencies to trade accuracy against speed.

On the other hand, organisms are faced with many decisions where the evidence is noisy or arrives in piecemeal fashion over time. For decision-making under these conditions, accumulating evidence in favor of one choice or the other may be an optimal strategy, and may be well described by a bounded accumulation model. Ultimately, we would like to know how the brain combines evidence from multiple sources over time with factors associated with prior probability, predicted costs and benefits of the outcomes, and the cost of time. We would like to understand the neural mechanisms that underlie the incorporation of these factors into the decision process. We are optimistic that the principles of sequential analysis will guide this research program. Just how far we can push the kind of simple perceptual decisions described in this chapter toward achieving this understanding remains to be seen.

Appendix 10.1: Discrete Increments or Summation of Infinitesimals?

From one perspective, there is no particular reason to conceive of the accumulation of increments and decrements in discrete steps. According to this argument, each Δt is infinitesimally small: $\Delta t \to \delta t$. The random increments are drawn from a distribution with mean μ and variance $\sigma^2 \delta t$. Indeed, the process can be written as a stochastic differential equation for the change in the accumulation, Y:

$$\frac{dY}{dt} = \mu + N\left\{0, \sigma\sqrt{dt}\right\} \tag{10.48}$$

The second term is the noise term, a normal distribution with mean and standard deviation given by the arguments in the curly braces. The peculiar term for the standard deviation ensures that the variance of the accumulation is σ^2

when $t = 1$. Remember, it is the variance that accumulates, not the standard deviation. Equation (10.48) gives a glimpse of how one might set up a variety of accumulation problems, for example, those that involve some leakiness of the accumulation. For additional reading on this approach, we recommend [33, 34].

There are two important points to be made here. First, by moving to the infinitesimal, we tacitly assume that the random increments are drawn from a normal distribution. This is simply a consequence of the central limit theorem: in any finite Δt, there are so many infinitesimal increments that they must add to a random number that is Gaussian [33]. So, according to this formulation, we can forget about other distributions. In short, forget about generalizations revolving around θ_1; according to this formulation, there is only one formula for θ_1 (the one in equation (10.25)). The second point counters this position.

A common assumption behind all of the formulations we have considered is that the increments that are accumulated to form the random walk are independent of one another. That is why the variance of Y is the sum of the variances of the increments and not the sum of the covariances. This assumption is suspect in the brain, especially over very short time scales. Responses from neurons are weakly correlated over a time scale of $\sim$10 to 50 ms [3]. To obtain independent samples of the spike rate from an ensemble of neurons in the visual cortex, it is essential to wait a minimum of 10 ms between samples (see [21]). Over very short time scales, and certainly for infinitesimal increments, independent samples are unlikely to be available in the brain for accumulation. Therefore, when we map the momentary evidence to spike rates from ensembles of neurons in the brain, it is difficult to embrace the assumption of independence over very short time scales. For this reason, we think it is useful to consider the random walk process as if it occurs in discrete time with increments that are not necessarily drawn from a Gaussian distribution.

Acknowledgments

This study was supported by the Howard Hughes Medical Institute (HHMI) and the National Eye Institute. T.D.H. is also supported by a HHMI predoctoral fellowship.

References

[1] Albright TD (1993) Cortical processing of visual motion. In Miles FA, Wallman J, eds, *Visual Motion and Its Role in the Stabilization of Gaze*, pages 177-201, New York: Elsevier.

[2] Allman JM, Kaas JH (1971) A representation of the visual field in the caudal third of the middle temporal gyrus of the owl monkey (*Aotus trivirgatus*). *Brain Research*, 31:85-105.

[3] Bair W, Zohary E, Newsome WT (2001) Correlated firing in macaque visual area MT: time scales and relationship to behavior. *Journal of Neuroscience*, 21:1676-1697.

[4] Born RT, Bradley DC (2005) Structure and Function of Visual Area MT. *Annual Review of Neuroscience*, 28:157-189.

[5] Britten K (2003) The middle temporal area: motion processing and the link to perception. In Chalupa WJ, Werner JS, eds., *The Visual Neurosciences*, volume 2, pages 1203-1216, Cambridge, MA: MIT Press.

[6] Britten KH, Shadlen MN, Newsome WT, Movshon JA (1992) The analysis of visual motion: a comparison of neuronal and psychophysical performance. *Journal of Neuroscience*, 12:4745-4765.

[7] Britten KH, Shadlen MN, Newsome WT, Movshon JA (1993) Responses of neurons in macaque MT to stochastic motion signals. *Visual Neuroscience*, 10:1157-1169.

[8] Churchland AK, Kiani R, Tam M, Palmer J, Shadlen MN (2005) Responses of LIP neurons reflect accumulation of evidence in a multiple choice decision task. 2005 Abstract Viewer/Itinerary Planner Washington, DC: Society for Neuroscience Program No. 16.8.

[9] Cox D, Miller H (1965) *The theory of stochastic processes*. London: Chapman and Hall.

[10] Ditterich J (2006) Stochastic models of decisions about motion direction: Behavior and physiology. *Neural Networks*, in press.

[11] Ditterich J, Mazurek M, Shadlen MN (2003) Microstimulation of visual cortex affects the speed of perceptual decisions. *Nature Neuroscience*, 6:891-898.

[12] Dubner R, Zeki SM (1971) Response properties and receptive fields of cells in an anatomically defined region of the superior temporal sulcus. *Brain Research*, 35:528-532.

[13] Gnadt JW, Andersen RA (1988) Memory related motor planning activity in posterior parietal cortex of monkey. *Experimental Brain Research*, 70:216-220.

[14] Gold JI, Shadlen MN (2003) The influence of behavioral context on the representation of a perceptual decision in developing oculomotor commands. *Journal of Neuroscience*, 23:632-651.

[15] Karlin S, Taylor HM (1975) *A First Course in Stochastic Processes, 2nd edition*. Boston: Academic Press.

[16] Kohn A, Smith MA (2005) Stimulus dependence of neuronal correlation in primary visual cortex of the macaque. *Journal of Neuroscience*, 25:3661-3673.

[17] Laming DRJ (1968) *Information Theory of Choice-Reaction Times*. London: Academic Press.

[18] Lewis JW, Van Essen DC (2000) Corticocortical connections of visual, sensorimotor, and multimodal processing areas in the parietal lobe of the macaque monkey. *Journal of Comparative Neurology*, 428:112-137.

[19] Link SW (1992) *The Wave Theory of Difference and Similarity*. Hillsdale, NJ: Lawrence Erlbaum Associates.

[20] Link SW, Heath RA (1975) A sequential theory of psychological discrimination. *Psychometrika*, 40:77-105.

[21] Mazurek ME, Roitman JD, Ditterich J, Shadlen MN (2003) A role for neural integrators in perceptual decision making. *Cerebral Cortex*, 13:1257-1269.

[22] Newsome WT, Britten KH, Movshon JA (1989) Neuronal correlates of a perceptual decision. *Nature*, 341:52-54.

[23] Orban GA, Fize D, Peuskens H, Denys K, Nelissen K, Sunaert S, Todd J, Vanduffel W (2003) Similarities and differences in motion processing between the human and macaque brain: evidence from fMRI. *Neuropsychologia*, 41:1757-1768.

[24] Palmer J, Huk AC, Shadlen MN (2005) The effect of stimulus strength on the speed and accuracy of a perceptual decision. *Journal of Vision*, 5:376-404.

[25] Paré M, Wurtz RH (1997) Monkey posterior parietal cortex neurons antidromically activated from superior colliculus. *Journal of Neurophysiology*, 78:3493-3498.

[26] Ratcliff R, Rouder JN (1998) Modeling response times for two-choice decisions. *Psychological Science*, 9:347-356.

[27] Roitman JD, Shadlen MN (2002) Response of neurons in the lateral intraparietal area during a combined visual discrimination reaction time task. *Journal of Neuroscience*, 22:9475-9489.

[28] Salzman CD, Britten KH, Newsome WT (1990) Cortical microstimulation influences perceptual judgements of motion direction. *Nature*, 346:174-177.

[29] Sartre JP (1984) Existentialism and Human Emotions. New York: Carol Publishing Group.

[30] Shadlen MN, Gold JI (2004) The neurophysiology of decision-making as a window on cognition. In Gazzaniga MS, eds., *The Cognitive Neurosciences, 3rd edition*, pages 1229-1241, Cambridge, MA: MIT Press.

[31] Smith PL (1990) A note on the distribution of response times for a random walk with Gaussian increments. *Journal of Mathematical Psychology*, 34:445-459.

[32] Smith PL (1995) Psychophysically principled models of visual simple reaction time. *Psychological Review*, 102:567-593.

[33] Smith PL (2000) Stochastic dynamic models of response time and accuracy: A foundational primer. *Journal of Mathematical Psychology*, 44:408-463.

[34] Usher M, McClelland JL (2001) The time course of perceptual choice: the leaky, competing accumulator model. *Psychological Review*, 108:550-592.

[35] Usher M, Olami Z, McClelland JL (2002) Hick's law in a stochastic race model with speed-accuracy tradeoff. *Journal of Mathematical Psychology*, 46:704-715.

[36] Watson AB (1979) Probability summation over time. *Vision Research*, 19:515-522.

[37] Watson AB (1986) Temporal sensitivity. In Boff KR, Kaufman L, Thomas JP, eds., *Handbook of Perception and Human Performance*, pages 6.1-6.43, New York: Wiley.

[38] Zohary E, Shadlen MN, Newsome WT (1994) Correlated neuronal discharge rate and its implications for psychophysical performance. *Nature*, 370:140-143.

11 Neural Models of Bayesian Belief Propagation

Rajesh P. N. Rao

11.1 Introduction

Animals are constantly faced with the challenge of interpreting signals from noisy sensors and acting in the face of incomplete knowledge about the environment. A rigorous approach to handling uncertainty is to characterize and process information using probabilities. Having estimates of the probabilities of objects and events allows one to make intelligent decisions in the presence of uncertainty. A prey could decide whether to keep foraging or to flee based on the probability that an observed movement or sound was caused by a predator. Probabilistic estimates are also essential ingredients of more sophisticated decision-making routines such as those based on expected reward or utility. An important component of a probabilistic system is a method for reasoning based on combining prior knowledge about the world with current input data. Such methods are typically based on some form of Bayesian inference, involving the computation of the posterior probability distribution of one or more random variables of interest given input data.

In this chapter, we describe how neural circuits could implement a general algorithm for Bayesian inference known as belief propagation. The belief propagation algorithm involves passing "messages" (probabilities) between the nodes of a graphical model that captures the causal structure of the environment. We review the basic notion of graphical models and illustrate the belief propagation algorithm with an example. We investigate potential neural implementations of the algorithm based on networks of leaky integrator neurons and describe how such networks can perform sequential and hierarchical Bayesian inference. Simulation results are presented for comparison with neurobiological data. We conclude the chapter by discussing other recent models of inference in neural circuits and suggest directions for future research. Some of the ideas reviewed in this chapter have appeared in prior publications [30, 31, 32, 42]; these may be consulted for additional details and results not included in this chapter.

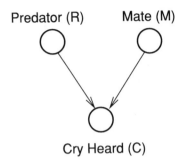

Predator (R)   Mate (M)

Cry Heard (C)

Figure 11.1 · An Example of a Graphical Model. Each circle represents a node denoting a random variable. Arrows represent probabilistic dependencies as specified by the probability table $P(C|R, M)$.

11.2   Bayesian Inference through Belief Propagation

Consider the problem of an animal deciding whether to flee or keep feeding based on the cry of another animal from a different species. Suppose it is often the case that the other animal emits the cry whenever there is a predator in the vicinity. However, the animal sometimes also emits the same cry when a potential mate is in the area. The probabilistic relationship between a cry and its probable causes can be captured using a *graphical model* as shown in figure 11.1. The circles (or nodes) represent the two causes and the observation as random variables R (Predator), M (Mate), and C (Cry heard). We assume these random variables are binary and can take on the values 1 and 0 (for "presence" and "absence" respectively), although this can be generalized to multiple values. The arcs connecting the nodes represent the probabilistic causal relationships as characterized by the probability table $P(C|R, M)$.

For the above problem, the decision to flee or not can be based on the posterior probability $P(R|C)$ of a predator given that a cry was heard ($C = 1$). This probability can be calculated directly as:

$$P(R = 1|C = 1) = \sum_M P(R = 1, M|C = 1)$$

$$= \sum_M kP(C = 1|R = 1, M)P(R = 1)P(M), \quad (11.1)$$

where we used Bayes rule to obtain the second equation from the first, with k being the normalization constant $1/\sum_{R,M} P(C = 1|R, M)P(R)P(M)$.

The above calculation required summing over the random variable M that was irrelevant to the problem at hand. In a general scenario, one would need to sum over all irrelevant random variables, an operation which scales exponentially with the total number of variables, quickly becoming intractable. Fortunately, there exists an alternate method known as *belief propagation* (or probability propagation) [26] that involves passing messages (probability vectors) between the nodes of the graphical model and summing over local products of messages, an operation that can be tractable. The belief propagation algorithm involves two types of computation: marginalization (summation over local joint distributions) and multiplication of local marginal probabilities. Because the operations are local, the algorithm is also well suited to neural implementation, as we shall discuss below. The algorithm is provably correct for singly connected graphs (i.e., no undirected cycles) [26], although it has been used with some success in some graphical models with cycles as well [25].

11.2.1   A Simple Example

We illustrate the belief propagation algorithm using the feed-or-flee problem above. The nodes R and M first generate the messages $P(R)$ and $P(M)$ respectively, which are vectors of length two storing the prior probabilities for $R = 0$ and 1, and $M = 0$ and 1 respectively. These messages are sent to node C. Since a cry was heard, the value of C is known ($C = 1$) and therefore, the messages from R and M do not affect node C. We are interested in computing the marginal probabilities for the two hidden nodes R and M. The node C generates the message $\mathbf{m}_{C \to R} = \mathbf{m}_{C \to M} = (0, 1)$, i.e., probability of absence of a cry is 0 and probability of presence of a cry is 1 (since a cry was heard). This message is passed on to the nodes R and M.

Each node performs a marginalization over variables other than itself using the local conditional probability table and the incoming messages. For example, in the case of node R, this is $\sum_{M,C} P(C|R, M)P(M)P(C) = \sum_M P(C = 1|R, M)P(M)$ since C is known to be 1. Similarly, the node M performs the marginalization $\sum_{R,C} P(C|R, M)P(R)P(C) = \sum_R P(C = 1|R, M)P(R)$. The final step involves multiplying these marginalized probabilities with other messages received, in this case, $P(R)$ and $P(M)$ respectively, to yield, after normalization, the posterior probability of R and M given the observation $C = 1$:

$$P(R|C = 1) \quad = \quad \alpha \Big(\sum_M P(C = 1|R, M)P(M) \Big) P(R) \qquad (11.2)$$

$$P(M|C = 1) \quad = \quad \beta \Big(\sum_R P(C = 1|R, M)P(R) \Big) P(M), \qquad (11.3)$$

where α and β are normalization constants. Note that equation (11.2) above yields the same expression for $P(R = 1|C = 1)$ as equation (11.1) that was derived using Bayes rule. In general, belief propagation allows efficient computation of the posterior probabilities of unknown random variables in singly connected graphical models, given any available evidence in the form of observed values for any subset of the random variables.

11.2.2   Belief Propagation over Time

Belief propagation can also be applied to graphical models evolving over time. A simple but widely used model is the hidden Markov model (HMM) shown in figure 11.2A. The input that is observed at time t ($= 1, 2, \ldots$) is represented by the random variable $\mathbf{I}(t)$, which can either be discrete-valued or a real-valued vector such as an image or a speech signal. The input is assumed to be generated by a hidden cause or "state" $\theta(t)$, which can assume one of N discrete values $1, \ldots, N$. The state $\theta(t)$ evolves over time in a Markovian manner, depending only on the previous state according to the transition probabilities given by $P(\theta(t) = i|\theta(t-1) = j) = P(\theta_i^t|\theta_j^{t-1})$ for $i, j = 1 \ldots N$. The observation $\mathbf{I}(t)$ is generated according to the probability $P(\mathbf{I}(t)|\theta(t))$.

The belief propagation algorithm can be used to compute the posterior probability of the state given current and past inputs (we consider here only the "forward" propagation case, corresponding to on-line state estimation). As in the previous example, the node θ^t performs a marginalization over neighboring variables, in this case θ^{t-1} and $\mathbf{I}(t)$. The first marginalization results in a probability vector whose ith component is $\sum_j P(\theta_i^t|\theta_j^{t-1})m_j^{t-1,t}$ where $m_j^{t-1,t}$ is the jth component of the message from node θ^{t-1} to θ^t. The second marginalization is from node $\mathbf{I}(t)$ and is given by $\sum_{\mathbf{I}(t)} P(\mathbf{I}(t)|\theta_i^t)P(\mathbf{I}(t))$. If a particular input $\mathbf{I}'$ is observed, this sum becomes $\sum_{\mathbf{I}(t)} P(\mathbf{I}(t)|\theta_i^t)\delta(\mathbf{I}(t), \mathbf{I}') = P(\mathbf{I}'|\theta_i^t)$, where δ is the delta function which evaluates to 1 if its two arguments are equal and 0 otherwise. The two "messages" resulting from the marginalization along the arcs from θ^{t-1} and $\mathbf{I}(t)$ can be multiplied at node θ^t to yield the following message to θ^{t+1}:

$$m_i^{t,t+1} = P(\mathbf{I}'|\theta_i^t) \sum_j P(\theta_i^t|\theta_j^{t-1})m_j^{t-1,t} \tag{11.4}$$

If $m_i^{0,1} = P(\theta_i)$ (the prior distribution over states), then it is easy to show using Bayes rule that $m_i^{t,t+1} = P(\theta_i^t, \mathbf{I}(t), \ldots, \mathbf{I}(1))$.

Rather than computing the joint probability, one is typically interested in calculating the posterior probability of the state, given current and past inputs, i.e., $P(\theta_i^t|\mathbf{I}(t), \ldots, \mathbf{I}(1))$. This can be done by incorporating a normalization step at each time step. Define (for $t = 1, 2, \ldots$):

$$m_i^t = P(\mathbf{I}'|\theta_i^t) \sum_j P(\theta_i^t|\theta_j^{t-1})m_j^{t-1,t} \tag{11.5}$$

$$m_i^{t,t+1} = m_i^t/n^t, \tag{11.6}$$

where $n^t = \sum_j m_j^t$. If $m_i^{0,1} = P(\theta_i)$ (the prior distribution over states), then it is easy to see that:

$$m_i^{t,t+1} = P(\theta_i^t|\mathbf{I}(t), \ldots, \mathbf{I}(1)) \tag{11.7}$$

This method has the additional advantage that the normalization at each time step promotes stability, an important consideration for recurrent neuronal networks, and allows the likelihood function $P(\mathbf{I}'|\theta_i^t)$ to be defined in proportional terms without the need for explicitly calculating its normalization factor (see section 11.4 for an example).

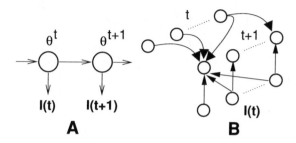

Figure 11.2 Graphical Model for a HMM and its Neural Implementation. (A) Dynamic graphical model for a hidden Markov model (HMM). Each circle represents a node denoting the state variable θ^t which can take on values $1, \ldots, N$. (B) Recurrent network for implementing on-line belief propagation for the graphical model in (A). Each circle represents a neuron encoding a state i. Arrows represent synaptic connections. The probability distribution over state values at each time step is represented by the entire population.

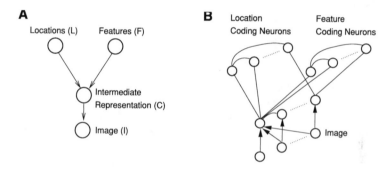

Figure 11.3 A Hierarchical Graphical Model for Images and its Neural Implementation. (A) Three-level graphical model for generating simple images containing one of many possible features at a particular location. (B) Three-level network for implementing on-line belief propagation for the graphical model in (A). Arrows represent synaptic connections in the direction pointed by the arrow heads. Lines without arrow heads represent bidirectional connections.

11.2.3 Hierarchical Belief Propagation

As a third example of belief propagation, consider the three-level graphical model shown in figure 11.3A. The model describes a simple process for generating images based on two random variables: L, denoting spatial locations, and F, denoting visual features (a more realistic model would involve a hierarchy of such features, sub-features, and locations). Both random variables are assumed to be discrete, with L assuming one of n values $L_1, \ldots, L_n$, and F assuming one of m different values $F_1, \ldots, F_m$. The node C denotes different combinations of features and locations, each of its values $C_1, \ldots, C_p$ encoding a specific feature at a specific location. Representing all possible combinations is infeasible but it is sufficient to represent those that occur frequently and to map each feature-location (L, F) combination to the closest C_i using an appropriate distribution $P(C_i|L, F)$ (see section 11.4 for an example). An image with a specific feature at a specific location is generated according to the image likelihood $P(I|C)$.

Given the above graphical model for images, we are interested in computing the posterior probabilities of features (more generally, objects or object parts) and their locations in an input image. This can be done using belief propagation. Given the model in figure 11.3A and a specific input image $I = I'$, belief propagation prescribes that the following "messages" (probabilities) be transmitted from one node to another, as given by the arrows in the subscripts:

$$m_{L \to C} = P(L) \tag{11.8}$$

$$m_{F \to C} = P(F) \tag{11.9}$$

$$m_{I \to C} = P(I = I'|C) \tag{11.10}$$

$$m_{C \to L} = \sum_F \sum_C P(C|L, F)P(F)P(I = I'|C) \tag{11.11}$$

$$m_{C \to F} = \sum_L \sum_C P(C|L, F)P(L)P(I = I'|C) \tag{11.12}$$

The first three messages above are simply prior probabilities encoding beliefs about locations and features before a sensory input becomes available. The posterior probabilities of the unknown variables C, L, and F given the input image I, are calculated by combining the messages at each node as follows:

$$P(C|I = I') = \alpha m_{I \to C} \sum_F \sum_L P(C|L, F) m_{L \to C} m_{F \to C} \tag{11.13}$$

$$P(L|I = I') = \beta m_{C \to L} P(L) \tag{11.14}$$

$$P(F|I = I') = \gamma m_{C \to F} P(F), \tag{11.15}$$

where α, β, and γ are normalization constants that make each of the above probabilities sum to 1. Note how the prior $P(L)$ multiplicatively modulates the posterior probability of a feature in equation 11.15 via equation 11.12. This observation plays an important role in section 11.4 below where we simulate spatial attention by increasing $P(L)$ for a desired location.

11.3   Neural Implementations of Belief Propagation

11.3.1   Approximate Inference in Linear Recurrent Networks

We begin by considering a commonly used neural architecture for modeling cortical response properties, namely, a linear recurrent network with firing-rate dynamics (see, for example, [5]). Let $\mathbf{I}$ denote the vector of input firing rates to the network and let $\mathbf{v}$ represent the output firing rates of N recurrently connected neurons in the network. Let $\mathbf{W}$ represent the feedforward synaptic weight matrix and $\mathbf{M}$ the recurrent weight matrix. The following equation describes the dynamics of the network:

$$\tau \frac{d\mathbf{v}}{dt} = -\mathbf{v} + \mathbf{W}\mathbf{I} + \mathbf{U}\mathbf{v}, \tag{11.16}$$

where τ is a time constant. The equation can be written in a discrete form as follows:

$$v_i(t+1) \quad = \quad v_i(t) + \epsilon(-v_i(t) + \mathbf{w}_i\mathbf{I}(t) + \sum_j u_{ij}v_j(t)), \tag{11.17}$$

where ϵ is the integration rate, v_i is the ith component of the vector $\mathbf{v}$, $\mathbf{w}_i$ is the ith row of the matrix $\mathbf{W}$, and u_{ij} is the element of $\mathbf{U}$ in the ith row and jth column. The above equation can be rewritten as:

$$v_i(t+1) \quad = \quad \epsilon\mathbf{w}_i\mathbf{I}(t) + \sum_j U_{ij}v_j(t), \tag{11.18}$$

where $U_{ij} = \epsilon u_{ij}$ for $i \neq j$ and $U_{ii} = 1 + \epsilon(u_{ii} - 1)$. Comparing the belief propagation equation (11.5) for a HMM with equation (11.18) above, it can be seen that both involve propagation of quantities over time with contributions from the input and activity from the previous time step. However, the belief propagation equation involves multiplication of these contributions while the leaky integrator equation above involves addition.

Now consider belief propagation in the log domain. Taking the logarithm of both sides of equation (11.5), we get:

$$\log m_i^t = \log P(\mathbf{I}'|\theta_i^t) + \log \sum_j P(\theta_i^t|\theta_j^{t-1})m_j^{t-1,t} \tag{11.19}$$

This equation is much more conducive to neural implementation via equation (11.18). In particular, equation (11.18) can implement equation (11.19) if:

$$v_i(t+1) \quad = \quad \log m_i^t \tag{11.20}$$
$$\epsilon\mathbf{w}_i\mathbf{I}(t) \quad = \quad \log P(\mathbf{I}'|\theta_i^t) \tag{11.21}$$
$$\sum_j U_{ij}v_j(t) \quad = \quad \log \sum_j P(\theta_i^t|\theta_j^{t-1})m_j^{t-1,t} \tag{11.22}$$

The normalization step (equation (11.6)) can be computed by a separate group of neurons representing $m_i^{t,t+1}$ that receive as excitatory input $\log m_i^t$ and inhibitory input $\log n^t = \log \sum_j m_j^t$:

$$\log m_i^{t,t+1} \quad = \quad \log m_i^t - \log n^t \tag{11.23}$$

These neurons convey the normalized posterior probabilities $m_i^{t,t+1}$ back to the neurons implementing equation (11.19) so that m_i^{t+1} may be computed at the next time step. Note the the normalization step makes the overall network nonlinear.

In equation (11.21), the log-likelihood $\log P(\mathbf{I}'|\theta_i^t)$ is calculated using a linear operation $\epsilon \mathbf{w}_i \mathbf{I}(t)$ (see also [45]). Since the messages are normalized at each time step, one can relax the equality in equation (11.21) and make $\log P(\mathbf{I}'|\theta_i^t) \propto \mathbf{F}(\theta_i)\mathbf{I}(t)$ for some linear filter $\mathbf{F}(\theta_i) = \epsilon \mathbf{w}_i$. This avoids the problem of calculating the normalization factor for $P(\mathbf{I}'|\theta_i^t)$, which can be especially hard when $\mathbf{I}'$ takes on continuous values such as in an image. A more challenging problem is to pick recurrent weights U_{ij} such that equation (11.22) holds true. For equation (11.22) to hold true, we need to approximate a *log-sum* with a *sum-of-logs*. One approach is to generate a set of random probabilities $x_j(t)$ for $t = 1, \dots, T$ and find a set of weights U_{ij} that satisfy:

$$\sum_j U_{ij} \log x_j(t) \approx \log\left[\sum_j P(\theta_i^t|\theta_j^{t-1})x_j(t)\right] \tag{11.24}$$

for all i and t. This can be done by minimizing the squared error in equation (11.24) with respect to the recurrent weights U_{ij}. This empirical approach, followed in [30], is used in some of the experiments below. An alternative approach is to exploit the nonlinear properties of dendrites as suggested in the following section.

11.3.2   Exact Inference in Nonlinear Networks

A firing rate model that takes into account some of the effects of nonlinear filtering in dendrites can be obtained by generalizing equation (11.18) as follows:

$$v_i(t+1) = f\big(\mathbf{w}_i \mathbf{I}(t)\big) + g\Big(\sum_j U_{ij} v_j(t)\Big), \tag{11.25}$$

where f and g model nonlinear dendritic filtering functions for feedforward and recurrent inputs. By comparing this equation with the belief propagation equation in the log domain (equation (11.19)), it can be seen that the first equation can implement the second if:

$$v_i(t+1) = \log m_i^t \tag{11.26}$$

$$f\big(\mathbf{w}_i \mathbf{I}(t)\big) = \log P(\mathbf{I}'|\theta_i^t) \tag{11.27}$$

$$g\Big(\sum_j U_{ij} v_j(t)\Big) = \log \sum_j P(\theta_i^t|\theta_j^{t-1})m_j^{t-1,t} \tag{11.28}$$

In this model (figure 11.2B), N neurons represent $\log m_i^t$ ($i = 1, \dots, N$) in their firing rates. The dendritic filtering functions f and g approximate the logarithm function, the feedforward weights $\mathbf{w}_i$ act as a linear filter on the input to yield the likelihood $P(\mathbf{I}'|\theta_i^t)$ and the recurrent synaptic weights U_{ij} directly encode the transition probabilities $P(\theta_i^t|\theta_j^{t-1})$. The normalization step is computed as in equation (11.23) using a separate group of neurons that represent log posterior probabilities $\log m_i^{t,t+1}$ and that convey these probabilities for use in equation (11.28) by the neurons computing $\log m_i^{t+1}$.

11.3.3   Inference Using Noisy Spiking Neurons

Spiking Neuron Model

The models above were based on firing rates of neurons, but a slight modification allows an interpretation in terms of noisy spiking neurons. Consider a variant of equation (11.16) where $\mathbf{v}$ represents the membrane potential values of neurons rather than their firing rates. We then obtain the classic equation describing the dynamics of the membrane potential v_i of neuron i in a recurrent network of leaky integrate-and-fire neurons:

$$\tau \frac{dv_i}{dt} = -v_i + \sum_j w_{ij} I_j + \sum_j u_{ij} v'_j, \tag{11.29}$$

where τ is the membrane time constant, I_j denotes the synaptic current due to input neuron j, w_{ij} represents the strength of the synapse from input j to recurrent neuron i, v'_j denotes the synaptic current due to recurrent neuron j, and u_{ij} represents the corresponding synaptic strength. If v_i crosses a threshold T, the neuron fires a spike and v_i is reset to the potential v_{reset}. Equation (11.29) can be rewritten in discrete form as:

$$v_i(t+1) \quad = \quad v_i(t) + \epsilon(-v_i(t) + \sum_j w_{ij} I_j(t)) + \sum_j u_{ij} v'_j(t)) \tag{11.30}$$

i.e. $\quad v_i(t+1) \quad = \quad \epsilon \sum_j w_{ij} I_j(t) + \sum_j U_{ij} v'_j(t), \tag{11.31}$

where ϵ is the integration rate, $U_{ii} = 1 + \epsilon(u_{ii} - 1)$ and for $i \neq j$, $U_{ij} = \epsilon u_{ij}$. The nonlinear variant of the above equation that includes dendritic filtering of input currents in the dynamics of the membrane potential is given by:

$$v_i(t+1) = f\left(\sum_j w_{ij} I_j(t)\right) + g\left(\sum_j U_{ij} v'_j(t)\right), \tag{11.32}$$

where f and g are nonlinear dendritic filtering functions for feedforward and recurrent inputs.

We can model the effects of background inputs and the random openings of membrane channels by adding a Gaussian white noise term to the right-hand side of equations (11.31) and (11.32). This makes the spiking of neurons in the recurrent network stochastic. Plesser and Gerstner [27] and Gerstner [11] have shown that under reasonable assumptions, the probability of spiking in such noisy neurons can be approximated by an "escape function" (or hazard function) that depends only on the distance between the (noise-free) membrane potential v_i and the threshold T. Several different escape functions were found to yield similar results. We use the following exponential function suggested in [11] for noisy integrate-and-fire networks:

$$P(\text{neuron } i \text{ spikes at time } t) = k e^{(v_i(t) - T)}, \tag{11.33}$$

where k is an arbitrary constant. We use a model that combines equations (11.32) and (11.33) to generate spikes.

Inference in Spiking Networks

By comparing the membrane potential equation (11.32) with the belief propagation equation in the log domain (equation (11.19)), we can postulate the following correspondences:

$$v_i(t+1) \;=\; \log m_i^t \tag{11.34}$$

$$f\Big(\sum_j w_{ij} I_j(t)\Big) \;=\; \log P(\mathbf{I'}|\theta_i^t) \tag{11.35}$$

$$g\Big(\sum_j U_{ij} v_j'(t)\Big) \;=\; \log \sum_j P(\theta_i^t|\theta_j^{t-1}) m_j^{t-1,t} \tag{11.36}$$

The dendritic filtering functions f and g approximate the logarithm function, the synaptic currents $I_j(t)$ and $v_j'(t)$ are approximated by the corresponding instantaneous firing rates, and the recurrent synaptic weights U_{ij} encode the transition probabilities $P(\theta_i^t|\theta_j^{t-1})$.

Since the membrane potential $v_i(t+1)$ is assumed to be equal to $\log m_i^t$ (equation (11.34)), we can use equation (11.33) to calculate the probability of spiking for each neuron i as:

$$P(\text{neuron } i \text{ spikes at time } t+1) \;\propto\; e^{(v_i(t+1)-T)} \tag{11.37}$$

$$\propto\; e^{(\log m_i^t - T)} \tag{11.38}$$

$$\propto\; m_i^t \tag{11.39}$$

Thus, the probability of spiking (or, equivalently, the instantaneous firing rate) for neuron i in the recurrent network is directly proportional to the message m_i^t, which is the posterior probability of the neuron's preferred state and current input given past inputs. Similarly, the instantaneous firing rates of the group of neurons representing $\log m_i^{t,t+1}$ is proportional to $m_i^{t,t+1}$, which is the precisely the input required by equation (11.36).

11.4 Results

11.4.1 Example 1: Detecting Visual Motion

We first illustrate the application of the linear firing rate-based model (section 11.3.1) to the problem of detecting visual motion. A prominent property of visual cortical cells in areas such as V1 and MT is selectivity to the direction of visual motion. We show how the activity of such cells can be interpreted as representing the posterior probability of stimulus motion in a particular direction, given a series of input images. For simplicity, we focus on the case of 1D motion in an image consisting of X pixels with two possible motion directions: leftward (L) or rightward (R).

Let the state θ_{ij} represent a motion direction $j \in \{L, R\}$ at spatial location i. Consider a network of N neurons, each representing a particular state θ_{ij} (figure 11.4A). The feedforward weights are assumed to be Gaussians, i.e. $\mathbf{F}(\theta_{iR}) = \mathbf{F}(\theta_{iL}) = \mathbf{F}(\theta_i) =$ Gaussian centered at location i with a standard

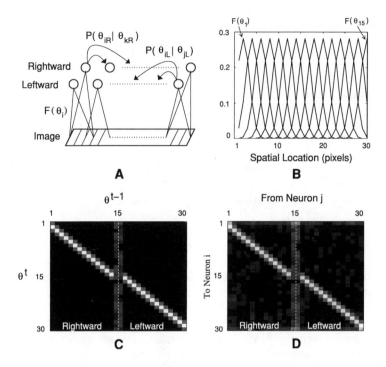

Figure 11.4   Recurrent Network for Motion Detection (from [30]). (A) depicts a recurrent network of neurons, shown for clarity as two chains selective for leftward and rightward motion respectively. The feedforward synaptic weights for neuron i (in the leftward or rightward chain) are determined by $\mathbf{F}(\theta_i)$. The recurrent weights reflect the transition probabilities $P(\theta_{iR}|\theta_{kR})$ and $P(\theta_{iL}|\theta_{jL})$. (B) Feedforward weights $\mathbf{F}(\theta_i)$ for neurons $i = 1, \ldots, 15$ (rightward chain). The feedforward weights for neurons $i = 15, \ldots, 30$ (leftward chain) are identical. (C) Transition probabilities $P(\theta^t|\theta^{t-1})$. Probability values are proportional to pixel brightness. (D) Recurrent weights U_{ij} computed from the transition probabilities in (C) using Equation 11.24.

deviation σ. Figure 11.4B depicts the feedforward weights for a network of 30 neurons, 15 encoding leftward and 15 encoding rightward motion.

We model visual motion using an HMM. The transition probabilities $P(\theta_{ij}|\theta_{kl})$ are selected to reflect both the direction of motion and speed of the moving stimulus. The transition probabilities for rightward motion from the state θ_{kR} (i.e. $P(\theta_{iR}|\theta_{kR})$) were set according to a Gaussian centered at location $k + x$, where x is a parameter determined by stimulus speed. The transition probabilities for leftward motion from the state θ_{kL} were likewise set to Gaussian values centered at $k - x$. The transition probabilities from states near the two boundaries ($i = 1$ and $i = X$) were chosen to be uniformly random values. Figure 11.4C shows the matrix of transition probabilities.

Recurrent Network Model

To detect motion using Bayesian inference in the above HMM, consider first a model based on the linear recurrent network as in equation (11.18) but with normalization as in equation (11.23) (which makes the network nonlinear). We can compute the recurrent weights m_{ij} for the transition probabilities given above using the approximation method in equation (11.24) (see figure 11.4D). The resulting network then implements approximate belief propagation for the HMM based on equation (11.20-11.23). Figure 11.5 shows the output of the network in the middle of a sequence of input images depicting a bar moving either leftward or rightward. As shown in the figure, for a leftward-moving bar at a particular location i, the highest network output is for the neuron representing location i and direction L, while for a rightward-moving bar, the neuron representing location i and direction R has the highest output. The output firing rates were computed from the log probabilities $\log m_i^{t,t+1}$ using a simple linear encoding model: $f_i = [c \cdot v_i + F]^+$ where c is a positive constant ($= 12$ for this plot), F is the maximum firing rate of the neuron ($= 100$ in this example), and $+$ denotes rectification. Note that even though the log-likelihoods are the same for leftward- and rightward-moving inputs, the asymmetric recurrent weights (which represent the transition probabilities) allow the network to distinguish between leftward- and rightward-moving stimuli. The posterior probabilities $m_i^{t,t+1}$ are shown in figure 11.5 (lowest panels). The network correctly computes posterior probabilities close to 1 for the states θ_{iL} and θ_{iR} for leftward and rightward motion respectively at location i.

Nonlinear Spiking Model

The motion detection task can also be solved using a nonlinear network with spiking neurons as described in section 11.3.3. A single-level recurrent network of 30 neurons as in the previous section was used. The feedforward weights were the same as in figure 11.4B. The recurrent connections directly encoded transition probabilities for leftward motion (see figure 11.4C). As seen in figure 11.6A, neurons in the network exhibited direction selectivity. Furthermore, the spiking probability of neurons reflects the probability m_i^t of motion direction at a given location as in equation (11.39) (figure 11.6B), suggesting a probabilistic interpretation of direction-selective spiking responses in visual cortical areas such as V1 and MT.

11.4.2   Example 2: Bayesian Decision-Making in a Random-Dots Task

To establish a connection to behavioral data, we consider the well-known random dots motion discrimination task (see, for example, [41]). The stimulus consists of an image sequence showing a group of moving dots, a fixed fraction of which are randomly selected at each frame and moved in a fixed direction (for example, either left or right). The rest of the dots are moved in random directions. The fraction of dots moving in the same direction is called

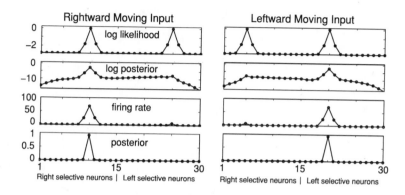

Figure 11.5 Network Output for a Moving Stimulus (from [30]). (Left Panel) The four plots depict respectively the log likelihoods, log posteriors, neural firing rates, and posterior probabilities observed in the network for a rightward moving bar when it arrives at the central image location. Note that the log likelihoods are the same for the rightward and leftward selective neurons (the first 15 and last 15 neurons respectively, as dictated by the feedforward weights in Figure 11.4B) but the outputs of these neurons correctly reflect the direction of motion as a result of recurrent interactions. (Right Panel) The same four plots for a leftward moving bar as it reaches the central location.

the *coherence* of the stimulus. Figure 11.7A depicts the stimulus for two different levels of coherence. The task is to decide the direction of motion of the coherently moving dots for a given input sequence. A wealth of data exists on the psychophysical performance of humans and monkeys as well as the neural responses in brain areas such as the middle temporal (MT) and lateral intraparietal areas (LIP) in monkeys performing the task (see [41] and references therein). Our goal is to explore the extent to which the proposed models for neural belief propagation can explain the existing data for this task.

The nonlinear motion detection network in the previous section computes the posterior probabilities $P(\theta_{iL}|\mathbf{I}(t),\ldots,\mathbf{I}(1))$ and $P(\theta_{iR}|\mathbf{I}(t),\ldots,\mathbf{I}(1))$ of leftward and rightward motion at different locations i. These outputs can be used to decide the direction of coherent motion by computing the posterior probabilities for leftward and rightward motion irrespective of location, given the input images. These probabilities can be computed by marginalizing the posterior distribution computed by the neurons for leftward (L) and rightward (R) motion over all spatial positions i:

$$P(L|\mathbf{I}(t),\ldots,\mathbf{I}(1)) \;=\; \sum_i P(\theta_{iL}|\mathbf{I}(t),\ldots,\mathbf{I}(1)) \qquad (11.40)$$

$$P(R|\mathbf{I}(t),\ldots,\mathbf{I}(1)) \;=\; \sum_i P(\theta_{iR}|\mathbf{I}(t),\ldots,\mathbf{I}(1)) \qquad (11.41)$$

To decide the overall direction of motion in a random-dots stimulus, there exist two options: (1) view the decision process as a "race" between the two

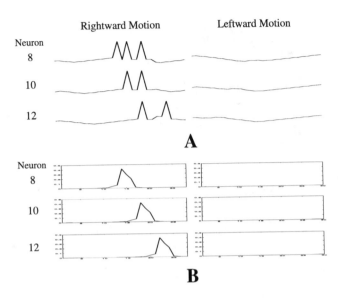

A

B

Figure 11.6 Responses from the Spiking Motion Detection Network. (A) Spiking responses of three of the first 15 neurons in the recurrent network (neurons 8, 10, and 12). As is evident, these neurons have become selective for rightward motion as a consequence of the recurrent connections (= transition probabilities) specified in Figure 11.4C. (B) Posterior probabilities over time of motion direction (at a given location) encoded by the three neurons for rightward and leftward motion.

probabilities above to a prechosen threshold (this also generalizes to more than two choices); or (2) compute the log of the ratio between the two probabilities above and compare this log-posterior ratio to a prechosen threshold. We use the latter method to allow comparison to the results of Shadlen and colleagues, who postulate a ratio-based model in area LIP in primate parietal cortex [12]. The log-posterior ratio $r(t)$ of leftward over rightward motion can be defined as:

$$r(t) \;=\; \log P(L|\mathbf{I}(t),\dots,\mathbf{I}(1)) - \log P(R|\mathbf{I}(t),\dots,\mathbf{I}(1)) \tag{11.42}$$

$$\;=\; \log \frac{P(L|\mathbf{I}(t),\dots,\mathbf{I}(1))}{P(R|\mathbf{I}(t),\dots,\mathbf{I}(1))} \tag{11.43}$$

If $r(t) > 0$, the evidence seen so far favors leftward motion and vice versa for $r(t) < 0$. The instantaneous ratio $r(t)$ is susceptible to rapid fluctuations due to the noisy stimulus. We therefore use the following decision variable $d_L(t)$ to track the running average of the log posterior ratio of L over R:

$$d_L(t+1) \;=\; d_L(t) + \alpha(r(t) - d_L(t)) \tag{11.44}$$

and likewise for $d_R(t)$ (the parameter α is between 0 and 1). We assume that the decision variables are computed by a separate set of "decision neurons" that receive inputs from the motion detection network. These neurons are once again leaky-integrator neurons as described by Equation 11.44, with the driving inputs $r(t)$ being determined by inhibition between the summed inputs from the two chains in the motion detection network (as in equation (11.42)). The output of the model is "L" if $d_L(t) > c$ and "R" if $d_R(t) > c$, where c is a "confidence threshold" that depends on task constraints (for example, accuracy vs. speed requirements) [35].

Figure 11.7B and C shows the responses of the two decision neurons over time for two different directions of motion and two levels of coherence. Besides correctly computing the direction of coherent motion in each case, the model also responds faster when the stimulus has higher coherence. This phenomenon can be appreciated more clearly in figure 11.7D, which predicts progressively shorter reaction times for increasingly coherent stimuli (dotted arrows).

Comparison to Neurophysiological Data

The relationship between faster rates of evidence accumulation and shorter reaction times has received experimental support from a number of studies. Figure 11.7E shows the activity of a neuron in the frontal eye fields (FEF) for fast, medium, and slow responses to a visual target [39, 40]. Schall and collaborators have shown that the distribution of monkey response times can be reproduced using the time taken by neural activity in FEF to reach a fixed threshold [15]. A similar rise-to-threshold model by Carpenter and colleagues has received strong support in human psychophysical experiments that manipulate the prior probabilities of targets [3] and the urgency of the task [35].

In the case of the random-dots task, Shadlen and collaborators have shown that in primates, one of the cortical areas involved in making the decision regarding coherent motion direction is area LIP. The activities of many neurons in this area progressively increase during the motion-viewing period, with faster rates of rise for more coherent stimuli (see figure 11.7F) [37]. This behavior is similar to the responses of "decision neurons" in the model (figure 11.7B–D), suggesting that the outputs of the recorded LIP neurons could be interpreted as representing the log-posterior ratio of one task alternative over another (see [3, 12] for related suggestions).

11.4.3 Example 3: Attention in the Visual Cortex

The responses of neurons in cortical areas V2 and V4 can be significantly modulated by attention to particular locations within an input image. McAdams and Maunsell [23] showed that the tuning curve of a neuron in cortical area V4 is multiplied by an approximately constant factor when the monkey focuses attention on a stimulus within the neuron's receptive field. Reynolds et al. [36] have shown that focusing attention on a target in the presence of distractors causes the response of a V2 or V4 neuron to closely approximate the response elicited when the target appears alone. Finally, a study by Connor et al. [4]

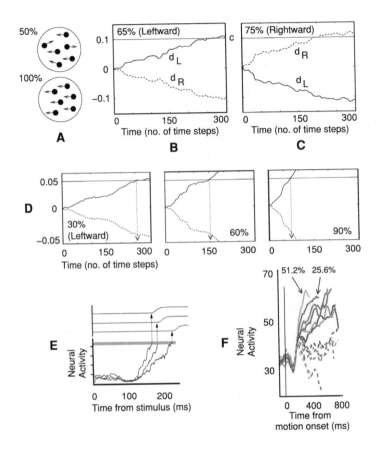

Figure 11.7   Output of Decision Neurons in the Model. (A) Depiction of the random dots task. Two different levels of motion coherence (50% and 100%) are shown. A 1-D version of this stimulus was used in the model simulations. (B) & (C) Outputs $d_L(t)$ and $d_R(t)$ of model decision neurons for two different directions of motion. The decision threshold is labeled "c." (D) Outputs of decision neurons for three different levels of motion coherence. Note the increase in rate of evidence accumulation at higher coherencies. For a fixed decision threshold, the model predicts faster reaction times for higher coherencies (dotted arrows). (E) Activity of a neuron in area FEF for a monkey performing an eye movement task (from [40] with permission). Faster reaction times were associated with a more rapid rise to a fixed threshold (see the three different neural activity profiles). The arrows point to the initiation of eye movements, which are depicted at the top. (F) Averaged firing rate over time of 54 neurons in area LIP during the random dots task, plotted as a function of motion coherence (from [37] with permission). Solid and dashed curves represent trials in which the monkey judged motion direction toward and away from the receptive field of a given neuron, respectively. The slope of the response is affected by motion coherence (compare, for example, responses for 51.2% and 25.6%) in a manner similar to the model responses shown in (D).

demonstrated that responses to unattended stimuli can be affected by spatial attention to nearby locations.

All three types of response modulation described above can be explained in terms of Bayesian inference using the hierarchical graphical model for images given in section 11.2.3 (figure 11.3). Each V4 neuron is assumed to encode a feature F_i as its preferred stimulus. A separate group of neurons (e.g., in the parietal cortex) is assumed to encode spatial locations (and potentially other spatiotemporal transformations) irrespective of feature values. Lower-level neurons (for example, in V2 and V1) are assumed to represent the intermediate representations C_i. Figure 11.3B depicts the corresponding network for neural belief propagation. Note that this network architecture mimics the division of labor between the ventral object processing ("what") stream and the dorsal spatial processing ("where") stream in the visual cortex [24].

The initial firing rates of location- and feature-coding neurons represent prior probabilities $P(L)$ and $P(F)$ respectively, assumed to be set by task-dependent feedback from higher areas such as those in prefrontal cortex. The input likelihood $P(I = I'|C)$ is set to $\sum_j w_{ij} I_j$, where the weights w_{ij} represent the attributes of C_i (specific feature at a specific location). Here, we set these weights to spatially localized oriented Gabor filters. equation (11.11) and (11.12) are assumed to be computed by feedforward neurons in the location-coding and feature-coding parts of the network, with their synapses encoding $P(C|L, F)$. Taking the logarithm of both sides of equations (11.13-11.15), we obtain equations that can be computed using leaky integrator neurons as in equation (11.32) (f and g are assumed to approximate a logarithmic transformation). Recurrent connections in equation (11.32) are used to implement the inhibitory component corresponding to the negative logarithm of the normalization constants. Furthermore, since the membrane potential $v_i(t)$ is now equal to the log of the posterior probability, i.e., $v_i(t) = \log P(F|I = I')$ (and similarly for L and C), we obtain, using equation (11.33):

$$P(\text{feature coding neuron } i \text{ spikes at time } t) \propto P(F|I = I') \qquad (11.45)$$

This provides a new interpretation of the spiking probability (or instantaneous firing rate) of a V4 neuron as representing the posterior probability of a preferred feature in an image (irrespective of spatial location).

To model the three primate experiments discussed above [4, 23, 36], we used horizontal and vertical bars that could appear at nine different locations in the input image (figure 11.8A). All results were obtained using a network with a single set of parameters. $P(C|L, F)$ was chosen such that for any given value of L and F, say location L_j and feature F_k, the value of C closest to the combination (L_j, F_k) received the highest probability, with decreasing probabilities for neighboring locations (see figure 11.8B).

Multiplicative Modulation of Responses

We simulated the attentional task of McAdams and Maunsell [23] by presenting a vertical bar and a horizontal bar simultaneously in an input image. "At-

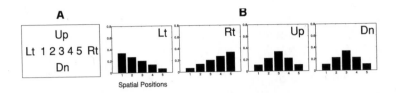

Figure 11.8   Input Image Configuration and Conditional Probabilities used in the Attention Experiments. (A) Example image locations (labeled 1-5 and Up, Dn, Lt, and Rt
for up, down, left, and right) relevant to the experiments discussed in the paper. (B)
Each bar plot shows $P(C_i|L, F)$ for a fixed value of L (= Lt, Rt, Up, or Dn) and for an
arbitrary fixed value of F. Each bar represents the probability for the feature-location
combination C_i encoding one of the locations 1-5.

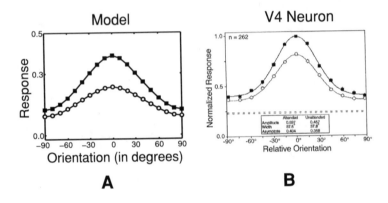

Figure 11.9   Multiplicative Modulation due to Attention. (A) Orientation tuning curve
of a feature coding model neuron with a preferred stimulus orientation of 0 degrees
with (filled squares) and without (unfilled circles) attention (from [31]). (B) Orientation tuning curves of a V4 neuron with (filled squares) and without attention (unfilled
circles) (from [23]).

tention" to a location L_i containing one of the bars was simulated by setting
a high value for $P(L_i)$, corresponding to a higher firing rate for the neuron
coding for that location.

Figure 11.9A depicts the orientation tuning curves of the vertical feature coding model V4 neuron in the presence and absence of attention (squares and
circles respectively). The plotted points represent the neuron's firing rate, en-
coding the posterior probability $P(F|I = I')$, F being the vertical feature. At-
tention in the model approximately multiplies the "unattended" responses by
a constant factor, similar to V4 neurons (figure 11.9B). This is due to the change
in the prior $P(L)$ between the two modes, which affects equation (11.12) and
(11.15) multiplicatively.

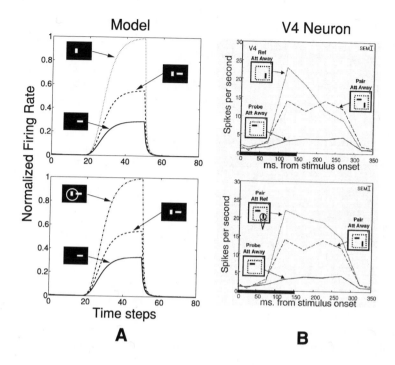

Figure 11.10 Attentional Response Restoration in the presence of Distractors. (A) (Top Panel) The three line plots represent the vertical feature coding neuron's response to a vertical bar ("Reference"), a horizontal bar at a different position ("Probe"), and both bars presented simultaneously ("Pair"). In each case, the input lasted 30 time steps, beginning at time step 20. (Bottom Panel) When "attention" (depicted as a white oval) is focused on the vertical bar, the firing rate for the Pair stimulus approximates the firing rate obtained for the Reference alone (from [31]). (B) (Top Panel) Responses from a V4 neuron without attention. (Bottom Panel) Responses from the same neuron when attending to the vertical bar (see condition Pair Att Ref) (from [36]).

Effects of Attention on Responses in the Presence of Distractors

To simulate the experiments of Reynolds et al. [36], a single vertical bar ("Reference") were presented in the input image and the responses of the vertical feature coding model neuron were recorded over time. As seen in figure 11.10A (top panel, dotted line), the neuron's firing rate reflects a posterior probability close to 1 for the vertical stimulus. When a horizontal bar ("Probe") alone is presented at a different location, the neuron's response drops dramatically (solid line) since its preferred stimulus is a vertical bar, not a horizontal bar. When the horizontal and vertical bars are simultaneously presented ("Pair"), the firing rate drops to almost half the value elicited for the vertical bar alone (dashed line), signaling increased uncertainty about the stimulus compared to the Reference-only case. However, when "attention" is turned on by increasing $P(L)$ for the vertical bar location (figure 11.10A, bottom panel), the firing rate is restored back to its original value and a posterior probability close to 1 is signaled (topmost plot, dot-dashed line). Thus, attention acts to reduce uncertainty about the stimulus given a location of interest. Such behavior closely mimics the effect of spatial attention in areas V2 and V4 [36] (figure 11.10B).

Effects of Attention on Neighboring Spatial Locations

We simulated the experiments of Connor et al. [4] using an input image containing four fixed horizontal bars as shown in figure 11.11A. A vertical bar was flashed at one of five different locations in the center (figure 11.11A, 1-5). Each bar plot in figure 11.11B shows the responses of the vertical feature coding model V4 neuron as a function of vertical bar location (bar positions 1 through 5) when attention is focused on one of the horizontal bars (left, right, upper, or lower). Attention was again simulated by assigning a high prior probability for the location of interest.

As seen in figure 11.11B, there is a pronounced effect of proximity to the locus of attention: the unattended stimulus (vertical bar) produces higher responses when it is closer to the attended location than further away (see, for example, "Attend Left"). This effect is due to the spatial spread in the conditional probability $P(C|L, F)$ (see figure 11.8B), and its effect on equation (11.12) and (11.15). The larger responses near the attended location reflect a reduction in uncertainty at locations closer to the focus of attention compared to locations farther away. For comparison, the responses from a V4 neuron are shown in figure 11.11C (from [4]).

11.5   Discussion

This chapter described models for neurally implementing the belief propagation algorithm for Bayesian inference in arbitrary graphical models. Linear and nonlinear models based on firing rate dynamics, as well as a model based on noisy spiking neurons, were presented. We illustrated the suggested approach in two domains: (1) inference over time using an HMM and its application to visual motion detection and decision-making, and (2) inference in a hierarchical graphical model and its application to understanding attentional effects in the primate visual cortex.

The approach suggests an interpretation of cortical neurons as computing the posterior probability of their preferred state, given current and past inputs. In particular, the spiking probability (or instantaneous firing rate) of a neuron can be shown to be directly proportional to the posterior probability of the preferred state. The model also ascribes a functional role to local recurrent connections (lateral/horizontal connections) in the neocortex: connections from excitatory neurons are assumed to encode transition probabilities between states from one time step to the next, while inhibitory connections are

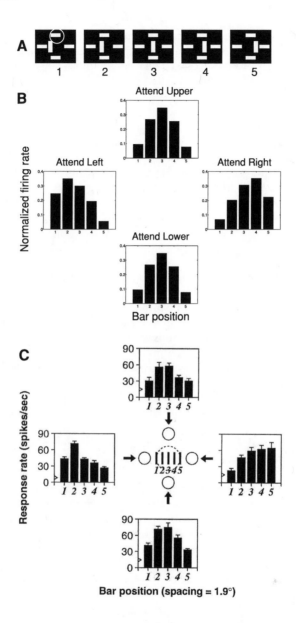

Figure 11.11 Spatial Distribution of Attention. (A) Example trial based on Connor et al.'s experiments [4] showing five images, each containing four horizontal bars and one vertical bar. Attention was focused on a horizontal bar (upper, lower, left, or right) while the vertical bar's position was varied. (B) Responses of the vertical feature coding model neuron. Each plot shows five responses, one for each location of the vertical bar, as attention was focused on the upper, lower, left, or right horizontal bar (from [31]). (C) Responses of a V4 neuron (from [4]).

used for probability normalization (see equation (11.23)). Similarly, feedback connections from higher to lower areas are assumed to convey prior probabilities reflecting prior knowledge or task constraints, as used in the attention model in section 11.4.3.

11.5.1   Related Models

A number of models have been proposed for probabilistic computation in networks of neuron-like elements. These range from early models based on statistical mechanics (such as the Boltzmann machine [19, 20]) to more recent models that explicitly rely on probabilistic generative or causal models [6, 10, 29, 33, 43, 44, 45]. We review in more detail some of the models that are closely related to the approach presented in this chapter.

Models based on Log-Likelihood Ratios

Gold and Shadlen [12] have proposed a model for neurons in area LIP that interprets their responses as representing the log-likelihood ratio between two alternatives. Their model is inspired by neurophysiological results from Shadlen's group and others showing that the responses of neurons in area LIP exhibit a behavior similar to a random walk to a fixed threshold. The neuron's response increases given evidence in favor of the neuron's preferred hypothesis and decreases when given evidence against that hypothesis, resulting in an evidence accumulation process similar to computing a log-likelihood ratio over time (see section 11.4.2). Gold and Shadlen develop a mathematical model [12] to formalize this intuition. They show how the log-likelihood ratio can be propagated over time as evidence trickles in at each time instant. This model is similar to the one proposed above involving log-posterior ratios for decision-making. The main difference is in the representation of probabilities. While we explicitly maintain a representation of probability distributions of relevant states using populations of neurons, the model of Gold and Shadlen relies on the argument that input firing rates can be directly interpreted as log-likelihood ratios without the need for explicit representation of probabilities.

An extension of the Gold and Shadlen model to the case of spiking neurons was recently proposed by Deneve [8]. In this model, each neuron is assumed to represent the log-"odds" ratio for a preferred binary-valued state, i.e., the logarithm of the probability that the preferred state is 1 over the probability that the preferred state is 0, given all inputs seen thus far. To promote efficiency, each neuron fires only when the difference between its log-odds ratio and a prediction of the log-odds ratio (based on the output spikes emitted thus far) reaches a certain threshold.

Models based on log-probability ratios such as the ones described above have several favorable properties. First, since only ratios are represented, one may not need to normalize responses at each step to ensure probabilities sum to 1 as in an explicit probability code. Second, the ratio representation lends itself naturally to some decision-making procedures such as the one postulated by Gold and Shadlen. However, the log-probability ratio representation also suffers from some potential shortcomings. Because it is a ratio, it is susceptible to instability when the probability in the denominator approaches zero (a log probability code also suffers from a similar problem), although this can be handled using bounds on what can be represented by the neural code. Also, the approach becomes inefficient when the number of hypotheses being considered is large, given the large number of ratios that may need to be represented corresponding to different combinations of hypotheses. Finally, the lack of an explicit probability representation means that many useful operations in probability calculus, such as marginalization or uncertainty estimation in specific dimensions, could become complicated to implement.

Inference Using Distributional Codes

There has been considerable research on methods for encoding and decoding information from populations of neurons. One class of methods uses basis functions (or "kernels") to represent probability distributions within neuronal ensembles [1, 2, 9]. In this approach, a distribution $P(\mathbf{x})$ over stimulus $\mathbf{x}$ is represented using a linear combination of basis functions:

$$P(\mathbf{x}) = \sum_i r_i b_i(\mathbf{x}), \tag{11.46}$$

where r_i is the normalized response (firing rate) and b_i the implicit basis function associated with neuron i in the population. The basis function of each neuron is assumed to be linearly related to the tuning function of the neuron as measured in physiological experiments. The basis function approach is similar to the approach described in this chapter in that the stimulus space is spanned by a limited number of neurons with preferred stimuli or state vectors. The two approaches differ in how probability distributions are represented by neural responses, one using an additive method and the other using a logarithmic transformation either in the firing rate representation (sections 11.3.1 and 11.3.2) or in the membrane potential representation (section 11.3.3).

   A limitation of the basis function approach is that due to its additive nature, it cannot represent distributions that are sharper than the component distributions. A second class of models addresses this problem using a generative approach, where an encoding model (e.g., Poisson) is first assumed and a Bayesian decoding model is used to estimate the stimulus $\mathbf{x}$ (or its distribution), given a set of responses r_i [28, 46, 48, 49, 51]. For example, in the distributional population coding (DPC) method [48, 49], the responses are assumed to depend on general distributions $P(\mathbf{x})$ and a maximimum a posteriori (MAP) probability distribution over possible distributions over $\mathbf{x}$ is computed. The best estimate in this method is not a single value of $\mathbf{x}$ but an entire distribution over $\mathbf{x}$, which is assumed to be represented by the neural population. The underlying goal of representing entire distributions within neural populations is common to both the DPC approach and the models presented in this chapter. However, the approaches differ in how they achieve this goal: the DPC method assumes prespecified tuning functions for the neurons and a sophisticated, non-neural decoding operation, whereas the method introduced in this chapter directly instantiates a probabilistic generative model with an exponential or linear decoding operation. Sahani and Dayan have recently extended the DPC method to the case where there is uncertainty as well as simultaneous multiple stimuli present in the input [38]. Their approach, known as doubly distributional population coding (DDPC), is based on encoding probability distributions over a function $m(\mathbf{x})$ of the input x rather than distributions over x itself. Needless to say, the greater representational capacity of this method comes at the expense of more complex encoding and decoding schemes.

The distributional coding models discussed above were geared primarily toward representing probability distributions. More recent work by Zemel and colleagues [50] has explored how distributional codes could be used for inference as well. In their approach, a recurrent network of leaky integrate-and-fire neurons is trained to capture the probabilistic dynamics of a hidden variable $X(t)$ by minimizing the Kullback-Leibler (KL) divergence between an input encoding distribution $P(X(t)|\mathbf{R}(t))$ and an output decoding distribution $Q(X(t)|\mathbf{S}(t))$, where $\mathbf{R}(t)$ and $\mathbf{S}(t)$ are the input and output spike trains respectively. The advantage of this approach over the models presented in this chapter is that the decoding process may allow a higher-fidelity representation of the output distribution than the direct representational scheme used in this chapter. On the other hand, since the probability representation is implicit in the neural population, it becomes harder to map inference algorithms such as belief propagation to neural circuitry.

Hierarchical Inference

There has been considerable interest in neural implementation of hierarchical models for inference. Part of this interest stems from the fact that hierarchical models often capture the multiscale structure of input signals such as images in a very natural way (e.g., objects are composed of parts, which are composed of subparts,..., which are composed of edges). A hierarchical decomposition often results in greater efficiency, both in terms of representation (e.g., a large number of objects can be represented by combining the same set of parts in many different ways) and in terms of learning. A second motivation for hierarchical models has been the evidence from anatomical and physiological studies that many regions of the primate cortex are hierarchically organized (e.g., the visual cortex, motor cortex, etc.).

Hinton and colleagues investigated a hierarchical network called the Helmholtz machine [16] that uses feedback connections from higher to lower levels to instantiate a probabilistic generative model of its inputs (see also [18]). An interesting learning algorithm termed the "wake-sleep" algorithm was proposed that involved learning the feedback weights during a "wake" phase based on inputs and the feedforward weights in the "sleep" phase based on "fantasy" data produced by the feedback model. Although the model employs feedback connections, these are used only for bootstrapping the learning of the feedforward weights (via fantasy data). Perception involves a single feedforward pass through the network and the feedback connections are not used for inference or top-down modulation of lower-level activities.

A hierarchical network that does employ feedback for inference was explored by Lewicki and Sejnowski [22] (see also [17] for a related model). The Lewicki-Sejnowski model is a Bayesian belief network where each unit encodes a binary state and the probability that a unit's state S_i is equal to 1 depends on the states of its parents pa$[S_i]$ via:

$$P(S_i = 1|\text{pa}[S_i], W) = h(\sum_j w_{ji}S_j),$$ (11.47)

where W is the matrix of weights, w_{ji} is the weight from S_j to S_i ($w_{ji} = 0$ for $j < i$), and h is the noisy OR function $h(x) = 1 - e^{-x}$ ($x \geq 0$). Rather than inferring a posterior distribution over states as in the models presented in this chapter, Gibbs sampling is used to obtain samples of states from the posterior; the sampled states are then used to learn the weights w_{ji}.

Rao and Ballard proposed a hierarchical generative model for images and explored an implementation of inference in this model based on predictive coding [34]. Unlike the models presented in this chapter, the predictive coding model focuses on estimating the MAP value of states rather than an entire distribution. More recently, Lee and Mumford sketched an abstract hierarchical model [21] for probabilistic inference in the visual cortex based on an inference method known as particle filtering. The model is similar to our approach in that inference involves message passing between different levels, but whereas the particle-filtering method assumes continuous random variables, our approach uses discrete random variables. The latter choice allows a concrete model for neural representation and processing of probabilities, while it is unclear how a biologically plausible network of neurons can implement the different components of the particle filtering algorithm.

The hierarchical model for attention described in section 11.4.3 bears some similarities to a recent Bayesian model proposed by Yu and Dayan [47] (see also [7, 32]). Yu and Dayan use a five-layer neural architecture and a log probability encoding scheme as in [30] to model reaction time effects and multiplicative response modulation. Their model, however, does not use an intermediate representation to factor input images into separate feature and location attributes. It therefore cannot explain effects such as the influence of attention on neighboring unattended locations [4]. A number of other neural models exist for attention, e.g., models by Grossberg and colleagues [13, 14], that are much more detailed in specifying how various components of the model fit with cortical architecture and circuitry. The approach presented in this chapter may be viewed as a first step toward bridging the gap between detailed neural models and more abstract Bayesian theories of perception.

11.5.2   Open Problems and Future Challenges

An important open problem not addressed in this chapter is learning and adaptation. How are the various conditional probability distributions in a graphical model learned by a network implementing Bayesian inference? For instance, in the case of the HMM model used in section 11.4.1, how can the transition probabilities between states from one time step to the next be learned? Can well-known biologically plausible learning rules such as Hebbian learning or the Bienenstock-Cooper-Munro (BCM) rule (e.g., see [5]) be used to learn conditional probabilities? What are the implications of spike-timing dependent plasticity (STDP) and short-term plasticity on probabilistic representations in neural populations?

A second open question is the use of spikes in probabilistic representations. The models described above were based directly or indirectly on instantaneous firing rates. Even the noisy spiking model proposed in section 11.3.3 can be regarded as encoding posterior probabilities in terms of instantaneous firing rates. Spikes in this model are used only as a mechanism for communicating information about firing rate over long distances. An intriguing alternate possibility that is worth exploring is whether probability distributions can be encoded using spike timing-based codes. Such codes may be intimately linked to timing-based learning mechanisms such as STDP.

Another interesting issue is how the dendritic nonlinearities known to exist in cortical neurons could be exploited to implement belief propagation as in equation (11.19). This could be studied systematically with a biophysical compartmental model of a cortical neuron by varying the distribution and densities of various ionic channels along the dendrites.

Finally, this chapter explored neural implementations of Bayesian inference in only two simple graphical models (HMMs and a three-level hierarchical model). Neuroanatomical data gathered over the past several decades provide a rich set of clues regarding the types of graphical models implicit in brain structure. For instance, the fact that visual processing in the primate brain involves two hierarchical but interconnected pathways devoted to spatial and object vision (the "what" and "where" streams) [24] suggests a multilevel graphical model wherein the input image is factored into progressively complex sets of object features and their transformations. Similarly, the existence of multimodal areas in the inferotemporal cortex suggests graphical models that incorporate a common modality-independent representation at the highest level that is causally related to modality-dependent representations at lower levels. Exploring such graphical models that are inspired by neurobiology could not only shed new light on brain function but also furnish novel architectures for solving fundamental problems in machine vision and robotics.

Acknowledgments This work was supported by grants from the ONR Adaptive Neural Systems program, NSF, NGA, the Sloan Foundation, and the Packard Foundation.

References

[1] Anderson CH (1995) Unifying perspectives on neuronal codes and processing. In *19th International Workshop on Condensed Matter Theories*. Caracas, Venezuela.

[2] Anderson CH, Van Essen DC (1994) Neurobiological computational systems. In Zurada JM, Marks II RJ, Robinson CJ, eds., *Computational Intelligence: Imitating Life*, pages 213–222, New York: IEEE Press.

[3] Carpenter RHS, Williams MLL (1995) Neural computation of log likelihood in control of saccadic eye movements. *Nature*, 377:59–62.

[4] Connor CE, Preddie DC, Gallant JL, Van Essen DC (1997) Spatial attention effects in macaque area V4. *Journal of Neuroscience*, 17:3201–3214.

[5] Dayan P, Abbott LF (2001) *Theoretical Neuroscience: Computational and Mathematical Modeling of Neural Systems*. Cambridge, MA: MIT Press.

[6] Dayan P, Hinton G, Neal R, Zemel R (1995) The Helmholtz machine. *Neural Computation*, 7:889–904.

[7] Dayan P, Zemel R (1999) Statistical models and sensory attention. In Willshaw D, Murray A, eds., *Proceedings of the International Conference on Artificial Neural Networks (ICANN)*, pages 1017–1022, London: IEEE Press.

[8] Deneve S (2005) Bayesian inference in spiking neurons. In Saul LK, Weiss Y, Bottou L, eds., *Advances in Neural Information Processing Systems 17*, pages 353–360, Cambridge, MA: MIT Press.

[9] Eliasmith C, Anderson CH (2003) *Neural Engineering: Computation, Representation, and Dynamics in Neurobiological Systems*. Cambridge, MA: MIT Press.

[10] Freeman WT, Haddon J, Pasztor EC (2002) Learning motion analysis. In Rao RPN, Olshausen BA, Lewicki MS, eds., *Probabilistic Models of the Brain: Perception and Neural Function*, pages 97–115, Cambridge, MA: MIT Press.

[11] Gerstner W (2000) Population dynamics of spiking neurons: Fast transients, asynchronous states, and locking. *Neural Computation*, 12(1):43–89.

[12] Gold JI, Shadlen MN (2001) Neural computations that underlie decisions about sensory stimuli. *Trends in Cognitive Sciences*, 5(1):10–16.

[13] Grossberg S (2005) Linking attention to learning, expectation, competition, and consciousness. In Itti L, Rees G, Tsotsos JK, eds., *Neurobiology of Attention*, pages 652–662. San Diego: Elsevier.

[14] Grossberg S, Raizada R (2000) Contrast-sensitive perceptual grouping and object-based attention in the laminar circuits of primary visual cortex. *Vision Research*, 40:1413–1432.

[15] Hanes DP, Schall JD (1996) Neural control of voluntary movement initiation. *Science*, 274:427–430.

[16] Hinton G, Dayan P, Frey B, Neal R (1995) The wake-sleep algorithm for unsupervised neural networks. *Science*, 268:1158–1161.

[17] Hinton G, Ghahramani Z (1997) Generative models for discovering sparse distributed representations. *Philosophical Transactions of the Royal Society of London, Series B.*, 352:1177–1190.

[18] Hinton G, Osindero S, Teh Y (2006) A fast learning algorithm for deep belief nets. *Neural Computation*, 18:1527–1554.

[19] Hinton G, Sejnowski T (1983) Optimal perceptual inference. In *Proceedings of the IEEE Conference on Computer Vision and Pattern Recognition*, pages 448–453, Washington DC 1983, New York: IEEE Press.

[20] Hinton G, Sejnowski T (1986) Learning and relearning in Boltzmann machines. In Rumelhart D, McClelland J, eds., *Parallel Distributed Processing*, volume 1, chapter 7, pages 282–317, Cambridge, MA: MIT Press.

[21] Lee TS, Mumford D (2003) Hierarchical Bayesian inference in the visual cortex. *Journal of the Optical Society of America A*, 20(7):1434–1448.

[22] Lewicki MS, Sejnowski TJ (1997) Bayesian unsupervised learning of higher order structure. In Mozer M, Jordan M, Petsche T, eds., *Advances in Neural Information Processing Systems 9*, pages 529–535, Cambridge, MA: MIT Press.

[23] McAdams CJ, Maunsell JHR (1999) Effects of attention on orientation-tuning functions of single neurons in macaque cortical area V4. *Journal of Neuroscience*, 19:431–441.

[24] Mishkin M, Ungerleider LG, Macko KA (1983) Object vision and spatial vision: two cortical pathways. *Trends in Neuroscience*, 6:414–417.

[25] Murphy K, Weiss Y, Jordan M (1999) Loopy belief propagation for approximate inference: an empirical study. In Laskey K, Prade H eds., *Proceedings of UAI (Uncertainty in AI)*, pages 467–475, San Francisco: Morgan Kaufmann.

[26] Pearl J (1988) *Probabilistic Reasoning in Intelligent Systems: Networks of Plausible Inference*. San Mateo: CA,Morgan Kaufmann.

[27] Plesser HE, Gerstner W (2000) Noise in integrate-and-fire neurons: from stochastic input to escape rates. *Neural Computation*, 12(2):367–384, .

[28] Pouget A, Zhang K, Deneve S, Latham PE (1998) Statistically efficient estimation using population coding. *Neural Computation*, 10(2):373–401.

[29] Rao RPN (1999) An optimal estimation approach to visual perception and learning. *Vision Research*, 39(11):1963–1989.

[30] Rao RPN (2004) Bayesian computation in recurrent neural circuits. *Neural Computation*, 16(1):1–38.

[31] Rao RPN (2005) Bayesian inference and attentional modulation in the visual cortex. *Neuroreport*, 16(16):1843–1848.

[32] Rao RPN (2005) Hierarchical Bayesian inference in networks of spiking neurons. In Saul LK, Weiss Y, Bottou L, eds., *Advances in Neural Information Processing Systems 17*, pages 1113–1120, Cambridge, MA: MIT Press.

[33] Rao RPN, Ballard DH (1997) Dynamic model of visual recognition predicts neural response properties in the visual cortex. *Neural Computation*, 9(4):721–763.

[34] Rao RPN, Ballard DH (1999) Predictive coding in the visual cortex: a functional interpretation of some extra-classical receptive field effects. *Nature Neuroscience*, 2(1):79–87.

[35] Reddi BA, Carpenter RH (2000) The influence of urgency on decision time. *Nature Neuroscience*, 3(8):827–830.

[36] Reynolds JH, Chelazzi L, Desimone R (1999) Competitive mechanisms subserve attention in macaque areas V2 and V4. *Journal of Neuroscience*, 19:1736–1753.

[37] Roitman JD, Shadlen MN (2002) Response of neurons in the lateral intraparietal area during a combined visual discrimination reaction time task. *Journal of Neuroscience*, 22:9475–9489.

[38] Sahani M, Dayan P (2003) Doubly distributional population codes: simultaneous representation of uncertainty and multiplicity. *Neural Computation*, 15:2255–2279.

[39] Schall JD, Hanes DP (1998) Neural mechanisms of selection and control of visually guided eye movements. *Neural Networks*, 11:1241–1251.

[40] Schall JD, Thompson KG (1999) Neural selection and control of visually guided eye movements. *Annual Review of Neuroscience*, 22:241–259.

[41] Shadlen MN, Newsome WT (2001) Neural basis of a perceptual decision in the parietal cortex (area LIP) of the rhesus monkey. *Journal of Neurophysiology*, 86(4):1916–1936.

[42] Shon AP, Rao RPN (2005) Implementing belief propagation in neural circuits. *Neurocomputing*, 65-66:393–399.

[43] Simoncelli EP (1993) *Distributed Representation and Analysis of Visual Motion*. PhD thesis, Department of Electrical Engineering and Computer Science, MIT, Cambridge, MA.

[44] Weiss Y, Fleet DJ (2002) Velocity likelihoods in biological and machine vision. In Rao RPN, Olshausen BA, Lewicki MS, eds., *Probabilistic Models of the Brain: Perception and Neural Function*, pages 77–96, Cambridge, MA: MIT Press.

[45] Weiss Y, Simoncelli EP, Adelson EH (2002) Motion illusions as optimal percepts. *Nature Neuroscience*, 5(6):598–604.

[46] Wu S, Chen D, Niranjan M, Amari SI (2003) Sequential Bayesian decoding with a population of neurons. *Neural Computation*, 15(5): 993–1012.

[47] Yu A, Dayan P (2005) Inference, attention, and decision in a Bayesian neural architecture. In Saul LK, Weiss Y, Bottou L, eds., *Advances in Neural Information Processing Systems 17*, pages 1577–1584. Cambridge, MA: MIT Press, 2005.

[48] Zemel RS, Dayan P (1999) Distributional population codes and multiple motion models. In Kearns MS, Solla SA, Cohn DA, eds., *Advances in Neural Information Processing Systems 11*, pages 174–180, Cambridge, MA: MIT Press.

[49] Zemel RS, Dayan P, Pouget A (1998) Probabilistic interpretation of population codes. *Neural Computation*, 10(2):403–430.

[50] Zemel RS, Huys QJM, Natarajan R, Dayan P (2005) Probabilistic computation in spiking populations. In Saul LK, Weiss Y, Bottou L, eds., *Advances in Neural Information Processing Systems 17*, pages 1609–1616. Cambridge, MA: MIT Press.

[51] Zhang K, Ginzburg I, McNaughton BL, Sejnowski TJ (1998) Interpreting neuronal population activity by reconstruction: A unified framework with application to hippocampal place cells. *Journal of Neurophysiology*, 79(2):1017–1044.

12 Optimal Control Theory

Emanuel Todorov

Optimal control theory is a mature mathematical discipline with numerous applications in both science and engineering. It is emerging as the computational framework of choice for studying the neural control of movement, in much the same way that probabilistic inference is emerging as the computational framework of choice for studying sensory information processing. Despite the growing popularity of optimal control models, however, the elaborate mathematical machinery behind them is rarely exposed and the big picture is hard to grasp without reading a few technical books on the subject. While this chapter cannot replace such books, it aims to provide a self-contained mathematical introduction to optimal control theory that is sufficiently broad and yet sufficiently detailed when it comes to key concepts. The text is not tailored to the field of motor control (apart from section 12.7 and the overall emphasis on systems with continuous state) so it will hopefully be of interest to a wider audience. Of special interest in the context of this book is the material on the duality of optimal control and probabilistic inference; such duality suggests that neural information processing in sensory and motor areas may be more similar than currently thought. The chapter is organized in the following sections:

1. Dynamic programming, Bellman equations, optimal value functions, value and policy iteration, shortest paths, Markov decision processes

2. Hamilton-Jacobi-Bellman equations, approximation methods, finite and infinite horizon formulations, basics of stochastic calculus

3. Pontryagin's maximum principle, ordinary differential equation and gradient descent methods, relationship to classical mechanics

4. Linear-quadratic-Gaussian control, Riccati equations, iterative linear approximations to nonlinear problems

5. Optimal recursive estimation, Kalman filter, Zakai equation

6. Duality of optimal control and optimal estimation (including new results)

7. Optimality models in motor control, promising research directions

12.1   Discrete Control: Bellman Equations

Let $x \in \mathcal{X}$ denote the state of an agent's environment, and $u \in \mathcal{U}(x)$ the action (or control) which the agent chooses while at state x. For now both $\mathcal{X}$ and $\mathcal{U}(x)$ are finite sets. Let $next(x, u) \in \mathcal{X}$ denote the state which results from applying action u in state x, and $cost(x, u) \geq 0$ the cost of applying action u in state x. As an example, x may be the city where we are now, u the flight we choose to take, $next(x, u)$ the city where that flight lands, and $cost(x, u)$ the price of the ticket. We can now pose a simple yet practical optimal control problem: find the cheapest way to fly to your destination. This problem can be formalized as follows: find an action sequence $(u_0, u_1, \cdots u_{n-1})$ and corresponding state sequence $(x_0, x_1, \cdots x_n)$ minimizing the total cost

$$ J(x., u.) = \sum_{k=0}^{n-1} cost(x_k, u_k), $$

where $x_{k+1} = next(x_k, u_k)$ and $u_k \in \mathcal{U}(x_k)$. The initial state $x_0 = x^{\text{init}}$ and destination state $x_n = x^{\text{dest}}$ are given. We can visualize this setting with a directed graph where the states are nodes and the actions are arrows connecting the nodes. If $cost(x, u) = 1$ for all (x, u) the problem reduces to finding the shortest path from x^{init} to x^{dest} in the graph.

12.1.1   Dynamic Programming

Optimization problems such as the one stated above are efficiently solved via *dynamic programming* (DP). DP relies on the following obvious fact: if a given state-action sequence is optimal, and we were to remove the first state and action, the remaining sequence is also optimal (with the second state of the original sequence now acting as initial state). This is the *Bellman optimality principle*. Note the close resemblance to the Markov property of stochastic processes (a process is Markov if its future is conditionally independent of the past given the present state). The optimality principle can be reworded in similar language: the choice of optimal actions in the future is independent of the past actions which led to the present state. Thus optimal state-action sequences can be constructed by starting at the final state and extending backward. Key to this procedure is the *optimal value function* (or optimal cost-to-go function):

$v(x) = $ "minimal total cost for completing the task starting from state x"

This function captures the long-term cost for starting from a given state, and makes it possible to find optimal actions through the following algorithm:

Consider every action available at the current state,
add its immediate cost to the optimal value of the resulting next state,
and choose an action for which the sum is minimal.

The above algorithm is "greedy" in the sense that actions are chosen based on local information, without explicit consideration of all future scenarios. And yet the resulting actions are optimal. This is possible because the optimal value function contains all information about future scenarios that is relevant to the present choice of action. Thus the optimal value function is an extremely useful quantity, and indeed its calculation is at the heart of many methods for optimal control.

The above algorithm yields an optimal action $u = \pi(x) \in \mathcal{U}(x)$ for every state x. A mapping from states to actions is called *control law* or control policy. Once we have a control law $\pi : \mathcal{X} \rightarrow \mathcal{U}(\mathcal{X})$ we can start at any state x_0, generate action $u_0 = \pi(x_0)$, transition to state $x_1 = next(x_0, u_0)$, generate action $u_1 = \pi(x_1)$, and keep going until we reach x^{dest}.

Formally, an optimal control law π satisfies

$$\pi(x) = \arg\min_{u \in \mathcal{U}(x)} \{cost(x, u) + v(next(x, u))\} \tag{12.1}$$

The minimum in equation (12.1) may be achieved for multiple actions in the set $\mathcal{U}(x)$, which is why π may not be unique. However the optimal value function v is always uniquely defined, and satisfies

$$v(x) = \min_{u \in \mathcal{U}(x)} \{cost(x, u) + v(next(x, u))\} \tag{12.2}$$

Equations (12.1) and (12.2) are the *Bellman equations* .

If for some x we already know $v(next(x, u))$ for all $u \in \mathcal{U}(x)$, then we can apply the Bellman equations directly and compute $\pi(x)$ and $v(x)$. Thus dynamic programming is particularly simple in acyclic graphs where we can start from x^{dest} with $v(x^{\text{dest}}) = 0$, and perform a backward pass in which every state is visited after all its successor states have been visited. It is straightforward to extend the algorithm to the case where we are given nonzero final costs for a number of destination states (or absorbing states).

12.1.2   Value Iteration and Policy Iteration

The situation is more complex in graphs with cycles. Here the Bellman equations are still valid, but we cannot apply them in a single pass. This is because the presence of cycles makes it impossible to visit each state only after all its successors have been visited. Instead, the Bellman equations are treated as consistency conditions and used to design iterative relaxation schemes – much like partial differential equations (PDEs) are treated as consistency conditions and solved with corresponding relaxation schemes. By "relaxation scheme" we mean guessing the solution, and iteratively improving the guess so as to make it more compatible with the consistency condition.

The two main relaxation schemes are *value iteration* and *policy iteration* . Value iteration uses only equation (12.2). We start with a guess $v^{(0)}$ of the optimal value function, and construct a sequence of improved guesses:

$$v^{(i+1)}(x) = \min_{u \in \mathcal{U}(x)} \left\{ cost(x, u) + v^{(i)}(next(x, u)) \right\} \tag{12.3}$$

This process is guaranteed to converge to the optimal value function v in a finite number of iterations. The proof relies on the important idea of contraction mappings : one defines the approximation error $e\left(v^{(i)}\right) = \max_x \left| v^{(i)}\left(x\right) - v\left(x\right)\right|$, and shows that the above iteration causes $e\left(v^{(i)}\right)$ to decrease as i increases. In other words, the mapping $v^{(i)} \rightarrow v^{(i+1)}$ given by equation (12.3) contracts the "size" of $v^{(i)}$ as measured by the error norm $e\left(v^{(i)}\right)$.

Policy iteration uses both equation (12.1) and (12.2). It starts with a guess $\pi^{(0)}$ of the optimal control law, and constructs a sequence of improved guesses:

$$v^{\pi^{(i)}}\left(x\right) = cost\left(x, \pi^{(i)}\left(x\right)\right) + v^{\pi^{(i)}}\left(next\left(x, \pi^{(i)}\left(x\right)\right)\right) \tag{12.4}$$

$$\pi^{(i+1)}\left(x\right) = \arg\min_{u\in\mathcal{U}(x)}\left\{cost\left(x, u\right) + v^{\pi^{(i)}}\left(next\left(x, u\right)\right)\right\}$$

The first line of equation (12.4) requires a separate relaxation to compute the value function $v^{\pi^{(i)}}$ for the control law $\pi^{(i)}$. This function is defined as the total cost for starting at state x and acting according to $\pi^{(i)}$ thereafter. Policy iteration can also be proven to converge in a finite number of iterations. It is not obvious which algorithm is better, because each of the two nested relaxations in policy iteration converges faster than the single relaxation in value iteration. In practice, both algorithms are used depending on the problem at hand.

12.1.3   Markov Decision Processes

The problems considered thus far are deterministic, in the sense that applying action u at state x always yields the same next state $next\left(x, u\right)$. Dynamic programming easily generalizes to the stochastic case where we have a probability distribution over possible next states:

$$p\left(y|x, u\right) = \text{"probability that } next\left(x, u\right) = y\text{"}$$

In order to qualify as a probability distribution the function p must satisfy

$$\sum_{y\in\mathcal{X}} p\left(y|x, u\right) = 1$$

$$p\left(y|x, u\right) \geq 0$$

In the stochastic case the value function from equation (12.2) becomes

$$v\left(x\right) = \min_{u\in\mathcal{U}(x)}\left\{cost\left(x, u\right) + E\left[v\left(next\left(x, u\right)\right)\right]\right\}, \tag{12.5}$$

where E denotes expectation over $next\left(x, u\right)$, and is computed as

$$E\left[v\left(next\left(x, u\right)\right)\right] = \sum_{y\in\mathcal{X}} p\left(y|x, u\right) v\left(y\right)$$

Equations (12.1), (12.3), and (12.4) generalize to the stochastic case in the same way as equation (12.2) does.

An optimal control problem with discrete states and actions and probabilistic state transitions is called a *Markov decision process* (MDP). MDPs are extensively studied in Reinforcement Learning – which is a subfield of Machine Learning focusing on optimal control problems with discrete state. In contrast, optimal control theory focuses on problems with continuous state and exploits their rich differential structure.

12.2   Continuous Control: Hamilton-Jacobi-Bellman Equations

We now turn to optimal control problems where the state $\mathbf{x} \in \mathbb{R}^{n_x}$ and control $\mathbf{u} \in \mathcal{U}(\mathbf{x}) \subseteq \mathbb{R}^{n_u}$ are real-valued vectors. To simplify notation we will use the shortcut $\min_u$ instead of $\min_{u \in \mathcal{U}(\mathbf{x})}$, although the latter is implied unless noted otherwise. Consider the stochastic differential equation

$$d\mathbf{x} = \mathbf{f}(\mathbf{x}, \mathbf{u}) \, dt + F(\mathbf{x}, \mathbf{u}) \, d\mathbf{w}, \tag{12.6}$$

where $d\mathbf{w}$ is n_w-dimensional Brownian motion. This is sometimes called a *controlled Ito diffusion*, with $\mathbf{f}(\mathbf{x}, \mathbf{u})$ being the drift and $F(\mathbf{x}, \mathbf{u})$ the diffusion coefficient. In the absence of noise, i.e. when $F(\mathbf{x}, \mathbf{u}) = 0$, we can simply write $\dot{\mathbf{x}} = \mathbf{f}(\mathbf{x}, \mathbf{u})$. However in the stochastic case this would be meaningless because the sample paths of Brownian motion are not differentiable (the term $d\mathbf{w}/dt$ is infinite). What equation (12.6) really means is that the integral of the left-hand side is equal to the integral of the right-hand side:

$$\mathbf{x}(t) = \mathbf{x}(0) + \int_0^t \mathbf{f}(\mathbf{x}(s), \mathbf{u}(s)) \, ds + \int_0^t F(\mathbf{x}(s), \mathbf{u}(s)) \, d\mathbf{w}(s)$$

The last term is an Ito integral, defined for square-integrable functions $g(t)$ as

$$\int_0^t g(s) \, dw(s) = \lim_{n \to \infty} \sum_{k=0}^{n-1} g(s_k) \left(w(s_{k+1}) - w(s_k) \right)$$
$$\text{where } 0 = s_0 < s_2 < \cdots < s_n = t$$

We will stay away from the complexities of stochastic calculus to the extent possible. Instead we will discretize the time axis and obtain results for the continuous-time case in the limit of infinitely small time step.

The appropriate Euler discretization of equation (12.6) is

$$\mathbf{x}_{k+1} = \mathbf{x}_k + \Delta \mathbf{f}(\mathbf{x}_k, \mathbf{u}_k) + \sqrt{\Delta} F(\mathbf{x}_k, \mathbf{u}_k) \, \varepsilon_k,$$

where Δ is the time step, $\varepsilon_k \sim \mathcal{N}(0, I^{n_w})$ and $\mathbf{x}_k = \mathbf{x}(k\Delta)$. The $\sqrt{\Delta}$ term appears because the variance of Brownian motion grows linearly with time, and thus the standard deviation of the discrete-time noise should scale as $\sqrt{\Delta}$.

To define an optimal control problem we also need a cost function. In finite-horizon problems, i.e. when a final time t_f is specified, it is natural to separate the total cost into a time-integral of a *cost rate* $\ell(\mathbf{x}, \mathbf{u}, t) \geq 0$, and a *final cost*

$h(\mathbf{x}) \geq 0$ which is only evaluated at the final state $\mathbf{x}(t_f)$. Thus the total cost for a given state-control trajectory $\{\mathbf{x}(t), \mathbf{u}(t) : 0 \leq t \leq t_f\}$ is defined as

$$J(\mathbf{x}(\cdot), \mathbf{u}(\cdot)) = h(\mathbf{x}(t_f)) + \int_0^{t_f} \ell(\mathbf{x}(t), \mathbf{u}(t), t)\, dt$$

Keep in mind that we are dealing with a stochastic system. Our objective is to find a control law $\mathbf{u} = \pi(\mathbf{x}, t)$ which minimizes the *expected* total cost for starting at a given $(\mathbf{x}, t)$ and acting according to π thereafter.

In discrete time the total cost becomes

$$J(\mathbf{x}., \mathbf{u}.) = h(\mathbf{x}_n) + \Delta \sum_{k=0}^{n-1} \ell(\mathbf{x}_k, \mathbf{u}_k, k\Delta),$$

where $n = t_f/\Delta$ is the number of time steps (assume that t_f/Δ is integer).

12.2.1   Derivation of the HJB Equations

We are now ready to apply dynamic programming to the time-discretized stochastic problem. The development is similar to the MDP case except that the state space is now infinite: it consists of $n + 1$ copies of $\mathbb{R}^{n_x}$. The reason we need multiple copies of $\mathbb{R}^{n_x}$ is that we have a finite-horizon problem, and therefore the time when a given $\mathbf{x} \in \mathbb{R}^{n_x}$ is reached makes a difference.

The state transitions are now stochastic: the probability distribution of $\mathbf{x}_{k+1}$ given $\mathbf{x}_k, \mathbf{u}_k$ is the multivariate Gaussian

$$\mathbf{x}_{k+1} \sim \mathcal{N}(\mathbf{x}_k + \Delta \mathbf{f}(\mathbf{x}_k, \mathbf{u}_k), \ \Delta S(\mathbf{x}_k, \mathbf{u}_k)),$$

where $S(\mathbf{x}, \mathbf{u}) = F(\mathbf{x}, \mathbf{u}) F(\mathbf{x}, \mathbf{u})^\mathsf{T}$.

The Bellman equation for the optimal value function v is similar to equation (12.5), except that v is now a function of space and time. We have

$$v(\mathbf{x}, k) = \min_{\mathbf{u}} \{\Delta \ell(\mathbf{x}, \mathbf{u}, k\Delta) + E[v(\mathbf{x} + \Delta \mathbf{f}(\mathbf{x}, \mathbf{u}) + \xi, \ k+1)]\}, \qquad (12.7)$$

where $\xi \sim \mathcal{N}(0, \ \Delta S(\mathbf{x}, \mathbf{u}))$ and $v(\mathbf{x}, n) = h(\mathbf{x})$.

Consider the second-order Taylor-series expansion of v, with the time index $k + 1$ suppressed for clarity:

$$v(\mathbf{x} + \delta) = v(\mathbf{x}) + \delta^\mathsf{T} v_\mathbf{x}(\mathbf{x}) + \tfrac{1}{2}\delta^\mathsf{T} v_{\mathbf{xx}}(\mathbf{x})\, \delta + o(\delta^3).$$

$$\text{where } \delta = \Delta \mathbf{f}(\mathbf{x}, \mathbf{u}) + \xi, \ v_\mathbf{x} = \tfrac{\partial}{\partial \mathbf{x}} v, \ v_{\mathbf{xx}} = \tfrac{\partial^2}{\partial \mathbf{x} \partial \mathbf{x}} v.$$

Now compute the expectation of the optimal value function at the next state, using the above Taylor-series expansion and only keeping terms up to first order in Δ. The result is:

$$E[v] = v(\mathbf{x}) + \Delta \mathbf{f}(\mathbf{x}, \mathbf{u})^\mathsf{T} v_\mathbf{x}(\mathbf{x}) + \tfrac{1}{2} \operatorname{tr}(\Delta S(\mathbf{x}, \mathbf{u}) v_{\mathbf{xx}}(\mathbf{x})) + o(\Delta^2)$$

The trace term appears because

$$E\left[\xi^{\mathsf{T}} v_{\mathbf{xx}} \xi\right] = E\left[\operatorname{tr}\left(\xi\xi^{\mathsf{T}} v_{\mathbf{xx}}\right)\right] = \operatorname{tr}\left(\operatorname{Cov}\left[\xi\right] v_{\mathbf{xx}}\right) = \operatorname{tr}\left(\Delta S v_{\mathbf{xx}}\right).$$

Note the second-order derivative $v_{\mathbf{xx}}$ in the first-order approximation to $E\left[v\right]$. This is a recurrent theme in stochastic calculus. It is directly related to *Ito's lemma*, which states that if $x\left(t\right)$ is an Ito diffusion with coefficient σ, then

$$dg\left(x\left(t\right)\right) = g_x\left(x\left(t\right)\right) dx\left(t\right) + \tfrac{1}{2}\sigma^2 g_{xx}\left(x\left(t\right)\right) dt.$$

Coming back to the derivation, we substitute the expression for $E\left[v\right]$ in equation (12.7), move the term $v\left(\mathbf{x}\right)$ outside the minimization operator (since it does not depend on $\mathbf{u}$), and divide by Δ. Suppressing $\mathbf{x}, \mathbf{u}, k$ on the right-hand side, we have

$$\frac{v\left(\mathbf{x}, k\right) - v\left(\mathbf{x}, k+1\right)}{\Delta} = \min_{\mathbf{u}}\left\{\ell + \mathbf{f}^{\mathsf{T}} v_{\mathbf{x}} + \tfrac{1}{2}\operatorname{tr}\left(S v_{\mathbf{xx}}\right) + o\left(\Delta\right)\right\}$$

Recall that $t = k\Delta$, and consider the optimal value function $v\left(\mathbf{x}, t\right)$ defined in continuous time. The left hand side in the above equation is then

$$\frac{v\left(\mathbf{x}, t\right) - v\left(\mathbf{x}, t+\Delta\right)}{\Delta}$$

In the limit $\Delta \to 0$ the latter expression becomes $-\frac{\partial}{\partial t} v$, which we denote $-v_t$. Thus for $0 \le t \le t_f$ and $v\left(\mathbf{x}, t_f\right) = h\left(\mathbf{x}\right)$, the following holds:

$$-v_t\left(\mathbf{x}, t\right) = \min_{\mathbf{u} \in \mathcal{U}(\mathbf{x})}\left\{\ell\left(\mathbf{x}, \mathbf{u}, t\right) + \mathbf{f}\left(\mathbf{x}, \mathbf{u}\right)^{\mathsf{T}} v_{\mathbf{x}}\left(\mathbf{x}, t\right) + \tfrac{1}{2}\operatorname{tr}\left(S\left(\mathbf{x}, \mathbf{u}\right) v_{\mathbf{xx}}\left(\mathbf{x}, t\right)\right)\right\}$$

$$(12.8)$$

Similarly to the discrete case, an optimal control $\pi\left(\mathbf{x}, t\right)$ is a value of $\mathbf{u}$ which achieves the minimum in equation (12.8):

$$\pi\left(\mathbf{x}, t\right) = \arg\min_{\mathbf{u} \in \mathcal{U}(\mathbf{x})}\left\{\ell\left(\mathbf{x}, \mathbf{u}, t\right) + \mathbf{f}\left(\mathbf{x}, \mathbf{u}\right)^{\mathsf{T}} v_{\mathbf{x}}\left(\mathbf{x}, t\right) + \tfrac{1}{2}\operatorname{tr}\left(S\left(\mathbf{x}, \mathbf{u}\right) v_{\mathbf{xx}}\left(\mathbf{x}, t\right)\right)\right\}$$

$$(12.9)$$

Equations (12.8) and (12.9) are the *Hamilton-Jacobi-Bellman* (HJB) equations .

12.2.2   Numerical Solutions of the HJB Equations

The HJB equation (12.8) is a nonlinear (due to the min operator) second-order PDE with respect to the unknown function v. If a differentiable function v satisfying equation (12.8) for all $(\mathbf{x}, t)$ exists, then it is the unique optimal value function. However, nonlinear differential equations do not always have classic solutions which satisfy them everywhere. For example, consider the equation

$|\dot{g}(t)| = 1$ with boundary conditions $g(0) = g(1) = 0$. The slope of g is either $+1$ or -1, and so g has to change slope (discontinuously) somewhere in the interval $0 \le t \le 1$ in order to satisfy the boundary conditions. At the points where that occurs the derivative $\dot{g}(t)$ is undefined. If we decide to admit such "weak" solutions, we are faced with infinitely many solutions to the same differential equation. In particular when equation (12.8) does not have a classic solution, the optimal value function is a weak solution but there are many other weak solutions. How can we then solve the optimal control problem? The recent development of nonsmooth analysis and the idea of *viscosity solutions* provide a reassuring answer. It can be summarized as follows: (i) "viscosity" provides a specific criterion for selecting a single weak solution; (ii) the optimal value function is a viscosity solution to the HJB equation (and thus it is the only viscosity solution); (iii) numerical approximation schemes which take the limit of solutions to discretized problems converge to a viscosity solution (and therefore to the optimal value function). The bottom line is that in practice one need not worry about the absence of classic solutions.

Unfortunately there are other practical issues to worry about. The only numerical methods guaranteed to converge to the optimal value function rely on discretizations of the state space, and the required number of discrete states is exponential in the state-space dimensionality n_x. Bellman called this the *curse of dimensionality*. It is a problem which most likely does not have a general solution. Nevertheless, the HJB equations have motivated a number of methods for approximate solution. Such methods rely on parametric models of the optimal value function, or the optimal control law, or both. Below we outline one such method.

Consider an approximation $\tilde{v}(\mathbf{x}, t; \theta)$ to the optimal value function, where θ is some vector of parameters. Particularly convenient are models of the form

$$\tilde{v}(\mathbf{x}, t; \theta) = \sum_i \phi^i(\mathbf{x}, t) \theta_i,$$

where $\phi^i(\mathbf{x}, t)$ are some predefined basis functions, and the unknown parameters θ appear linearly. Linearity in θ simplifies the calculation of derivatives:

$$\tilde{v}_{\mathbf{x}}(\mathbf{x}, t; \theta) = \sum_i \phi_{\mathbf{x}}^i(\mathbf{x}, t) \theta_i$$

and similarly for $\tilde{v}_{\mathbf{xx}}$ and $\tilde{v}_t$. Now choose a large enough set of states $(\mathbf{x}, t)$ and evaluate the right-hand side of equation (12.8) at those states (using the approximation to v and minimizing over $\mathbf{u}$). This procedure yields target values for the left hand side of equation (12.8). Then adjust the parameters θ so that $-\tilde{v}_t(\mathbf{x}, t; \theta)$ gets closer to these target values. The discrepancy being minimized by the parameter adjustment procedure is the *Bellman error*.

12.2.3   Infinite-Horizon Formulations

Thus far we focused on finite-horizon problems. There are two infinite-horizon formulations used in practice, both of which yield time-invariant forms of the

HJB equations. One is the discounted-cost formulation, where the total cost for an (infinitely long) state-control trajectory is defined as

$$J\left(\mathbf{x}\left(\cdot\right),\mathbf{u}\left(\cdot\right)\right) = \int_0^\infty \exp\left(-\alpha t\right) \ell\left(\mathbf{x}\left(t\right),\mathbf{u}\left(t\right)\right) dt$$

with $\alpha > 0$ being the discount factor. Intuitively this says that future costs are less costly (whatever that means). Here we do not have a final cost $h\left(\mathbf{x}\right)$, and the cost rate $\ell\left(\mathbf{x},\mathbf{u}\right)$ no longer depends on time explicitly. The HJB equation for the optimal value function becomes

$$\alpha v\left(\mathbf{x}\right) = \min_{\mathbf{u}\in\mathcal{U}(\mathbf{x})} \left\{\ell\left(\mathbf{x},\mathbf{u}\right) + \mathbf{f}\left(\mathbf{x},\mathbf{u}\right)^{\mathsf{T}} v_{\mathbf{x}}\left(\mathbf{x}\right) + \tfrac{1}{2}\operatorname{tr}\left(S\left(\mathbf{x},\mathbf{u}\right) v_{\mathbf{xx}}\left(\mathbf{x}\right)\right)\right\} \quad (12.10)$$

Another alternative is the average-cost-per-stage formulation, with total cost

$$J\left(\mathbf{x}\left(\cdot\right),\mathbf{u}\left(\cdot\right)\right) = \lim_{t_f\to\infty} \frac{1}{t_f} \int_0^{t_f} \ell\left(\mathbf{x}\left(t\right),\mathbf{u}\left(t\right)\right) dt$$

In this case the HJB equation for the optimal value function is

$$\lambda = \min_{\mathbf{u}\in\mathcal{U}(\mathbf{x})} \left\{\ell\left(\mathbf{x},\mathbf{u}\right) + \mathbf{f}\left(\mathbf{x},\mathbf{u}\right)^{\mathsf{T}} v_{\mathbf{x}}\left(\mathbf{x}\right) + \tfrac{1}{2}\operatorname{tr}\left(S\left(\mathbf{x},\mathbf{u}\right) v_{\mathbf{xx}}\left(\mathbf{x}\right)\right)\right\} \quad (12.11)$$

where $\lambda \geq 0$ is the average cost per stage, and v now has the meaning of a differential value function.

Equations (12.10) and (12.11) do not depend on time, which makes them more amenable to numerical approximations in the sense that we do not need to store a copy of the optimal value function at each point in time. From another point of view, however, equation (12.8) may be easier to solve numerically. This is because dynamic programming can be performed in a single backward pass through time: initialize $v\left(\mathbf{x},t_f\right) = h\left(\mathbf{x}\right)$ and simply integrate equation (12.8) backward in time, computing the spatial derivatives numerically along the way. In contrast, equation (12.10) and (12.11) call for relaxation methods (such as value iteration or policy iteration) which in the continuous-state case may take an arbitrary number of iterations to converge. Relaxation methods are of course guaranteed to converge in a finite number of iterations for any finite state approximation, but that number may increase rapidly as the discretization of the continuous state space is refined.

12.3   Deterministic Control: Pontryagin's Maximum Principle

Optimal control theory is based on two fundamental ideas. One is dynamic programming and the associated optimality principle, introduced by Bellman in the United States. The other is the *maximum principle*, introduced by Pontryagin in the Soviet Union. The maximum principle applies only to deterministic problems, and yields the same solutions as dynamic programming. Unlike dynamic programming, however, the maximum principle avoids the curse of dimensionality. Here we derive the maximum principle indirectly via the HJB equation, and directly via Lagrange multipliers. We also clarify its relationship to classical mechanics.

12.3.1   Derivation via the HJB Equations

For deterministic dynamics $\dot{\mathbf{x}} = \mathbf{f}(\mathbf{x}, \mathbf{u})$ the finite-horizon HJB equation (12.8) becomes

$$-v_t(\mathbf{x}, t) = \min_{\mathbf{u}} \left\{ \ell(\mathbf{x}, \mathbf{u}, t) + \mathbf{f}(\mathbf{x}, \mathbf{u})^\mathsf{T} v_{\mathbf{x}}(\mathbf{x}, t) \right\} \tag{12.12}$$

Suppose a solution to the minimization problem in equation (12.12) is given by an optimal control law $\pi(\mathbf{x}, t)$ which is differentiable in $\mathbf{x}$. Setting $\mathbf{u} = \pi(\mathbf{x}, t)$ we can drop the min operator in equation (12.12) and write

$$0 = v_t(\mathbf{x}, t) + \ell(\mathbf{x}, \pi(\mathbf{x}, t), t) + \mathbf{f}(\mathbf{x}, \pi(\mathbf{x}, t))^\mathsf{T} v_{\mathbf{x}}(\mathbf{x}, t)$$

This equation is valid for all $\mathbf{x}$, and therefore can be differentiated w.r.t. $\mathbf{x}$ to obtain (in shortcut notation)

$$0 = v_{t\mathbf{x}} + \ell_{\mathbf{x}} + \pi_{\mathbf{x}}^\mathsf{T}\ell_{\mathbf{u}} + \left(\mathbf{f}_{\mathbf{x}}^\mathsf{T} + \pi_{\mathbf{x}}^\mathsf{T}\mathbf{f}_{\mathbf{u}}^\mathsf{T}\right) v_{\mathbf{x}} + v_{\mathbf{x}\mathbf{x}}\mathbf{f}$$

Regrouping terms, and using the identity $\dot{v}_{\mathbf{x}} = v_{\mathbf{x}\mathbf{x}}\dot{\mathbf{x}} + v_{t\mathbf{x}} = v_{\mathbf{x}\mathbf{x}}\mathbf{f} + v_{t\mathbf{x}}$, yields

$$0 = \dot{v}_{\mathbf{x}} + \ell_{\mathbf{x}} + \mathbf{f}_{\mathbf{x}}^\mathsf{T} v_{\mathbf{x}} + \pi_{\mathbf{x}}^\mathsf{T}\left(\ell_{\mathbf{u}} + \mathbf{f}_{\mathbf{u}}^\mathsf{T} v_{\mathbf{x}}\right)$$

We now make a key observation: the term in the brackets is the gradient w.r.t. $\mathbf{u}$ of the quantity being minimized w.r.t. $\mathbf{u}$ in equation (12.12). That gradient is zero (assuming unconstrained minimization), which leaves us with

$$-\dot{v}_{\mathbf{x}}(\mathbf{x}, t) = \ell_{\mathbf{x}}(\mathbf{x}, \pi(\mathbf{x}, t), t) + \mathbf{f}_{\mathbf{x}}^\mathsf{T}(\mathbf{x}, \pi(\mathbf{x}, t)) v_{\mathbf{x}}(\mathbf{x}, t) \tag{12.13}$$

This may look like a PDE for v, but if we think of $v_{\mathbf{x}}$ as a vector $\mathbf{p}$ instead of a gradient of a function which depends on $\mathbf{x}$, then equation (12.13) is an ordinary differential equation (ODE) for $\mathbf{p}$. That equation holds along any trajectory generated by $\pi(\mathbf{x}, t)$. The vector $\mathbf{p}$ is called the *costate* vector.

We are now ready to formulate the maximum principle. It states that if $\{\mathbf{x}(t), \mathbf{u}(t) : 0 \le t \le t_f\}$ is an optimal state-control trajectory (i.e. a trajectory obtained by initializing $\mathbf{x}(0)$ and controlling the system optimally until t_f), then there exists a costate trajectory $\mathbf{p}(t)$ such that equation (12.13) holds with $\mathbf{p}$ in place of $v_{\mathbf{x}}$ and $\mathbf{u}$ in place of π. The conditions on $\{\mathbf{x}(t), \mathbf{u}(t), \mathbf{p}(t)\}$ are

$$\dot{\mathbf{x}}(t) = \mathbf{f}(\mathbf{x}(t), \mathbf{u}(t)) \tag{12.14}$$

$$-\dot{\mathbf{p}}(t) = \ell_{\mathbf{x}}(\mathbf{x}(t), \mathbf{u}(t), t) + \mathbf{f}_{\mathbf{x}}^\mathsf{T}(\mathbf{x}(t), \mathbf{u}(t)) \mathbf{p}(t)$$

$$\mathbf{u}(t) = \arg\min_{\underline{\mathbf{u}}} \left\{ \ell(\mathbf{x}(t), \underline{\mathbf{u}}, t) + \mathbf{f}(\mathbf{x}(t), \underline{\mathbf{u}})^\mathsf{T} \mathbf{p}(t) \right\}$$

The boundary condition is $\mathbf{p}\left(t_f\right) = h_{\mathbf{x}}\left(\mathbf{x}\left(t_f\right)\right)$, and $\mathbf{x}\left(0\right), t_f$ are given. Clearly the costate is equal to the gradient of the optimal value function evaluated along the optimal trajectory.

The maximum principle can be written in more compact and symmetric form with the help of the *Hamiltonian* function

$$H\left(\mathbf{x}, \mathbf{u}, \mathbf{p}, t\right) = \ell\left(\mathbf{x}, \mathbf{u}, t\right) + \mathbf{f}\left(\mathbf{x}, \mathbf{u}\right)^{\mathsf{T}} \mathbf{p} \tag{12.15}$$

which is the quantity we have been minimizing w.r.t. $\mathbf{u}$ all along (it was about time we gave it a name). With this definition, equation (12.14) becomes

$$\dot{\mathbf{x}}\left(t\right) = \tfrac{\partial}{\partial \mathbf{p}} H\left(\mathbf{x}\left(t\right), \mathbf{u}\left(t\right), \mathbf{p}\left(t\right), t\right) \tag{12.16}$$
$$-\dot{\mathbf{p}}\left(t\right) = \tfrac{\partial}{\partial \mathbf{x}} H\left(\mathbf{x}\left(t\right), \mathbf{u}\left(t\right), \mathbf{p}\left(t\right), t\right)$$
$$\mathbf{u}\left(t\right) = \arg\min_{\underline{\mathbf{u}}} H\left(\mathbf{x}\left(t\right), \underline{\mathbf{u}}, \mathbf{p}\left(t\right), t\right)$$

The remarkable property of the maximum principle is that it is an ODE, even though we derived it starting from a PDE. An ODE is a consistency condition which singles out specific trajectories without reference to neighboring trajectories (as would be the case in a PDE). This is possible because the *extremal* trajectories which solve equation (12.14) make $H_{\mathbf{u}} = \ell_{\mathbf{u}} + \mathbf{f}_{\mathbf{u}}^{\mathsf{T}}\mathbf{p}$ vanish, which in turn removes the dependence on neighboring trajectories. The ODE (12.14) is a system of $2n_x$ scalar equations subject to $2n_x$ scalar boundary conditions. Therefore we can solve this system with standard boundary-value solvers (such as Matlab's `bvp4c`). The only complication is that we would have to minimize the Hamiltonian repeatedly. This complication is avoided for a class of problems where the control appears linearly in the dynamics and quadratically in the cost rate:

dynamics: $\dot{\mathbf{x}} = \mathbf{a}\left(\mathbf{x}\right) + B\left(\mathbf{x}\right)\mathbf{u}$

cost rate: $\ell\left(\mathbf{x}, \mathbf{u}, t\right) = \tfrac{1}{2}\mathbf{u}^{\mathsf{T}} R\left(\mathbf{x}\right)\mathbf{u} + q\left(\mathbf{x}, t\right)$

In such problems the Hamiltonian is quadratic in $\mathbf{u}$ and can be minimized explicitly:

$$H\left(\mathbf{x}, \mathbf{u}, \mathbf{p}, t\right) = \tfrac{1}{2}\mathbf{u}^{\mathsf{T}} R\left(\mathbf{x}\right)\mathbf{u} + q\left(\mathbf{x}, t\right) + \left(\mathbf{a}\left(\mathbf{x}\right) + B\left(\mathbf{x}\right)\mathbf{u}\right)^{\mathsf{T}} \mathbf{p}$$
$$\arg\min_{\mathbf{u}} H = -R\left(\mathbf{x}\right)^{-1} B\left(\mathbf{x}\right)^{\mathsf{T}} \mathbf{p}$$

The computational complexity (or at least the storage requirement) for ODE solutions based on the maximum principle grows linearly with the state dimensionality n_x, and so the curse of dimensionality is avoided. One drawback is that equation (12.14) could have multiple solutions (one of which is the optimal solution) but in practice that does not appear to be a serious problem. Another drawback of course is that the solution to equation (12.14) is valid for a single initial state, and if the initial state were to change we would have to solve the problem again. If the state change is small, however, the solution change should also be small, and so we can speed up the search by initializing the ODE solver with the previous solution.

The maximum principle can be generalized in a number of ways, including terminal state constraints instead of "soft" final costs; state constraints at intermediate points along the trajectory; free (i.e. optimized) final time; first exit time; control constraints. It can also be applied in *model-predictive control* settings where one seeks an optimal state-control trajectory up to a fixed time horizon (and approximates the optimal value function at the horizon). The initial portion of this trajectory is used to control the system, and then a new optimal trajectory is computed. This is closely related to the idea of a *rollout policy* – which is essential in computer chess programs for example.

12.3.2   Derivation via Lagrange Multipliers

The maximum principle can also be derived for discrete-time systems, as we show next. Note that the following derivation is actually the more standard one (in continuous time it relies on the calculus of variations). Consider the discrete-time optimal control problem

dynamics: $\mathbf{x}_{k+1} = \mathbf{f}(\mathbf{x}_k, \mathbf{u}_k)$

cost rate: $\ell(\mathbf{x}_k, \mathbf{u}_k, k)$

final cost: $h(\mathbf{x}_n)$

with given initial state $\mathbf{x}_0$ and final time n. We can approach this as a regular constrained optimization problem: find sequences $(\mathbf{u}_0, \mathbf{u}_1, \cdots \mathbf{u}_{n-1})$ and $(\mathbf{x}_0, \mathbf{x}_1, \cdots \mathbf{x}_n)$ minimizing J subject to constraints $\mathbf{x}_{k+1} = \mathbf{f}(\mathbf{x}_k, \mathbf{u}_k)$. Constrained optimization problems can be solved with the method of Lagrange multipliers . As a reminder, in order to minimize a scalar function $g(\mathbf{x})$ subject to $c(\mathbf{x}) = 0$, we form the Lagrangian $L(\mathbf{x}, \lambda) = g(\mathbf{x}) + \lambda c(\mathbf{x})$ and look for a pair $(\mathbf{x}, \lambda)$ such that $\frac{\partial}{\partial \mathbf{x}} L = 0$ and $\frac{\partial}{\partial \lambda} L = 0$.

In our case there are n constraints, so we need a sequence of n Lagrange multipliers $(\lambda_1, \lambda_2, \cdots \lambda_n)$. The Lagrangian is

$$L(\mathbf{x}., \mathbf{u}., \lambda.) = h(\mathbf{x}_n) + \sum_{k=0}^{n-1} \left(\ell(\mathbf{x}_k, \mathbf{u}_k, k) + (\mathbf{f}(\mathbf{x}_k, \mathbf{u}_k) - \mathbf{x}_{k+1})^\mathsf{T} \lambda_{k+1} \right)$$

Define the discrete-time Hamiltonian

$$H^{(k)}(\mathbf{x}, \mathbf{u}, \lambda) = \ell(\mathbf{x}, \mathbf{u}, k) + \mathbf{f}(\mathbf{x}, \mathbf{u})^\mathsf{T} \lambda$$

and rearrange the terms in the Lagrangian to obtain

$$L = h(\mathbf{x}_n) - \mathbf{x}_n^\mathsf{T} \lambda_n + \mathbf{x}_0^\mathsf{T} \lambda_0 + \sum_{k=0}^{n-1} \left(H^{(k)}(\mathbf{x}_k, \mathbf{u}_k, \lambda_{k+1}) - \mathbf{x}_k^\mathsf{T} \lambda_k \right).$$

Now consider differential changes in L due to changes in $\mathbf{u}$ which in turn lead to changes in **x**. We have

$$dL = \left(h_{\mathbf{x}} \left(\mathbf{x}_n \right) - \lambda_n \right)^{\mathsf{T}} d\mathbf{x}_n + \lambda_0^{\mathsf{T}} d\mathbf{x}_0 +$$
$$+ \sum_{k=0}^{n-1} \left(\left(\tfrac{\partial}{\partial \mathbf{x}} H^{(k)} - \lambda_k \right)^{\mathsf{T}} d\mathbf{x}_k + \left(\tfrac{\partial}{\partial \mathbf{u}} H^{(k)} \right)^{\mathsf{T}} d\mathbf{u}_k \right).$$

In order to satisfy $\frac{\partial}{\partial \mathbf{x}_k} L = 0$ we choose the Lagrange multipliers λ to be

$$\lambda_k = \tfrac{\partial}{\partial \mathbf{x}} H^{(k)} = \ell_{\mathbf{x}} \left(\mathbf{x}_k, \mathbf{u}_k, k \right) + \mathbf{f}_{\mathbf{x}}^{\mathsf{T}} \left(\mathbf{x}_k, \mathbf{u}_k \right) \lambda_{k+1}, \quad 0 \le k < n$$
$$\lambda_n = h_{\mathbf{x}} \left(\mathbf{x}_n \right).$$

For this choice of λ the differential dL becomes

$$dL = \lambda_0^{\mathsf{T}} d\mathbf{x}_0 + \sum_{k=0}^{n-1} \left(\tfrac{\partial}{\partial \mathbf{u}} H^{(k)} \right)^{\mathsf{T}} d\mathbf{u}_k. \tag{12.17}$$

The first term in equation (12.17) is 0 because $\mathbf{x}_0$ is fixed. The second term becomes 0 when $\mathbf{u}_k$ is the (unconstrained) minimum of $H^{(k)}$. Summarizing the conditions for an optimal solution, we arrive at the discrete-time maximum principle:

$$\mathbf{x}_{k+1} = \mathbf{f} \left(\mathbf{x}_k, \mathbf{u}_k \right) \tag{12.18}$$
$$\lambda_k = \ell_{\mathbf{x}} \left(\mathbf{x}_k, \mathbf{u}_k, k \right) + \mathbf{f}_{\mathbf{x}}^{\mathsf{T}} \left(\mathbf{x}_k, \mathbf{u}_k \right) \lambda_{k+1}$$
$$\mathbf{u}_k = \arg \min_{\underline{\mathbf{u}}} H^{(k)} \left(\mathbf{x}_k, \underline{\mathbf{u}}, \lambda_{k+1} \right)$$

with $\lambda_n = h_{\mathbf{x}} \left(\mathbf{x}_n \right)$, and $\mathbf{x}_0, n$ given.

The similarity between the discrete-time (equation (12.18)) and the continuous-time (equation (12.14)) versions of the maximum principle is obvious. The costate **p**, which before was equal to the gradient $v_{\mathbf{x}}$ of the optimal value function, is now a Lagrange multiplier λ. Thus we have three different names for the same quantity. It actually has yet another name: *influence function*. This is because λ_0 is the gradient of the minimal total cost w.r.t. the initial condition $\mathbf{x}_0$ (as can be seen from equation (12.17)) and so λ_0 tells us how changes in the initial condition influence the total cost. The minimal total cost is of course equal to the optimal-value function, thus λ is the gradient of the optimal value function.

12.3.3   Numerical Optimization via Gradient Descent

From equation (12.17) it is clear that the quantity

$$\tfrac{\partial}{\partial \mathbf{u}} H^{(k)} = \ell_{\mathbf{u}} \left(\mathbf{x}_k, \mathbf{u}_k, k \right) + \mathbf{f}_{\mathbf{u}}^{\mathsf{T}} \left(\mathbf{x}_k, \mathbf{u}_k \right) \lambda_{k+1} \tag{12.19}$$

is the gradient of the total cost with respect to the control signal. This also holds in the continuous-time case. Once we have a gradient, we can optimize the (open-loop) control sequence for a given initial state via gradient descent. Here is the algorithm:

1. Given a control sequence, iterate the dynamics forward in time to find the corresponding state sequence. Then iterate equation (12.18) backward in time to find the Lagrange multiplier sequence. In the backward pass use the given control sequence instead of optimizing the Hamiltonian.

2. Evaluate the gradient using equation (12.19), and improve the control sequence with any gradient descent algorithm. Go back to step 1, or exit if converged.

As always, gradient descent in high-dimensional spaces is much more efficient if one uses a second-order method (conjugate gradient descent, Levenberg-Marquardt, Gauss-Newton, etc). Care should be taken to ensure stability. Stability of second-order optimization can be ensured via line-search or trust-region methods. To avoid local minima – which correspond to extremal trajectories that are not optimal – one could use multiple restarts with random initialization of the control sequence. Note that extremal trajectories satisfy the maximum principle, and so an ODE solver can get trapped in the same suboptimal solutions as a gradient descent method.

12.3.4   Relation to Classical Mechanics

We now return to the continuous-time maximum principle, and note that equation (12.16) resembles the Hamiltonian formulation of mechanics, with $\mathbf{p}$ being the generalized momentum (a fifth name for the same quantity). To see where the resemblance comes from, recall the Lagrange problem: given $\mathbf{x}\,(0)$ and $\mathbf{x}\,(t_f)$, find curves $\{\mathbf{x}\,(t)\,:\,0\le t\le t_f\}$ which optimize

$$J\left(\mathbf{x}\left(\cdot\right)\right)=\int_{0}^{t_f}L\left(\mathbf{x}\left(t\right),\dot{\mathbf{x}}\left(t\right)\right)dt. \tag{12.20}$$

Applying the calculus of variations, one finds that extremal curves (either maxima or minima of J) satisfy the *Euler-Lagrange equation*

$$\tfrac{d}{dt}\tfrac{\partial}{\partial\dot{\mathbf{x}}}L\left(\mathbf{x},\dot{\mathbf{x}}\right)-\tfrac{\partial}{\partial\mathbf{x}}L\left(\mathbf{x},\dot{\mathbf{x}}\right)=0$$

Its solutions are known to be equivalent to the solutions of *Hamilton's equation*:

$$\dot{\mathbf{x}}=\tfrac{\partial}{\partial\mathbf{p}}H\left(\mathbf{x},\mathbf{p}\right) \tag{12.21}$$

$$-\dot{\mathbf{p}}=\tfrac{\partial}{\partial\mathbf{x}}H\left(\mathbf{x},\mathbf{p}\right),$$

where the Hamiltonian is defined as

$$H\left(\mathbf{x},\mathbf{p}\right)=\mathbf{p}^{\mathsf{T}}\dot{\mathbf{x}}-L\left(\mathbf{x},\dot{\mathbf{x}}\right). \tag{12.22}$$

The change of coordinates $\mathbf{p}=\tfrac{\partial}{\partial\dot{\mathbf{x}}}L\left(\mathbf{x},\dot{\mathbf{x}}\right)$ is called a *Legendre transformation*. It may seem strange that $H\left(\mathbf{x},\mathbf{p}\right)$ depends on $\dot{\mathbf{x}}$ when $\dot{\mathbf{x}}$ is not explicitly an argument of H. This is because the Legendre transformation is invertible, i.e. $\dot{\mathbf{x}}$ can be recovered from $(\mathbf{x},\mathbf{p})$ as long as the matrix $\tfrac{\partial^2}{\partial\dot{\mathbf{x}}\partial\dot{\mathbf{x}}}L$ is nonsingular.

Thus the trajectories satisfying Hamilton's equation (12.21) are solutions to the Lagrange optimization problem. In order to explicitly transform equation (12.20) into an optimal control problem, define a control signal $\mathbf{u}$ and deterministic dynamics $\dot{\mathbf{x}} = \mathbf{f}(\mathbf{x}, \mathbf{u})$. Then the cost rate $\ell(\mathbf{x}, \mathbf{u}) = -L(\mathbf{x}, \mathbf{f}(\mathbf{x}, \mathbf{u})) = -L(\mathbf{x}, \dot{\mathbf{x}})$ yields an optimal control problem equivalent to equation (12.20). The Hamiltonian equation (12.22) becomes $H(\mathbf{x}, \mathbf{p}) = \mathbf{p}^\mathsf{T}\mathbf{f}(\mathbf{x}, \mathbf{u}) + \ell(\mathbf{x}, \mathbf{u})$, which is the optimal control Hamiltonian equation (12.15). Note that we can choose any dynamics $\mathbf{f}(\mathbf{x}, \mathbf{u})$, and then define the corresponding cost rate $\ell(\mathbf{x}, \mathbf{u})$ so as to make the optimal control problem equivalent to the Lagrange problem. The simplest choice is $\mathbf{f}(\mathbf{x}, \mathbf{u}) = \mathbf{u}$.

The function L is interpreted as an energy function. In mechanics it is

$$L(\mathbf{x}, \dot{\mathbf{x}}) = \tfrac{1}{2}\dot{\mathbf{x}}^\mathsf{T} M(\mathbf{x})\dot{\mathbf{x}} - g(\mathbf{x}).$$

The first term is kinetic energy (with $M(\mathbf{x})$ being the inertia matrix), and the second term is potential energy due to gravity or some other force field. When the inertia is constant, applying the Euler-Lagrange equation to the above L yields Newton's second law, $M\ddot{\mathbf{x}} = -g_{\mathbf{x}}(\mathbf{x})$, where the force $-g_{\mathbf{x}}(\mathbf{x})$ is the gradient of the potential field. If the inertia is not constant (joint-space inertia for a multijoint arm, for example), application of the Euler-Lagrange equation yields extra terms which capture nonlinear interaction forces. Geometrically, they contain Christoffel symbols of the Levi-Civita connection for the Riemannian metric given by $\langle \mathbf{y}, \mathbf{z}\rangle_{\mathbf{x}} = \mathbf{y}^\mathsf{T} M(\mathbf{x})\mathbf{z}$. We will not discuss differential geometry in any detail here, but it is worth noting that it affords a coordinate-free treatment, revealing intrinsic properties of the dynamical system that are invariant with respect to arbitrary smooth changes of coordinates. Such invariant quantities are called tensors. For example, the metric (inertia in our case) is a tensor.

12.4   Linear-Quadratic-Gaussian Control: Riccati Equations

Optimal control laws can rarely be obtained in closed form. One notable exception is the linear-quadratic Gaussian (LQG) case where the dynamics are linear, the costs are quadratic, and the noise (if present) is additive Gaussian. This makes the optimal value function quadratic, and allows minimization of the Hamiltonian in closed form. Here we derive the LQG optimal controller in continuous and discrete time.

12.4.1   Derivation via the HJB Equations

Consider the following stochastic optimal control problem:

$$\begin{aligned}
\text{dynamics:} \quad & d\mathbf{x} = (A\mathbf{x} + B\mathbf{u})\,dt + F d\mathbf{w} \\
\text{cost rate:} \quad & \ell(\mathbf{x}, \mathbf{u}) = \tfrac{1}{2}\mathbf{u}^\mathsf{T} R\mathbf{u} + \tfrac{1}{2}\mathbf{x}^\mathsf{T} Q\mathbf{x} \\
\text{final cost:} \quad & h(\mathbf{x}) = \tfrac{1}{2}\mathbf{x}^\mathsf{T} Q^f \mathbf{x}
\end{aligned}$$

where R is symmetric positive definite, Q and Q^f are symmetric positive semi-definite, and $\mathbf{u}$ is now unconstrained. We set $S = FF^\mathsf{T}$ as before. The matrices A, B, F, R, Q can be made time-varying without complicating the derivation below.

In order to solve for the optimal value function we will guess its parametric form, show that it satisfies the HJB equation (12.8), and obtain ODEs for its parameters. Our guess is

$$v(\mathbf{x}, t) = \tfrac{1}{2}\mathbf{x}^\mathsf{T} V(t)\mathbf{x} + a(t), \qquad\qquad (12.23)$$

where $V(t)$ is symmetric. The boundary condition $v(\mathbf{x}, t_f) = h(\mathbf{x})$ implies $V(t_f) = Q^f$ and $a(t_f) = 0$. From equation (12.23) we can compute the derivatives which enter into the HJB equation:

$$v_t(\mathbf{x}, t) = \tfrac{1}{2}\mathbf{x}^\mathsf{T} \dot{V}(t)\mathbf{x} + \dot{a}(t)$$
$$v_{\mathbf{x}}(\mathbf{x}, t) = V(t)\mathbf{x}$$
$$v_{\mathbf{xx}}(\mathbf{x}, t) = V(t)$$

Substituting these expressions in equation (12.8) yields

$$-\tfrac{1}{2}\mathbf{x}^\mathsf{T} \dot{V}(t)\mathbf{x} - \dot{a}(t) =$$
$$= \min_{\mathbf{u}} \left\{ \tfrac{1}{2}\mathbf{u}^\mathsf{T} R\mathbf{u} + \tfrac{1}{2}\mathbf{x}^\mathsf{T} Q\mathbf{x} + (A\mathbf{x} + B\mathbf{u})^\mathsf{T} V(t)\mathbf{x} + \tfrac{1}{2}\operatorname{tr}(SV(t)) \right\}$$

The Hamiltonian (i.e. the term inside the min operator) is quadratic in $\mathbf{u}$, and its Hessian R is positive definite, so the optimal control can be found analytically:

$$\mathbf{u} = -R^{-1}B^\mathsf{T} V(t)\mathbf{x} \qquad\qquad (12.24)$$

With this $\mathbf{u}$, the control-dependent part of the Hamiltonian becomes

$$\tfrac{1}{2}\mathbf{u}^\mathsf{T} R\mathbf{u} + (B\mathbf{u})^\mathsf{T} V(t)\mathbf{x} = -\tfrac{1}{2}\mathbf{x}^\mathsf{T} V(t) BR^{-1}B^\mathsf{T} V(t)\mathbf{x}$$

After grouping terms, the HJB equation reduces to

$$-\tfrac{1}{2}\mathbf{x}^\mathsf{T} \dot{V}(t)\mathbf{x} - \dot{a}(t) =$$
$$= -\tfrac{1}{2}\mathbf{x}^\mathsf{T} \left(Q + A^\mathsf{T} V(t) + V(t) A - V(t) BR^{-1}B^\mathsf{T} V(t) \right)\mathbf{x} + \tfrac{1}{2}\operatorname{tr}(SV(t))$$

where we replaced the term $2A^\mathsf{T} V$ with $A^\mathsf{T} V + VA$ to make the equation symmetric. This is justified because $\mathbf{x}^\mathsf{T} A^\mathsf{T} V\mathbf{x} = \mathbf{x}^\mathsf{T} V^\mathsf{T} A\mathbf{x} = \mathbf{x}^\mathsf{T} V A\mathbf{x}$.

Our guess of the optimal value function is correct if and only if the above equation holds for all $\mathbf{x}$, which is the case when the $\mathbf{x}$-dependent terms are matched:

$$-\dot{V}(t) = Q + A^\mathsf{T} V(t) + V(t) A - V(t) BR^{-1}B^\mathsf{T} V(t) \qquad (12.25)$$
$$-\dot{a}(t) = \tfrac{1}{2}\operatorname{trace}(SV(t))$$

Functions V, a satisfying equation (12.25) can obviously be found by initializing $V(t_f) = Q^f$, $a(t_f) = 0$ and integrating the ODE (12.25) backward in time. Thus equation (12.23) is the optimal value function with V, a given by equation (12.25), and equation (12.24) is the optimal control law (which in this case is unique).

The first line of equation (12.25) is called a *continuous-time Riccati equation*. Note that it does not depend on the noise covariance S. Consequently the optimal control law given by equation (12.24) is also independent of S. The only effect of S is on the total cost. As a corollary, the optimal control law remains the same in the deterministic case – called the *linear-quadratic regulator* (LQR).

12.4.2   Derivation via the Bellman Equations

In practice one usually works with discrete-time systems. To obtain an optimal control law for the discrete-time case one could use an Euler approximation to equation (12.25), but the resulting equation is missing terms quadratic in the time step Δ, as we will see below. Instead we apply dynamic programming directly, and obtain an exact solution to the discrete-time LQR problem. Dropping the (irrelevant) noise and discretizing the problem, we obtain

$$\begin{aligned} \text{dynamics:} \quad & \mathbf{x}_{k+1} = A\mathbf{x}_k + B\mathbf{u}_k \\ \text{cost rate:} \quad & \tfrac{1}{2}\mathbf{u}_k^\mathsf{T} R\mathbf{u}_k + \tfrac{1}{2}\mathbf{x}_k^\mathsf{T} Q\mathbf{x}_k \\ \text{final cost:} \quad & \tfrac{1}{2}\mathbf{x}_n^\mathsf{T} Q^f \mathbf{x}_n \end{aligned}$$

where $n = t_f/\Delta$ and the correspondence to the continuous-time problem is

$$\mathbf{x}_k \leftarrow \mathbf{x}(k\Delta), \ A \leftarrow (I + \Delta A), \ B \leftarrow \Delta B, \ R \leftarrow \Delta R, \ Q \leftarrow \Delta Q \qquad (12.26)$$

The guess for the optimal value function is again quadratic

$$v(\mathbf{x}, k) = \tfrac{1}{2}\mathbf{x}^\mathsf{T} V_k \mathbf{x}$$

with boundary condition $V_n = Q^f$. The Bellman equation (12.2) is

$$\tfrac{1}{2}\mathbf{x}^\mathsf{T} V_k \mathbf{x} = \min_{\mathbf{u}} \left\{ \tfrac{1}{2}\mathbf{u}^\mathsf{T} R\mathbf{u} + \tfrac{1}{2}\mathbf{x}^\mathsf{T} Q\mathbf{x} + \tfrac{1}{2}(A\mathbf{x} + B\mathbf{u})^\mathsf{T} V_{k+1}(A\mathbf{x} + B\mathbf{u}) \right\}.$$

As in the continuous-time case the Hamiltonian can be minimized analytically. The resulting optimal control law is

$$\mathbf{u} = -\left(R + B^\mathsf{T} V_{k+1} B\right)^{-1} B^\mathsf{T} V_{k+1} A\mathbf{x}.$$

Substituting this $\mathbf{u}$ in the Bellman equation, we obtain

$$V_k = Q + A^\mathsf{T} V_{k+1} A - A^\mathsf{T} V_{k+1} B \left(R + B^\mathsf{T} V_{k+1} B\right)^{-1} B^\mathsf{T} V_{k+1} A. \qquad (12.27)$$

This completes the proof that the optimal value function is in the assumed quadratic form. To compute V_k for all k we initialize $V_n = Q^f$ and iterate equation (12.27) backward in time.

The optimal control law is linear in $\mathbf{x}$, and is usually written as

$$\mathbf{u}_k = -L_k \mathbf{x}_k \tag{12.28}$$

where $L_k = \left(R + B^{\mathsf{T}} V_{k+1} B\right)^{-1} B^{\mathsf{T}} V_{k+1} A$.

The time-varying matrix L_k is called the *control gain*. It does not depend on the sequence of states, and therefore can be computed offline. Equation (12.27) is called a *discrete-time Riccati equation*. Clearly the discrete-time Riccati equation contains more terms that the continuous-time Riccati equation (12.25), and so the two are not identical. However one can verify that they become identical in the limit $\Delta \to 0$. To this end replace the matrices in equation (12.27) with their continuous-time analogs given by equation (12.26), and after rearrangement obtain

$$\frac{V_k - V_{k+1}}{\Delta} = Q + A^{\mathsf{T}} V_{k+1} + V_{k+1} A - V_{k+1} B \left(R + \Delta B^{\mathsf{T}} V_{k+1} B\right)^{-1} B^{\mathsf{T}} V_{k+1} + \frac{o\left(\Delta^2\right)}{\Delta},$$

where $o\left(\Delta^2\right)$ absorbs terms that are second-order in Δ. Taking the limit $\Delta \to 0$ yields the continuous-time Riccati equation (12.25).

12.4.3   Applications to Nonlinear Problems

Apart from solving LQG problems, the methodology described here can be adapted to yield approximate solutions to non-LQG optimal control problems. This is done iteratively, as follows:

1. Given a control sequence, apply it to the (nonlinear) dynamics and obtain a corresponding state sequence.

2. Construct a time-varying linear approximation to the dynamics and a time-varying quadratic approximation to the cost; both approximations are centered at the state-control sequence obtained in step 1. This yields an LQG optimal control problem with respect to the state and control deviations.

3. Solve the resulting LQG problem, obtain the control deviation sequence, and add it to the given control sequence. Go to step 1, or exit if converged. Note that multiplying the deviation sequence by a number smaller than 1 can be used to implement line-search.

Another possibility is to use *differential dynamic programming* (DDP), which is based on the same idea but involves a second-order rather than a first-order approximation to the dynamics. In that case the approximate problem is not LQG; however, one can assume a quadratic approximation to the optimal value function and derive Riccati-like equations for its parameters. DDP and iterative LQG (iLQG) have second-order convergence in the neighborhood of an optimal solution. They can be thought of as the analog of Newton's method in the domain of optimal control. Unlike general-purpose second order methods which construct Hessian approximations using gradient information, DDP and iLQG obtain the Hessian directly by exploiting the problem structure. For deterministic problems they converge to state-control trajectories which satisfy the maximum principle, but in addition, yield local feedback control laws. In our experience they are more efficient that either ODE or gradient descent methods. iLQG has been generalized to stochastic systems (including multiplicative noise) and to systems subject to control constraints.

12.5   Optimal Estimation: Kalman Filter

Optimal control is closely related to optimal estimation, for two reasons: (i) the only way to achieve optimal performance in the presence of sensor noise and delays is to incorporate an optimal estimator in the control system; (ii) the two problems are dual, as explained below. The most widely used optimal estimator is the *Kalman filter*. It is the dual of the linear-quadratic regulator – which in turn is the most widely used optimal controller.

12.5.1   The Kalman Filter

Consider the partially observable linear dynamical system:

$$
\begin{aligned}
\text{dynamics:} \qquad & \mathbf{x}_{k+1} = A\mathbf{x}_k + \mathbf{w}_k \\
\text{observation:} \qquad & \mathbf{y}_k = H\mathbf{x}_k + \mathbf{v}_k
\end{aligned}
\qquad (12.29)
$$

where $\mathbf{w}_k \sim \mathcal{N}(0, S)$ and $\mathbf{v}_k \sim \mathcal{N}(0, P)$ are independent Gaussian random variables, the initial state has a Gaussian prior distribution $\mathbf{x}_0 \sim \mathcal{N}(\widehat{\mathbf{x}}_0, \Sigma_0)$, and $A, H, S, P, \widehat{\mathbf{x}}_0, \Sigma_0$ are known. The states are hidden and all we have access to are the observations. The objective is to compute the posterior probability distribution $\widehat{p}_k$ of $\mathbf{x}_k$ given observations $\mathbf{y}_{k-1} \cdots \mathbf{y}_0$:

$$
\begin{aligned}
\widehat{p}_k &= p(\mathbf{x}_k | \mathbf{y}_{k-1} \cdots \mathbf{y}_0) \\
\widehat{p}_0 &= \mathcal{N}(\widehat{\mathbf{x}}_0, \Sigma_0)
\end{aligned}
$$

Note that our formulation is somewhat unusual: we are estimating $\mathbf{x}_k$ before $\mathbf{y}_k$ has been observed. This formulation is adopted here because it simplifies the results and also because most real-world sensors provide delayed measurements.

We will show by induction (moving forward in time) that $\widehat{p}_k$ is Gaussian for all k, and therefore can be represented by its mean $\widehat{\mathbf{x}}_k$ and covariance matrix Σ_k. This holds for $k = 0$ by definition. The Markov property of equation (12.29) implies that the posterior $\widehat{p}_k$ can be treated as prior over $\mathbf{x}_k$ for the purposes of estimation after time k. Since $\widehat{p}_k$ is Gaussian and equation (12.29) is linear-Gaussian, the joint distribution of $\mathbf{x}_{k+1}$ and $\mathbf{y}_k$ is also Gaussian. Its mean and covariance given the prior $\widehat{p}_k$ are easily computed:

$$E\begin{bmatrix} \mathbf{x}_{k+1} \\ \mathbf{y}_k \end{bmatrix} = \begin{bmatrix} A\widehat{\mathbf{x}}_k \\ H\widehat{\mathbf{x}}_k \end{bmatrix}, \quad \mathrm{Cov}\begin{bmatrix} \mathbf{x}_{k+1} \\ \mathbf{y}_k \end{bmatrix} = \begin{bmatrix} S + A\Sigma_k A^\mathsf{T} & A\Sigma_k H^\mathsf{T} \\ H\Sigma_k A^\mathsf{T} & P + H\Sigma_k H^\mathsf{T} \end{bmatrix}$$

Now we need to compute the probability of $\mathbf{x}_{k+1}$ conditional on the new observation $\mathbf{y}_k$. This is done using an important property of multivariate Gaussians summarized in the following lemma:

Let $\mathbf{p}$ and $\mathbf{q}$ be jointly Gaussian, with means $\bar{\mathbf{p}}$ and $\bar{\mathbf{q}}$ and covariances $\Sigma_{\mathbf{pp}}, \Sigma_{\mathbf{qq}}$ and $\Sigma_{\mathbf{pq}} = \Sigma_{\mathbf{qp}}^\mathsf{T}$. Then the conditional distribution of $\mathbf{p}$ given $\mathbf{q}$ is Gaussian, with mean and covariance

$$E[\mathbf{p}|\mathbf{q}] = \bar{\mathbf{p}} + \Sigma_{\mathbf{pq}}\Sigma_{\mathbf{qq}}^{-1}(\mathbf{q} - \bar{\mathbf{q}})$$
$$\mathrm{Cov}[\mathbf{p}|\mathbf{q}] = \Sigma_{\mathbf{pp}} - \Sigma_{\mathbf{pq}}\Sigma_{\mathbf{qq}}^{-1}\Sigma_{\mathbf{qp}}$$

Applying the lemma to our problem, we see that $\widehat{p}_{k+1}$ is Gaussian with mean

$$\widehat{\mathbf{x}}_{k+1} = A\widehat{\mathbf{x}}_k + A\Sigma_k H^\mathsf{T}\left(P + H\Sigma_k H^\mathsf{T}\right)^{-1}(\mathbf{y}_k - H\widehat{\mathbf{x}}_k) \qquad (12.30)$$

and covariance matrix

$$\Sigma_{k+1} = S + A\Sigma_k A^\mathsf{T} - A\Sigma_k H^\mathsf{T}\left(P + H\Sigma_k H^\mathsf{T}\right)^{-1}H\Sigma_k A^\mathsf{T}. \qquad (12.31)$$

This completes the induction proof. Equation (12.31) is a Riccati equation. Equation (12.30) is usually written as

$$\widehat{\mathbf{x}}_{k+1} = A\widehat{\mathbf{x}}_k + K_k(\mathbf{y}_k - H\widehat{\mathbf{x}}_k)$$
$$\text{where } K_k = A\Sigma_k H^\mathsf{T}\left(P + H\Sigma_k H^\mathsf{T}\right)^{-1}.$$

The time-varying matrix K_k is called the *filter gain*. It does not depend on the observation sequence and therefore can be computed offline. The quantity $\mathbf{y}_k - H\widehat{\mathbf{x}}_k$ is called the *innovation*. It is the mismatch between the observed and the expected measurement. The covariance Σ_k of the posterior probability distribution $p(\mathbf{x}_k|\mathbf{y}_{k-1}\cdots\mathbf{y}_0)$ is the *estimation error covariance*. The estimation error is $\mathbf{x}_k - \widehat{\mathbf{x}}_k$.

The above derivation corresponds to the discrete-time Kalman filter. A similar result holds in continuous time, and is called the *Kalman-Bucy filter*. It is possible to write down the Kalman filter in equivalent forms which have numerical advantages. One such approach is to propagate the matrix square root of Σ. This is called a *square-root filter*, and involves Riccati-like equations which are more stable because the dynamic range of the elements of Σ is reduced. Another approach is to propagate the inverse covariance Σ^{-1}. This is called an *information filter*, and again involves Riccati-like equations. The information filter can represent numerically very large covariances (and even infinite covariances – which are useful for specifying "noninformative" priors).

Instead of filtering one can do smoothing, i.e. obtain state estimates using observations from the past and from the future. In that case the posterior probability of each state given all observations is still Gaussian, and its parameters can be found by an additional backward pass known as *Rauch recursion*. The resulting *Kalman smoother* is closely related to the forward-backward algorithm for probabilistic inference in *hidden Markov models* (HMMs).

The Kalman filter is optimal in many ways. First of all it is a Bayesian filter, in the sense that it computes the posterior probability distribution over the hidden state. In addition, the mean $\hat{x}$ is the optimal point estimator with respect to multiple loss functions. Recall that optimality of point estimators is defined through a loss function $\ell(x, \hat{x})$ which quantifies how bad it is to estimate $\hat{x}$ when the true state is x. Some possible loss functions are $\|x - \hat{x}\|^2$, $\|x - \hat{x}\|$, $\delta(x - \hat{x})$, and the corresponding optimal estimators are the mean, median, and mode of the posterior probability distribution. If the posterior is Gaussian, then the mean, median, and mode coincide. If we choose an unusual loss function for which the optimal point estimator is not $\hat{x}$, even though the posterior is Gaussian, the information contained in $\hat{x}$ and Σ is still sufficient to compute the optimal point estimator. This is because $\hat{x}$ and Σ are *sufficient statistics* which fully describe the posterior probability distribution, which in turn captures all information about the state that is available in the observation sequence. The set of sufficient statistics can be thought of as an augmented state, with respect to which the partially observed process has a Markov property. It is called the *belief state* or, alternatively, the *information state*.

12.5.2   Beyond the Kalman Filter

When the estimation problem involves nonlinear dynamics or non-Gaussian noise the posterior probability distribution rarely has a finite set of sufficient statistics (although there are exceptions such as the *Benes* system). In that case one has to rely on numerical approximations. The most widely used approximation is the *extended Kalman filter* (EKF). It relies on local linearization centered at the current state estimate and closely resembles the LQG approximation to non-LQG optimal control problems. The EKF is not guaranteed to be optimal in any sense, but in practice if often yields good results – especially when the posterior is single-peaked. There is a recent improvement, called the *unscented filter*, which propagates the covariance using deterministic sampling instead of linearization of the system dynamics. The unscented filter tends to be superior to the EKF and requires a comparable amount of computation. An even more accurate, although computationally more expensive approach, is *particle filtering*. Instead of propagating a Gaussian approximation it propagates a cloud of points sampled from the posterior (without actually computing the posterior). Key to its success is the idea of *importance sampling*.

Even when the posterior does not have a finite set of sufficient statistics, it is still a well-defined scalar function over the state space, and as such must obey some equation. In discrete time this equation is simply a recursive version of Bayes' rule – which is not too revealing. In continuous time, however, the posterior satisfies a PDE which resembles the HJB equation. Before we present this result we need some notation. Consider the stochastic differential equations

$$d\mathbf{x} = \mathbf{f}(\mathbf{x})\,dt + F(\mathbf{x})\,d\mathbf{w} \tag{12.32}$$
$$d\mathbf{y} = \mathbf{h}(\mathbf{x})\,dt + d\mathbf{v}.$$

where $\mathbf{w}(t)$ and $\mathbf{v}(t)$ are Brownian motion processes, $\mathbf{x}(t)$ is the hidden state, and $\mathbf{y}(t)$ is the observation sequence. Define $S(\mathbf{x}) = F(\mathbf{x})F(\mathbf{x})^{\mathsf{T}}$ as before. One would normally think of the increments of $\mathbf{y}(t)$ as being the observations, but in continuous time these increments are infinite and so we work with their time-integral.

Let $p(\mathbf{x}, t)$ be the probability distribution of $\mathbf{x}(t)$ in the absence of any observations. At $t = 0$ it is initialized with a given prior $p(\mathbf{x}, 0)$. For $t > 0$ it is governed by the first line of equation (12.32), and can be shown to satisfy

$$p_t = -\mathbf{f}^{\mathsf{T}} p_{\mathbf{x}} + \tfrac{1}{2}\operatorname{tr}(S p_{\mathbf{x}\mathbf{x}}) + \left(-\sum_i \tfrac{\partial}{\partial x_i} f_i + \tfrac{1}{2}\sum_{ij} \tfrac{\partial^2}{\partial x_i \partial x_j} S_{ij}\right)p.$$

This is called the *forward Kolmogorov equation*, or alternatively the *Fokker-Planck equation*. We have written it in expanded form to emphasize the resemblance to the HJB equation. The more usual form is

$$\tfrac{\partial}{\partial t} p = -\sum_i \tfrac{\partial}{\partial x_i}(f_i p) + \tfrac{1}{2}\sum_{ij} \tfrac{\partial^2}{\partial x_i \partial x_j}(S_{ij} p).$$

Let $\tilde{p}(\mathbf{x}, t)$ be an unnormalized posterior over $\mathbf{x}(t)$ given the observations $\{\mathbf{y}(s) : 0 \le s \le t\}$; "unnormalized" means that the actual posterior $\hat{p}(\mathbf{x}, t)$ can be recovered by normalizing: $\hat{p}(\mathbf{x}, t) = \tilde{p}(\mathbf{x}, t)/\int \tilde{p}(\mathbf{z}, t)\,d\mathbf{z}$. It can be shown that some unnormalized posterior $\tilde{p}$ satisfies *Zakai's equation*:

$$d\tilde{p} = \left(-\sum_i \tfrac{\partial}{\partial x_i}(f_i \tilde{p}) + \tfrac{1}{2}\sum_{ij} \tfrac{\partial^2}{\partial x_i \partial x_j}(S_{ij}\tilde{p})\right)dt + \mathbf{h}^{\mathsf{T}}\tilde{p}\,d\mathbf{y}$$

The first term on the right reflects the prior and is the same as in the Kolmogorov equation (except that we have multiplied both sides by dt). The second term incorporates the observation and makes Zakai's equation a stochastic PDE. After certain manipulations (conversion to Stratonovich form and a gauge transformation) the second term can be integrated by parts, leading to a regular PDE. One can then approximate the solution to that PDE numerically via discretization methods. As in the HJB equation, however, such methods are only applicable in low-dimensional spaces due to the curse of dimensionality.

12.6   Duality of Optimal Control and Optimal Estimation

Optimal control and optimal estimation are closely related mathematical problems. The best-known example is the duality of the linear-quadratic regulator and the Kalman filter. To see that duality more clearly, we repeat the corresponding Riccati equations (12.27) and (12.31) side by side:

control: $V_k = Q + A^{\mathsf{T}}V_{k+1}A - A^{\mathsf{T}}V_{k+1}B\left(R + B^{\mathsf{T}}V_{k+1}B\right)^{-1}B^{\mathsf{T}}V_{k+1}A$

filtering: $\cdot\ \Sigma_{k+1} = S + A\Sigma_k A^{\mathsf{T}} - A\Sigma_k H^{\mathsf{T}}\left(P + H\Sigma_k H^{\mathsf{T}}\right)^{-1}H\Sigma_k A^{\mathsf{T}}$

These equations are identical up to a time reversal and some matrix transposes. The correspondence is given in the following table:

$$
\begin{array}{lcccccc}
\text{control:} & V & Q & A & B & R & k \\
& \updownarrow & & & & & \\
\text{filtering:} & \Sigma & S & A^{\mathsf{T}} & H^{\mathsf{T}} & P & n-k
\end{array}
\tag{12.33}
$$

The above duality was first described by Kalman in his seminal 1960 paper introducing the discrete-time Kalman filter, and is now mentioned in most books on estimation and control. However, its origin and meaning are not apparent. This is because the Kalman filter is optimal from multiple points of view and can be written in multiple forms, making it hard to tell which of its properties have a dual in the control domain.

Attempts to generalize the duality to non-LQG settings have revealed that the fundamental relationship is between the optimal value function and the negative log-posterior. This is actually inconsistent with equation (12.33), although the inconsistency has not been made explicit before. Recall that V is the Hessian of the optimal value function. The posterior is Gaussian with covariance matrix Σ, and thus the Hessian of the negative log-posterior is Σ^{-1}. However in equation (12.33) we have V corresponding to Σ and not to Σ^{-1}. Another problem is that while A^{T} in equation (12.33) makes sense for linear dynamics $\dot{x} = Ax$, the meaning of "transpose" for general nonlinear dynamics $\dot{x} = f(x)$ is unclear. Thus the duality described by Kalman is specific to LQG systems and does not generalize.

12.6.1   General Duality of Optimal Control and MAP Smoothing

We now discuss an alternative approach which does generalize. In fact we start with the general case and later specialize it to the LQG setting to obtain something known as a *minimum-energy* estimator . As far as we know, the general treatment presented here is a novel result. The duality we establish is between maximum a posteriori (MAP) smoothing and deterministic optimal control for systems with continuous state. For systems with discrete state (i.e. HMMs) an instance of such duality is the *Viterbi algorithm* – which finds the most likely state sequence using dynamic programming.

Consider the discrete-time partially observable system

$$
\begin{aligned}
p\left(\mathbf{x}_{k+1}|\mathbf{x}_k\right) &= \exp\left(-a\left(\mathbf{x}_{k+1}, \mathbf{x}_k\right)\right) \\
p\left(\mathbf{y}_k|\mathbf{x}_k\right) &= \exp\left(-b\left(\mathbf{y}_k, \mathbf{x}_k\right)\right) \\
p\left(\mathbf{x}_0\right) &= \exp\left(-c\left(\mathbf{x}_0\right)\right).
\end{aligned}
\tag{12.34}
$$

where a, b, c are the negative log-probabilities of the state transitions, observation emissions, and initial state respectively. The states are hidden and we only have access to the observations $(\mathbf{y}_1, \mathbf{y}_2, \cdots \mathbf{y}_n)$. Our objective is to find the most probable sequence of states $(\mathbf{x}_0, \mathbf{x}_1, \cdots \mathbf{x}_n)$, that is, the sequence which maximizes the posterior probability

$$p(\mathbf{x}.|\mathbf{y}.) = \frac{p(\mathbf{y}.|\mathbf{x}.)\,p(\mathbf{x}.)}{p(\mathbf{y}.)}.$$

The term $p(\mathbf{y}.)$ does not affect the maximization and so it can be dropped. Using the Markov property of equation (12.34) we have

$$p(\mathbf{y}.|\mathbf{x}.)\,p(\mathbf{x}.) = p(\mathbf{x}_0)\prod_{k=1}^{n} p(\mathbf{x}_k|\mathbf{x}_{k-1})\,p(\mathbf{y}_k|\mathbf{x}_k)$$

$$= \exp\left(-c(\mathbf{x}_0)\right)\prod_{k=1}^{n}\exp\left(-a(\mathbf{x}_k,\mathbf{x}_{k-1})\right)\exp\left(-b(\mathbf{y}_k,\mathbf{x}_k)\right)$$

$$= \exp\left(-c(\mathbf{x}_0) - \sum_{k=1}^{n}\left(a(\mathbf{x}_k,\mathbf{x}_{k-1}) + b(\mathbf{y}_k,\mathbf{x}_k)\right)\right).$$

Maximizing $\exp(-J)$ is equivalent to minimizing J. Therefore the most probable state sequence is the one which minimizes

$$J(\mathbf{x}.) = c(\mathbf{x}_0) + \sum_{k=1}^{n}\left(a(\mathbf{x}_k,\mathbf{x}_{k-1}) + b(\mathbf{y}_k,\mathbf{x}_k)\right). \qquad (12.35)$$

This is beginning to look like a total cost for a deterministic optimal control problem. However we are still missing a control signal. To remedy that we will define the passive dynamics as the expected state transition:

$$\mathbf{f}(\mathbf{x}_k) = E\left[\mathbf{x}_{k+1}|\mathbf{x}_k\right] = \int \mathbf{z}\exp\left(-a(\mathbf{z},\mathbf{x}_k)\right)d\mathbf{z}$$

and then define the control signal as the deviation from the expected state transition:

$$\mathbf{x}_{k+1} = \mathbf{f}(\mathbf{x}_k) + \mathbf{u}_k \qquad (12.36)$$

The control cost is now defined as

$$r(\mathbf{u}_k,\mathbf{x}_k) = a\left(\mathbf{f}(\mathbf{x}_k) + \mathbf{u}_k, \mathbf{x}_k\right), \quad 0 \le k < n$$

and the state cost is defined as

$$q(\mathbf{x}_0,0) = c(\mathbf{x}_0)$$
$$q(\mathbf{x}_k,k) = b(\mathbf{y}_k,\mathbf{x}_k), \quad 0 < k \le n$$

The observation sequence is fixed, and so q is well-defined as long as it depends explicitly on the time index k. Note that we could have chosen any $\mathbf{f}$; however, the present choice will make intuitive sense later.

With these definitions, the control system with dynamics (12.36), cost rate

$$\ell(\mathbf{x}_k,\mathbf{u}_k,k) = r(\mathbf{u}_k,\mathbf{x}_k) + q(\mathbf{x}_k,k), \quad 0 \le k < n$$

and final cost $q(\mathbf{x}_n,n)$ achieves total cost (12.35). Thus the MAP smoothing problem has been transformed into a deterministic optimal control problem. We can now bring any method for optimal control to bear on MAP smoothing. Of particular interest is the maximum principle – which can avoid the curse of dimensionality even when the posterior of the partially observable system does not have a finite set of sufficient statistics.

12.6.2   Duality of LQG Control and Kalman Smoothing

Let us now specialize these results to the LQG setting. Consider again the partially observable system (12.29) discussed earlier. The posterior is Gaussian, therefore the MAP smoother and the Kalman smoother yield identical state estimates. The negative log-probabilities from equation (12.34) now become

$$a\left(\mathbf{x}_k, \mathbf{x}_{k-1}\right) = \tfrac{1}{2}\left(\mathbf{x}_k - A\mathbf{x}_{k-1}\right)^{\mathsf{T}} S^{-1}\left(\mathbf{x}_k - A\mathbf{x}_{k-1}\right) + a_0$$

$$b\left(\mathbf{y}_k, \mathbf{x}_k\right) = \tfrac{1}{2}\left(\mathbf{y}_k - H\mathbf{x}_k\right)^{\mathsf{T}} P^{-1}\left(\mathbf{y}_k - H\mathbf{x}_k\right) + b_0$$

$$c\left(\mathbf{x}_0\right) = \tfrac{1}{2}\left(\mathbf{x}_0 - \widehat{\mathbf{x}}_0\right)^{\mathsf{T}} \Sigma_0^{-1}\left(\mathbf{x}_0 - \widehat{\mathbf{x}}_0\right) + c_0,$$

where a_0, b_0, c_0 are normalization constants. Dropping all terms that do not depend on $\mathbf{x}$, and using the fact that $\mathbf{x}_k - A\mathbf{x}_{k-1} = \mathbf{u}_{k-1}$ from equation (12.36), the quantity being minimized by the MAP smoother becomes

$$J\left(\mathbf{x}., \mathbf{u}.\right) = \sum_{k=0}^{n-1} \tfrac{1}{2}\mathbf{u}_k^{\mathsf{T}} R\mathbf{u}_k + \sum_{k=0}^{n} \left(\tfrac{1}{2}\mathbf{x}_k^{\mathsf{T}} Q_k \mathbf{x}_k + \mathbf{x}_k^{\mathsf{T}}\mathbf{q}_k\right),$$

where

$$R = S^{-1}$$

$$Q_0 = \Sigma_0^{-1}, \quad \mathbf{q}_0 = -\widehat{\mathbf{x}}_0$$

$$Q_k = H^{\mathsf{T}} P^{-1} H, \quad \mathbf{q}_k = -H^{\mathsf{T}} P^{-1} \mathbf{y}_k, \quad 0 < k \leq n.$$

Thus the linear-Gaussian MAP smoothing problem is equivalent to a linear-quadratic optimal control problem. The linear cost term $\mathbf{x}_k^{\mathsf{T}}\mathbf{q}_k$ was not previously included in the LQG derivation, but it is straightforward to do so.

Let us now compare this result to the Kalman duality (12.33). Here the estimation system has dynamics $\mathbf{x}_{k+1} = A\mathbf{x}_k + \mathbf{w}_k$ and the control system has dynamics $\mathbf{x}_{k+1} = A\mathbf{x}_k + \mathbf{u}_k$. Thus the time-reversal and the matrix transpose of A are no longer needed. Furthermore, the covariance matrices now appear inverted, and so we can directly relate costs to negative log-probabilities. Another difference is that in equation (12.33) we had $R \Longleftrightarrow P$ and $Q \Longleftrightarrow S$, while these two correspondences are now reversed.

A minimum-energy interpretation can help better understand the duality. From equation (12.29) we have $\mathbf{x}_k - A\mathbf{x}_{k-1} = \mathbf{w}_{k-1}$ and $\mathbf{y}_k - H\mathbf{x}_k = \mathbf{v}_k$. Thus the cost rate for the optimal control problem is of the form

$$\mathbf{w}^{\mathsf{T}} S^{-1} \mathbf{w} + \mathbf{v}^{\mathsf{T}} P^{-1} \mathbf{v}$$

This can be thought of as the energy of the noise signals $\mathbf{w}$ and $\mathbf{v}$. Note that an estimate for the states implies estimates for the two noise terms, and the likelihood of the estimated noise is a natural quantity to optimize. The first term above measures how far the estimated state is from the prior; it represents a control cost because the control signal pushes the estimate away from the prior. The second term measures how far the predicted observation (and thus the estimated state) is from the actual observation. One can think of this as a minimum-energy tracking problem with reference trajectory specified by the observations.

12.7   Optimal Control as a Theory of Biological Movement

To say that the brain generates the best behavior it can, subject to the constraints imposed by the body and environment, is almost trivial. After all,
the brain has evolved for the sole purpose of generating behavior advanta-
geous to the organism. It is then reasonable to expect that, at least in natural and well-practiced tasks, the observed behavior will be close to optimal.
This makes optimal control theory an appealing computational framework for
studying the neural control of movement. Optimal control is also a very successful framework in terms of explaining the details of observed movement.
We have recently reviewed this literature [12] and will not repeat the review
here. Instead we will briefly summarize existing optimal control models from
a methodological perspective, and then list some research directions which we
consider promising.

   Most optimality models of biological movement assume deterministic dynamics and impose state constraints at different points in time. These constraints can, for example, specify the initial and final posture of the body in
one step of locomotion, or the positions of a sequence of targets which the
hand has to pass through. Since the constraints guarantee accurate execution
of the task, there is no need for accuracy-related costs which specify what the
task is. The only cost is a cost rate which specifies the "style" of the movement.
It has been defined as (an approximation to) metabolic energy, or the squared
derivative of acceleration (i.e. jerk), or the squared derivative of joint torque.
The solution method is usually based on the maximum principle. Minimum-
energy models are explicitly formulated as optimal control problems, while
minimum-jerk and minimum-torque-change models are formulated in terms
of trajectory optimization. However, they can be easily transformed into optimal control problems by relating the derivative being minimized to a control
signal.

   Here is an example. Let $q(t)$ be the vector of generalized coordinates (e.g.
joint angles) for an articulated body such as the human arm. Let $\tau(t)$ be the
vector of generalized forces (e.g. joint torques). The equations of motion are

$$\tau = M(q)\ddot{q} + n(q, \dot{q}),$$

where $M(q)$ is the configuration-dependent inertia matrix, and $n(q, \dot{q})$ captures nonlinear interaction forces, gravity, and any external force fields that
depend on position or velocity. Unlike mechanical devices, the musculoskeletal system has order higher than two because the muscle actuators have their
own states. For simplicity assume that the torques τ correspond to the set of
muscle activations, and have dynamics

$$\dot{\tau} = \tfrac{1}{c}(u - \tau),$$

where $u(t)$ is the control signal sent by the nervous system, and c is the muscle
time constant (around 40 msc). The state vector of this system is

$$x = [q; \dot{q}; \tau].$$

We will use the subscript notation $\mathbf{x}_{[1]} = \mathbf{q}$, $\mathbf{x}_{[2]} = \dot{\mathbf{q}}$, $\mathbf{x}_{[3]} = \tau$. The general first-order dynamics $\mathbf{x} = \mathbf{f}(\mathbf{x}, \mathbf{u})$ are given by

$$\dot{\mathbf{x}}_{[1]} = \mathbf{x}_{[2]}$$
$$\dot{\mathbf{x}}_{[2]} = M\left(\mathbf{x}_{[1]}\right)^{-1}\left(\mathbf{x}_{[3]} - \mathbf{n}\left(\mathbf{x}_{[1]}, \mathbf{x}_{[2]}\right)\right)$$
$$\dot{\mathbf{x}}_{[3]} = \tfrac{1}{c}\left(\mathbf{u} - \mathbf{x}_{[3]}\right).$$

Note that these dynamics are affine in the control signal and can be written as

$$\dot{\mathbf{x}} = \mathbf{a}(\mathbf{x}) + B\mathbf{u}.$$

Now we can specify a desired movement time t_f, an initial state $\mathbf{x}_0$, and a final state $\mathbf{x}_f$. We can also specify a cost rate, such as

control energy: $\ell(\mathbf{x}, \mathbf{u}) = \tfrac{1}{2}\|\mathbf{u}\|^2$

torque-change: $\ell(\mathbf{x}, \mathbf{u}) = \tfrac{1}{2}\|\dot{\tau}\|^2 = \tfrac{1}{2c^2}\|\mathbf{u} - \mathbf{x}^{[3]}\|^2$

In both cases the cost is quadratic in $\mathbf{u}$ and the dynamics are affine in $\mathbf{u}$. Therefore the Hamiltonian can be minimized explicitly. Focusing on the minimum-energy model, we have

$$H(\mathbf{x}, \mathbf{u}, \mathbf{p}) = \tfrac{1}{2}\|\mathbf{u}\|^2 + (\mathbf{a}(\mathbf{x}) + B\mathbf{u})^{\mathsf{T}}\mathbf{p}$$
$$\pi(\mathbf{x}, \mathbf{p}) = \arg\min_{\mathbf{u}} H(\mathbf{x}, \mathbf{u}, \mathbf{p}) = -B^{\mathsf{T}}\mathbf{p}.$$

We can now apply the maximum principle, and obtain the ODE

$$\dot{\mathbf{x}} = \mathbf{a}(\mathbf{x}) - BB^{\mathsf{T}}\mathbf{p}$$
$$-\dot{\mathbf{p}} = \mathbf{a}_{\mathbf{x}}(\mathbf{x})^{\mathsf{T}}\mathbf{p}$$

with boundary conditions $\mathbf{x}(0) = \mathbf{x}_0$ and $\mathbf{x}(t_f) = \mathbf{x}_f$. If instead of a terminal constraint we wish to specify a final cost $h(\mathbf{x})$, then the boundary condition $\mathbf{x}(t_f) = \mathbf{x}_f$ is replaced with $\mathbf{p}(t_f) = \mathbf{h}_{\mathbf{x}}(\mathbf{x}(t_f))$. Either way we have as many scalar variables as boundary conditions, and the problem can be solved numerically using an ODE two-point boundary value solver. When a final cost is used the problem can also be solved using iterative LQG approximations.

Some optimal control models have considered stochastic dynamics, and used accuracy costs rather than state constraints to specify the task (state constraints cannot be enforced in a stochastic system). Such models have almost exclusively been formulated within the LQG setting. Control under sensory noise and delays has also been considered; in that case the model involves a sensorimotor loop composed of a Kalman filter and a linear-quadratic regulator. Of particular interest in stochastic models is control-multiplicative noise (also called signal-dependent noise). It is a well-established property of the motor system, and appears to be the reason for speed-accuracy tradeoffs such as Fitts' law. Control-multiplicative noise can be formalized as

$$d\mathbf{x} = (\mathbf{a}(\mathbf{x}) + B\mathbf{u})\, dt + \sigma BD(\mathbf{u})\, d\mathbf{w},$$

where $D(\mathbf{u})$ is a diagonal matrix with the components of $\mathbf{u}$ on its main diagonal. In this system, each component of the control signal is polluted with Gaussian noise whose standard deviation is proportional to that component. The noise covariance is then

$$S = \sigma^2 BD(\mathbf{u})D(\mathbf{u})^\mathsf{T} B^\mathsf{T}.$$

With these definitions, one can verify that

$$\mathrm{tr}(SX) = \sigma^2 \mathrm{tr}\left(D(\mathbf{u})^\mathsf{T} B^\mathsf{T} XBD(\mathbf{u})\right) = \sigma^2 \mathbf{u}^\mathsf{T} B^\mathsf{T} XB\mathbf{u}$$

for any matrix X. Now suppose the cost rate is

$$\ell(\mathbf{x},\mathbf{u}) = \tfrac{1}{2}\mathbf{u}^\mathsf{T} R\mathbf{u} + q(\mathbf{x},t).$$

Then the Hamiltonian for this stochastic optimal control problem is

$$\tfrac{1}{2}\mathbf{u}^\mathsf{T}\left(R + \sigma^2 B^\mathsf{T} v_{\mathbf{xx}}(\mathbf{x},t)B\right)\mathbf{u} + q(\mathbf{x},t) + (\mathbf{a}(\mathbf{x}) + B\mathbf{u})^\mathsf{T} v_{\mathbf{x}}(\mathbf{x},t).$$

If we think of the matrix $v_{\mathbf{xx}}(\mathbf{x},t)$ as a given, the above expression is the Hamiltonian for a deterministic optimal control problem with cost rate in the same form as above, and modified control-energy weighting matrix:

$$\widetilde{R}(\mathbf{x},t) = R + \sigma^2 B^\mathsf{T} v_{\mathbf{xx}}(\mathbf{x},t)B$$

Thus, incorporating control-multiplicative noise in an optimal control problem is equivalent to increasing the control energy cost. The cost increase required to make the two problems equivalent is, of course, impossible to compute without first solving the stochastic problem (since it depends on the unknown optimal value function). Nevertheless this analysis affords some insight into the effects of such noise. Note that in the LQG case v is quadratic, its Hessian $v_{\mathbf{xx}}$ is constant, and so the optimal control law under control-multiplicative noise can be found in closed form.

12.7.1 Promising Research Directions

There are plenty of examples where motor behavior is found to be optimal under a reasonable cost function. Similarly, there are plenty of examples where perceptual judgments are found to be optimal under a reasonable prior. There is little doubt that many additional examples will accumulate over time, and reinforce the principle of optimal sensorimotor processing. But can we expect future developments that are conceptually novel? Here we summarize four underexplored research directions which may lead to such developments.

Motor Learning and Adaptation

Optimal control has been used to model behavior in well-practiced tasks where performance is already stable. But the processes of motor learning and adaptation – which are responsible for reaching stable performance – have rarely been modeled from the viewpoint of optimality. Such modeling should be straight-forward given the numerous iterative algorithms for optimal controller design that exist.

Neural Implementation of Optimal Control Laws

Optimal control modeling has been restricted to the behavioral level of analysis; the control laws used to predict behavior are mathematical functions without an obvious neural implementation. In order to bridge the gap between behavior and single neurons, we will need realistic neural networks trained to mimic the input-output behavior of optimal control laws. Such networks will have to operate in closed loop with a simulated body.

Distributed and Hierarchical Control

Most existing models of movement control are monolithic. In contrast, the motor system is distributed and includes a number of anatomically distinct areas which presumably have distinct computational roles. To address this discrepancy, we have recently developed a hierarchical framework for approximately optimal control. In this framework, a low-level feedback controller transforms the musculoskeletal system into an augmented system for which high-level optimal control laws can be designed more efficiently [13].

Inverse Optimal Control

Optimal control models are presently constructed by guessing the cost function, obtaining the corresponding optimal control law, and comparing its predictions to experimental data. Ideally we would be able to do the opposite: record data, and automatically infer a cost function for which the observed behavior is optimal. There are reasons to believe that most sensible behaviors are optimal with respect to some cost function.

Recommended Further Reading

The mathematical ideas introduced in this chapter are developed in more depth in a number of well-written books. The standard reference on dynamic programming is Bertsekas [3]. Numerical approximations to dynamic programming, with emphasis on discrete state-action spaces, are introduced in Sutton and Barto [10] and formally described in Bertsekas and Tsitsiklis [2]. Discretization schemes for continuous stochastic optimal control problems are developed in Kushner and Dupuis [6]. The classic Bryson and Ho [5] remains one of the best treatments of the maximum principle and its applications (including applications to minimum-energy filters). A classic treatment of optimal estimation is Anderson and Moore [1]. A comprehensive text covering most aspects of continuous optimal control and estimation is Stengel [11]. The advanced subjects of nonsmooth analysis and viscosity solutions are covered in Vinter [14]. The differential-geometric approach to mechanics and control (including optimal control) is developed in Bloch [4]. An intuitive yet rigorous introduction to stochastic calculus can be found in Oksendal [7]. The applications of optimal control theory to biological movement are reviewed in Todorov [12] and also in Pandy [8]. The links to motor neurophysiology are explored in Scott [9]. A hierarchical framework for optimal control is presented in Todorov et al. [13].

Acknowledgments

This work was supported by US National Institutes of Health grant NS-045915, and US National Science Foundation grant ECS-0524761. Thanks to Weiwei Li for proofreading the manuscript.

References

[1]   Anderson B, Moore J (1979) *Optimal Filtering*. Englewood Cliffs, NJ: Prentice Hall.

[2]   Bertsekas D, Tsitsiklis J (1996) *Neuro-dynamic Programming*. Belmont, MA: Athena Scientific.

[3]   Bertsekas D. (2000) *Dynamic Programming and Optimal Control, 2nd edition*. Belmont, MA: Athena Scientific.

[4]   Bloch A (2003) *Nonholonomic Mechanics and Control*. New York: Springer-Verlag.

[5]   Bryson A, Ho Y (1969) *Applied Optimal Control*. Walthman, MA: Blaisdell Publishing.

[6]   Kushner H, Dupuis P (2001) *Numerical Methods for Stochastic Control Problems in Continuous Time, 2nd edition*. New York: Springer-Verlag.

[7]   Oksendal B (1995) *Stochastic Differential Equations, 4th edition*. Berlin: Springer-Verlag.

[8]   Pandy M (2001) Computer modeling and simulation of human movement. *Annual Review of Biomedical Engineering*, 3:245-273.

[9]   Scott S (2004) Optimal feedback control and the neural basis of volitional motor control. *Nature Reviews Neuroscience*, 5:534-546.

[10] Sutton R, Barto A (1998) *Reinforcement Learning: An Introduction*. Cambdrige, MA: MIT Press.

[11] Stengel R (1994) *Optimal Control and Estimation*. New York: Dover.

[12] Todorov E (2004) Optimality principles in sensorimotor control. *Nature Neuroscience*, 7:907-915.

[13] Todorov E, Li W, Pan X (2005) From task parameters to motor synergies: a hierarchical framework for approximately optimal control of redundant manipulators. *Journal of Robotic Systems*, 22:691-719.

[14] Vinter R (2000) *Optimal Control*. Cambdrige, MA: Birkhäuser Boston.

13 Bayesian Statistics and Utility Functions in Sensorimotor Control

Konrad P. Körding and Daniel M. Wolpert

13.1 Introduction

The primary output mechanism of the central nervous system is a signal that causes muscle contractions and ensuing movement. As such the purpose of the CNS is to compute motor commands that will allow us to thrive in an uncertain world. The determination of the appropriate motor command to generate is fundamentally a decision process–at each point in time we must select one particular motor command from all possible motor commands. Each decision we make has consequences in terms of the energy expended in the movement, the accuracy of the movement, or whether food or other rewards are acquired.

Much of economics research has addressed how people make decisions in a world full of uncertainty, risks, and rewards. Within the economics framework methods have been developed both to model the decision processes and to analyze how we actually make decisions.

Here we present how decision theory, the standard framework that is usually applied to the study of decisions in an economic setting, can be applied to the study of movement [35]. The decision-theoretic framework combines a probabilistic Bayesian model of the world with desires or goals of an agent that are formalized by a utility function. Within this framework it is possible to derive how we would expect people to move. It allows a characterization of the preferences we have as well as coherently phrasing the problem we are faced with when deciding how to move.

Decision theory relies on three parts. The first establishes a probabilistic relationship between our actions and the distribution of states we may achieve. The second is to quantify the values of being in each possible future state. Finally, these components can be combined to generate an optimal decision.

13.1.1 Uncertainty

In typical cases of decision-making we have only partial knowledge about the relevant variables. If we are buying a health insurance policy we do not know how healthy we will be in the future. We will, however, have some approximate knowledge about how healthy we are, and the effects of our current actions such as smoking, drinking, or snowboarding on future health. This would allow us to estimate a probability distribution of different levels of health in the future. Even if we do not know exactly how our action will affect the future state of the world we can report a probability distribution: $p\,(outcome|action)$ where $outcome$ is the state of the world (including our body's state) at the end of our choice and action is the course of action that we may choose to take.

We thus have to make such a decision in the presence of uncertainty about the outcomes of our decision. Many economic decisions inherently have this uncertainty property, and consequently economic theory has dealt extensively with the problem of describing decision-making in the presence of uncertainty. Fundamental to this process is the representation of this probabilistic relationship between actions and outcomes. Formalizing the way people make decisions should thus incorporate a description of the probabilistic nature of the knowledge they have. Bayesian statistics is the systematic way of estimating such probabilities. Within the Bayesian framework probabilities are assigned to the degree of belief. Numerous articles summarize the mathematical [7] and philosophical [13] ideas that are behind Bayesian statistics. Moreover, many studies phrase the problem of perception in a Bayesian framework [29, 15, 21]. The main focus of this chapter is on the concepts behind Bayesian decision-making and their application to decisions in human movement.

13.1.2   Utility

Knowledge about the world by itself is not sufficient to define how we should formalize decisions. To describe decision-making economists usually use the concept of a utility function [2, 4], a hypothesized function that increases with increasing desirability of the outcome. Although these concepts arose in economics, utility does not have to be directly related to money. For example, state of health, and even altruistic feelings of having helped others or having punished defectors [10], are assumed to influence utility. Mathematically, utility is defined as the value that we prescribe to each possible outcome of our decisions:

$$Utility = U\,(outcome) \tag{13.1}$$

Utility may have a complex relationship to quantity of rewarding stimuli. For example, if we invest well and double our money, we are now twice as well off with respect to the money we own but our utility may not increase by a factor of two as it may tend to saturate as our wealth increases. This effect is described in the framework of prospect theory [27]. While various deviations have been found that show that people do not seem to perform statistically optimally, the assumption of optimality can still typically explain much of the observed behavior. Because utility is such an important concept, different fields refer to the same idea using different names. Motor control often uses loss function as a name for the negative of the utility function. Neuroscience often refers to functions optimized by neurons as an objective function. And within a reinforcement learning framework utilities are often called rewards. Regardless of what they are called, utility functions serve to quantify the relative values of different decision outcomes.

13.1.3   Decision Theory

Decision theory quantifies how people should choose in the context of a given utility function and some partial knowledge of the world. The expected utility is defined as

$$E\left[Utility\right] \equiv \sum_{\substack{possible \\ outcomes,}} p(outcome)U(outcome) \qquad (13.2)$$

where p(*outcome*) is the probability of the outcome and U(outcome) is the utility associated with this outcome. According to decision theory people choose so as to maximize the expected value of utility. Choosing according to this criterion is the definition of choosing rationally. Within the framework of economics, numerous problems have been described in these terms. For example, people's decisions about the ratio of risky to nonrisky assets in their portfolio have been described in terms of people having partial knowledge about their future earnings while maximizing their future utility [19]. Companies' decisions about wages and employment of workers have been modeled in terms of the company having partial information about workers' ability and maximizing profits [16]. Moreover, the decisions of the central bank to increase or decrease interest rates has been modeled in terms of optimally reducing uncertainty about future inflation [3].

Economics tries to understand both how agents should optimally behave when deciding under uncertainty and how they actually behave in such cases. Bayesian decision-making is the systematic way of combining Bayesian estimates of probability with utility functions.

13.2   Motor Decisions

Movement decisions are inherently similar to economic decisions. When people make decisions about how to move, the same complicating factors exist as in other economic decision-making. There is uncertainty about how our actions will affect the future state of the world (in this case mostly our own body) and different movement outcomes will have different utility; movements come with risks and rewards. Both factors need to be considered to choose the best movement.

The sensors of humans are plagued by noise, and likewise our muscles produce noisy outputs. Even if we had perfect sensors they would only tell us about the part of the world that we can currently sense. Uncertainty that stems from noise or the lack of complete knowledge places estimation of attributes of the world and control of our actuators firmly within a statistical framework. In other words, the knowledge about movement outcomes must be described by a probability distribution.

Moreover, just like in economic decision-making, movement decisions also lead to meaningful losses and rewards; the cost of moving our muscles must constantly be weighed against the gains that can be obtained by moving. This means that in the framework of decision theory a utility function should quantify the overall desirability of the outcome of a movement decision. As in economic decision-making people should choose so that they maximize their expected utility. They should take into account both their uncertainty and their utility function to come up with an optimal solution. In the studies described in this chapter we review how human movement performance can be framed in terms of optimally combining probability estimates with utilities. The remainder of this chapter will examine whether people use Bayesian statistics to estimate important variables, how people's utility function is defined, and how people combine probabilities with utilities to choose how to move.

13.2.1   Estimation Using Bayes Rule

In many cases we will need to estimate the values of variables that are important to our movement decisions because our perceptual systems can not provide us with full information. If we want to choose where to run to when playing tennis we will try to run so that we are close to the place where the ball will hit the ground. The closer we are to the place where it will hit the ground, the better. For the moment we thus assume a very simple utility function which is just the mean-squared distance between us and the position where the ball will bounce. To calculate where we should run to we thus need to estimate where we should expect the ball to bounce. Because vision does not provide perfect information about the ball's speed there is uncertainty about where the ball will bounce. If we, however, have played a lot of tennis before, we can have knowledge about where our competitor is likely to play to. We want to combine this knowledge with what we see to obtain an optimal estimate of where the ball will hit the ground.

This example can be abstracted in the following way: The physical properties of the ball define the position x where the ball will hit the ground. The visual system, however, does not perceive where the ball will really hit the ground but rather some noisy version thereof, y. Knowing the uncertainties in the visual system we know how likely it is to perceive the ball being at y if it really is at x. This is called *likelihood* $((p(y|x)))$ and is sketched in red in figure 13.1A. Just based on this knowledge we could ignore any other knowledge we might have and our best estimate would be in the middle of the red cloud, at y. This procedure, however, ignores that we can have prior knowledge about the way our competitor plays. In particular, over the course of many matches the positions where the ball hits the ground will not be uniformly distributed

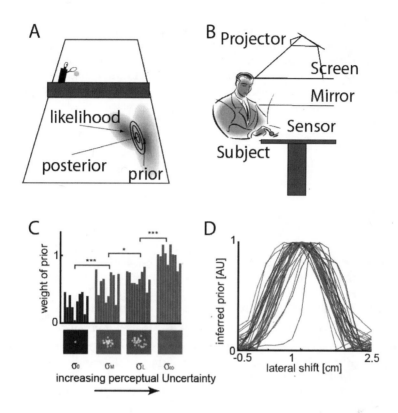

Figure 13.1   (A) Example: The other player is hitting the ball. Seeing the ball, we can estimate that it will land in the red region (with a likelihood proportional to the saturation). We have prior knowledge that the ball is likely to land in the green region (with a probability proportional to the saturation). The black ellipses denote the posterior, the region where the Bayesian estimate would predict the ball to land. (B) The experimental setup. (C) Human subjects' reliance on the prior as a function of increasing perceptual uncertainty. Replotted from Körding and Wolpert [33]). (D) The inferred prior for the different conditions and subjects. The real distribution is shown in red (see color insert).

but highly concentrated within the confines of the court and if our opponent is a good player the distribution may be highly peaked near the boundary lines where it is most difficult to return the ball. This distribution of positions where the ball hits the ground, p(x), is called the prior and could be learned through experience. We can apply Bayes rule to compute the posterior ($p(x|y)$), the probability of the ball bounce location taking into account the prior and the new evidence:

$$p(x|y) = p(y|x)\frac{p(x)}{p(y)}. \tag{13.3}$$

Our uncertainty about its position is thus set in terms of probability. Given our total knowledge, we can assign a probability to each possible bounce location of the ball. If we can assume that the prior distribution $p(x)$ is a symmetric two-dimensional Gaussian with variance σ_p^2 and mean $\hat{\mu}$ and that the likelihood $p(y|x)$ is also a symmetric two dimensional Gaussian with variance σ_V^2 and mean y, it is possible to compute the optimal estimate $(\hat{x})$ as

$$(\hat{x} =)\alpha y + (1-\alpha)\hat{\mu} \; , \tag{13.4}$$

where

$$\alpha = \frac{\sigma_p^2}{\sigma_p^2 + \sigma_V^2} . \tag{13.5}$$

Similar weighing can also be found as the optimal solution to the problem of combining two cues [14]. It is thus possible to define the optimal estimate given new and prior knowledge. It is not only possible to calculate what the optimal strategy is, but one can also calculate how much more precise the estimate is compared to a strategy ignoring prior knowledge: The variance of the estimate if only the visual feedback is used is σ_V^2, if, however, the prior is used, the variance is $\frac{\sigma_p^2}{\sigma_p^2 + \sigma_V^2}\sigma_V^2$, which is always less than the variance of the non-Bayesian estimate. If the prior has the same variance as the likelihood, then the variance of the Bayesian estimate has half the variance of the non-Bayesian estimate. Significant gains in precision are found whenever several sources of information are uncorrelated and have similar degrees of uncertainty.

In a recent experiment [33], we tested whether people use such a Bayesian strategy. The experiments consisted of trials, each of which started with the subject moving the index finger of their right hand to a defined position. They received feedback about the position of their finger in a virtual reality setting. Every time the subject started a new trial the cursor that is meant to indicate the position of the hand was displaced laterally by an amount that was fixed for the duration of the trial (figure 13.1B). The lateral displacement was independently drawn from a Gaussian distribution every trial. This means that the position of the cursor is not where the hand is. However, people are unaware of the fact that the cursor is shifted and assume that the errors they observe during their movement are due to motor errors they are making. The only way subjects get visual feedback is by seeing a representation of the cursor. At the end of the trial, subjects received visual feedback about the quality of their estimate of this lateral displacement. Subjects had to estimate this one-dimensional variable to perform well in the task. For this estimation they could use two sources of information: the distribution of displacements over the course of many trials, as well as what they see during the current trial. The displacement of a cursor relative to the hand in that experiment is thus in close analogy to estimating the position where the ball will bounce.

The experiment allowed a measurement of the subject's estimate of the displacement. Moreover, in the experiment the quality of the visual feedback was varied; in some cases a ball was shown at the position of the cursor giving very precise feedback, whereas in some other trials a large cloud was shown at the position of the cursor, making it much less precise to estimate where the cursor is (see figure 13.1C). The Bayesian estimation process defines how important the prior should be via the weighing α. It predicts that with decreasing quality of the feedback people should increasingly rely on the prior. This implies that with increasing uncertainty of their visual feedback they should use a larger weight of the prior compared to the weight of the visual feedback. Figure 13.1C shows that this strategy, which is predicted by Bayesian statistics, is indeed observed for the human subjects. Out of these data it is furthermore possible to infer the prior that people are using. If they ignore the prior information the prior should be flat. The data shown in figure 13.1D (blue) show that people used a prior that was very close to the optimal one (shown in red). This experiment thus showed that people can use Bayes rule to estimate the state of a variable.

As Bayesian statistics is such a powerful and versatile concept, we should expect people to resort to the use of Bayesian statistics in a large range of circumstances. Using very similar methods to the experiment described above it has been shown that people equally use a Bayesian strategy when they estimate a force [32]. Using a prior in a Bayesian way, however, is not only restricted to producing forces and movements. Some recent research used the same general framework to address information processing used in a timing task [37]. People see three LEDs, one activated after the other, and have to press a button at the time of seeing the third LED light up. The interval between the first two stimuli is identical to the interval between the second and third stimuli. To be able to press a button at the time of the third stimulus it is necessary to estimate the interval between the first two stimuli. The interval between the stimuli is drawn from a fixed Gaussian distribution each trial. Perception does not supply us with perfect knowledge about the timing of events, making it necessary to estimate the time interval between the events. In the timing domain it has also been shown that people's behavior is well predicted by the assumption that they use optimal Bayesian statistics as a strategy.

Bayesian statistics does not only specify how to combine new information, likelihood, and prior knowledge, but just as well how two sources of information should be combined into a joint estimate. Previous experiments have asked this question of how two sources of information are combined. For example, if we feel the size of an object (haptic information) and at the same time see this object we may want to combine the information of both sensors. This is most important if the uncertainty of both modalities is of a similar order of magnitude because then really both sources of information are valuable. A recent experiment thus showed that people use Bayesian methods to combine visual and haptic information by tuning the uncertainty of the visual input so that it roughly matches the uncertainty of the haptic input [9]. Many other phenomena have also been modeled assuming the same combination rules [14, 24, 52, 9, 1, 45]. Bayesian statistics is a general framework that states how people could optimally combine different sources of information into a

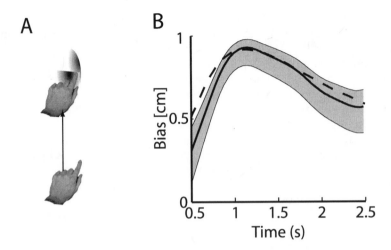

Figure 13.2   (A) Example: The hand is moving in the dark; we want to estimate where it is. The uncertainty about the state of the hand is sketched in red. (B) The error of the human estimates of traveled distance is shown as a function of the duration of the movement. The optimal (assuming overestimated force) Kalman controller predicts the red curve.

joint estimate. Human performance indicates that in many cases they operate very close to this theoretical optimum.

13.2.2   Kalman Controllers: Estimating Time-Varying Signals

In the above examples people did not need to integrate information over time. Either two signals had to be combined or one signal had to be combined with a prior that was assumed to be constant over the course of the experiment. In many cases, however, our estimate of the state of the world will depend on information we obtained about the world at a previous point in time. If we, for example, move our hand in the dark we have uncertainty about its exact position or velocity because our proprioceptive sensors are not perfect (figure 13.2A). To estimate the state of our hand optimally, proprioceptive information from previous time steps needs to be used. All the information that is obtained up to the point in time where the movement decision is made will be important for making an optimal decision. When moving their hand in the dark, people are faced with the problem of estimating the state of the hand, which is characterized by its position and velocity. From experience people know how the state of the hand changes over time. In particular they know that the position changes proportional to its velocity and that the velocity changes proportional to the force applied, although there might be noise in this process. This can be seen as a prior over the kinds of movements people make. Given this information subjects can combine knowledge that they accumulated up to a given point in time with the information gained at that time, the likelihood provided by their sensors to produce a better estimate of their state. In this case they thus constantly have to update their estimate, thus effectively using Bayes rule at every time step.

Assuming that the real state of our hand is x, then the perceived state y will be some noisy version thereof, and let u be the motor command we are sending to our muscles. We know something about the structure of the problem: the state of the hand at time t only depends on the state of the hand at time $t-1$ and the used motor command. This is what is a called Markov property: the state of the hand does not explicitly depend on the state of the hand at any but the preceding time. Using Bayes rule it is possible to obtain

$$p(x_t|x_{t-1}, y_t, u_t) \approx p(x_t|x_{t-1}, u_t)p(y_t|x_t), \tag{13.6}$$

where $p(x_t|x_{t-1}, u_t)$ is the probability of finding oneself in state x_t at time t after having been in state x_{t-1} at time $t-1$ and producing the motor command u_t. People can be expected to have a model for their hand in terms of these variables (called forward model) that they acquired from past experience. Assuming that random variables have n-dimensional Gaussian distributions, it is possible to calculate the optimal estimation strategy in an analytical fashion. The equations are called Kalman controller equations and it is possible to derive the optimal strategy [55] for predicting the state of the hand:

$$\dot{\hat{x}}(t) = \hat{A}\hat{x}(t) + \hat{B}u(t) + K(t)\left[y(t) - \hat{x}(t)\right], \tag{13.7}$$

where$(\hat{x})$is the current optimal estimate, $(\dot{\hat{x}})$ is the change of the optimal estimate, $\hat{A}$ is a matrix that characterizes how the hand moves without perturbation, $\hat{B}$ a matrix that characterizes how forces change the state of the hand, $K(t)$is the Kalman gain which is a function of the other matrices. The Kalman controller is a generalization of the Kalman filter [28] that does not allow a motor signal. Kalman filters are a standard technique used in engineering when the unknown state of a variable is to be tracked over time.

This idea was tested in a psychophysical experiment [55] to address which kinds of algorithms people use when estimating the state of their hand and to verify if people really use Bayesian strategies for motor control. Human volunteers moved their hands in the dark. After each movement they had to estimate where their hand was although the hand was not visible to them. Movements of varying temporal duration were done between 500 ms and 2500 ms. Subjects systematically estimated that their hand had moved farther than it actually had moved (figure 13.2C, gray). An optimal Kalman controller (figure 13.2C, red) produced very similar results if it was assumed that people systematically overestimate their forces. For small times the overestimation of distance increased with time. This was due to the overestimated forces. As times, however, increase, the likelihood becomes more important compared to the prior. The controller becomes more precise if the movement lasts a long period of time because the likelihood becomes more informative and the wrong

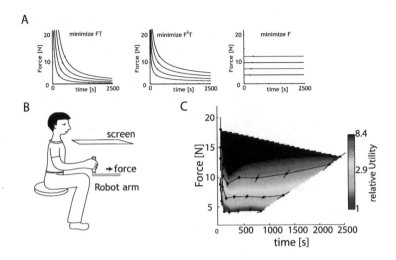

Figure 13.3 (A) Indifference curves in the force time space as predicted by different loss functions. (B) The experimental setup. The subject holds a robotic handle that produces forces that the subject has to hold. (C) The loss can be inferred from the subject's decisions. The hotter the color, the less desirable the force.

prior has a smaller effect. The optimal controller thus shows very similar errors to those made by human subjects. It thus seems that people are able to continuously update their estimates based on information coming in from the sensors in a way predicted by Bayesian statistics.

13.3   Utility: The Cost of Using our Muscles

In some cases, such as the position estimation experiments, people can be expected to move so that they are as precise as possible. It was implicitly assumed that people try and be as precise as possible in the sense of minimizing their mean squared errors. As the hand does not have to produce strong forces and the movements do not need to be very fast, the energy consumption of the muscles and most other parts of the utility function, apart from precision, can be expected to be minimal. In the general case, however, we will expect that costs of movement will have to be considered in addition to the cost of not being as precise as one would like to be and that several factors together define the utility function. Each movement, for example, while shaking hands with a robot (figure 13.3A) will require energy as we have to produce forces. It can be assumed that people will generally prefer less demanding movements – movements that put less strain on the muscles and can be executed using less energy. People are thus faced with the problem of selecting among the huge set of possible movements the one that minimizes their effort or loss and thus maximizes their utility.

A number of different loss functions have been proposed for pointing movements that do not involve producing large forces. It has been proposed that people move so that their movements are as smooth as possible [12]. In this framework it was possible to describe a large range of human movements as the optimal solution of minimizing a suitably chosen function of smoothness. More recently, evidence has been presented that not just a smooth trajectory is chosen but a trajectory that is smooth in the way that allows people to be as precise as possible in their pointing behavior [20]. In all these approaches it is assumed that there exists a utility function, or a loss function which measures how well a movement is performed. In the smoothness definition this function is the average squared third derivative of the position of the hand, the so-called jerk. In the precision case it is simply the variance of the endpoint error.

In the general case, however, we expect the loss function to depend on various parameters of the movement, for example, on the magnitude and the duration that subjects have to hold a force (figure 13.3B). If only the magnitude (F) and the duration (t) of a force are considered important, then the loss will be a function of these two parameters (Loss=f(F, t)). This function, however, is defined in our own head and it is not straightforward to measure it. The economists, however, are often faced with similar problems. Assume people have a fixed amount of money and can only buy apples and bananas, how many of each should they buy? The utility function determines the desirability of outcomes and is just the inverse of the loss.

A tool that is often used to study utility functions is called the indifference curve. An indifference curve is defined by the combinations of apples and bananas that yield the same utility. Elements in a set of combinations of apples and bananas can thus be equally desirable and people have no specific preference for any specific such combination. They could, for example, be equally content with having two bananas and three apples or three apples and two bananas. Measuring such indifference curves can often elucidate properties of the underlying utility function. Such curves can be inferred by asking people for judgments of preference, for example, would you rather have two bananas and three apples or one banana and four apples? A large number of such preference statements allow inferring the indifference curves and the utility function. The same concept can also be used for the study of loss functions in the sensorimotor system.

Various hypothesized utility functions predict different choices and thus different indifference lines. The first model we hypothesized was that subjects would minimize the integrated force they are using (FT). This predicts hyperbolas $F \sim 1/T$ as indifference lines (figure 13.3A, left). People could instead minimize the integrated squared force (F^2T) (figure 13.3A, middle). In this case they would prefer long-duration weak forces to short-duration strong forces of equal integrated force ($F \sim 1/\text{sqrt}(T)$). Another possible model would be that people just try to minimize the maximal force they have to produce, regardless of how long they have to hold it (F) (figure 13.3A, right).

In an experimental setting it was addressed which function of force people seem to be optimizing. Human volunteers had to produce forces of varying magnitude and duration [31, 41]. The experiment paradigm (figure 13.3B) asked subjects to hold hands with a robot that produces forces of different magnitude. The subjects had to counteract the forces of the robot and hold the handle of the robot approximately still. During each trial, the subjects' first experienced one force profile of a given duration and magnitude. They then experienced a second force profile with a different duration and a different magnitude. Finally, they got to decide which force profile to experience again. As they had to actively resist the forces there was an incentive for subjects to choose the less effortful force. From a large number of such comparisons it is possible to infer the indifference lines in the FT space, those lines along which the subjects have no relative preference (figure 13.3C). The indifference curves were surprisingly conserved between subjects. Finally, from these indifference curves it is possible to infer the loss function. For fundamental reasons it is only possible to determine the loss function up to an unknown constant. If, say, the loss function is multiplied by a factor of 2 for all magnitudes and durations, then the predictions with respect to the behavior would be exactly the same.

The loss function (figure 13.3C) for this task is relatively complicated and was different from the predictions made by any of the models we had originally considered. This is in contrast with previous theoretical explorations that have proposed relatively simple utility functions [20]. There is an interesting effect seen in the measured indifference curves; for long durations they actually increase. This means that subjects prefer to, say, hold a force of 10 N for 2 seconds to just holding it for 500 ms. While this is a really puzzling effect it can be explained by the assumption that the loss function is not just a force of maximal force and duration. All force profiles were scaled versions of one another. Therefore, short force profiles had larger transients than long times. When subjects experience long force profiles they can thus slowly ramp up their force, making sure that the robotic manipulandum does not move. If, however, the force profiles are very short, it is hard for subjects to produce a force that is so abrupt. These effects may thus explain the complicated structure of the measured loss function.

Methods from economics, in particular the method of indifference curves, allows measuring loss functions in potentially high dimensions. These techniques can thus be a step toward understanding which loss function people are really optimizing.

13.3.1 Utility: Internal Cost for Distance from Target

During our life we have to combine utility that stems from using our muscles, the cost of moving, with the potential rewards and punishments that come from performing a task of varying quality. When we think about the class of pointing movements there will be the cost of the forces we must generate but also a cost of missing the target. In such experiments the typical instruction is: "Move so that you are as precise as possible." While this is a typical instruc-

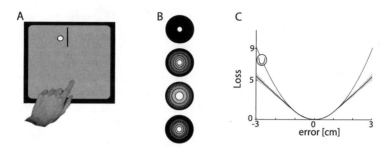

Figure 13.4   (A) Example: White spheres appear on a computer screen, one every 100 ms. Each sphere appears at a position drawn from a fixed probability distribution relative to the position of the hand. For example, the majority of positions might be slightly to the left of the hand while some are far to the right. The errors and their distribution, however, are controlled by a computer program. (B) An important question is how bad an error is compared to another error. Several possible ways how errors can be translated into loss are sketched. Hot colors indicate high loss while cold colors indicate low loss. (C) The loss function inferred in this experiment.

tion, it is not defined what this instruction will actually mean to the subjects. While they will assume that the farther away from the target they are the worse they are, it is not clear how the error they make will translate into the loss of utility. This loss of utility is an internal cost; subjects have a subjective internal valuation of how bad it is to make one kind of an error relative to another. If we are playing darts, then the dart board will assign a score to each of our throws. When we have to point to a position in space (figure 13.4A) we clearly want to point as precisely as possible. Because our sensorimotor system is not perfect we will nevertheless not be perfectly precise in pointing. We are nevertheless sometimes content or annoyed about a movement. Computationally, there must be some way how the brain assigns a loss to each possible movement outcome (figure 13.4B). For example, we could only count the number of hits or misses. Alternatively, the loss function could be linear in the error; an error that is twice as big might be twice as bad. Or people could minimize their mean-squared error and then an error that is twice as big is four times as bad. In other words there must be an "internal dartboard" that assigns a number to each error we are making. An important question is what this internal dartboard looks like and how bad, for example, it is to make an error of 2 cm compared to an error of 1 cm.

When people decide how to move they must combine their estimate of probabilities with the loss function. To measure the loss function in this case a different method from economics is used. In economics often people are given the choice between different probabilistic settings (cf. [26]). For example, "Would you rather have \$10 for sure or \$20 with 60% probability?" This is called the choice between two lotteries: (10,1) and (20,0.6). It is the choice between one probability distribution of outcomes vs. another probability distribution of outcomes. From the way people choose between different such lotteries, a lot can be learned about the way they calculate probabilities and utilities, in particular how they react to risk (e.g. [22]). To measure the loss function that people have with respect to deviations from a target that people aim at the following experiment was used [34]: Many dots like in figure 13.4A appeared on the screen, one after the other. The average position of the dots was determined by the position of the hand of the subject and a random factor. The dots varied around this average position in a way that was not symmetric but skewed. Each position of the hand thus corresponds to a different lottery, where the probability distribution over dot positions is different. From peoples' choices between these lotteries it is possible to infer the loss function, assuming that people use the decision-theoretic solution to maximize their utility.

To choose optimally people must choose the position of their hand x so that the expected utility is maximized or the loss is minimized. As position is a continuous variable, the sum over outcomes for the expected utility becomes an integral:

$$E\left[Utility|x\right] \equiv \int p(pos - x)U(pos)dpos \qquad (13.8)$$

Different loss functions predict different optimal behavior. Analyzing the way people actually moved, it was possible to infer the loss function they were using (figure 13.4C). The loss function is approximately quadratic for small errors and significantly less than quadratic for large errors. Estimation in this task is thus outlier insensitive. Such loss functions are very useful because a couple of outliers do not significantly influence the estimate. Consequently they are often used in artificial techniques, and a field called robust fitting [23] analyzes how such functions could best be built. In general, however, the loss function should be adapted to the kind of task that one wants to perform. While for pointing movements an outlier-insensitive loss function might be the optimal solution, it is not clear what the loss function should be for, say, moving a snowboard. A loss function is nevertheless a necessary factor to allow a system to learn in a world full of uncertainty.

13.3.2 Monetary Rewards

Probably the most salient rewards and punishments in our life are monetary. And most of economics studies how people make decisions in the context of monetary rewards and punishments. Usually experiments asking how people make decisions about monetary rewards are done in a setting where they have a lot of time to deliberate how they want to decide. Most everyday life decisions are done within parts of a second without even explicitly thinking about them [36]. Decisions about movements are almost always of this kind of fast simple decision type. It begs the question of how our movement system can incorporate monetary rewards or punishments for deciding how to move.

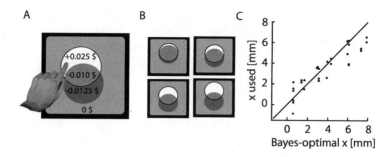

Figure 13.5 (A) Example: People rapidly move their hand to a computer screen to touch circles and gain rewards. The circles are quite small and they have to move so fast that they cannot be certain about their final finger position. (B) The relative position of the reward and punishment areas is varied in the experiment and the position where people touch the screen is recorded. (C) The positions toward which people moved are shown against the positions they should have pointed to assuming the use of Bayesian decision theory. Adapted with permission from (Trommershauser [51].

Taking this kind of an external reward as a substitute of the direct internal loss signal, a recent experiment tested if human subjects are able to use Bayesian decision theory to move [51] so as to maximize their monetary rewards. Subjects had to touch a touchscreen monitor very fast that displayed two circles, one defining a monetary loss, the other one a monetary gain (figure 13.5A). Because subjects had to move very fast there was a lot of variance associated with their movements. The deviations that people made over a set of repeated identical trials had an approximate distribution of a two-dimensional Gaussian with a standard deviation of a couple of millimeters. For this reason it was not possible to always get the reward and never get the punishment. If people aim at the reward they sometimes get the punishment. If people aim at a point that is far enough from the punishment so that they hardly ever get the punishment, then they also would not be getting much reward. The optimal position, according to decision theory, is to aim for a position that results in a large number of rewards and a relatively small number of punishments. In the experiment the position of the circle associated with reward relative to the circle associated with punishment was varied (figure 13.5B). In this experiment it was measured where on average subjects touched the screen. Assuming that people can vary the position they aim at but have no way of varying the noise in their movement, it is possible to mathematically calculate the optimal point where the subjects should hit the touchscreen, assuming that the utility is just the amount of money made:

$$E\left[Utility\right] \equiv \sum_{\text{targets } t} p(\text{hitting target } t | \text{aiming at } x) U (\text{hitting target } x) \quad (13.9)$$

Figure 13.5C shows the position where the screen was actually touched vs. the optimal position according to the theory. Subjects are very close to the optimal solution. This demonstrates that people can use Bayesian decision theory in the context of monetary rewards to move optimally.

13.4 Neurobiology

To make rational decisions in the sense of optimizing expected utility, the nervous system must supply a number of basic functional units. The nervous system must represent probabilities, compute with them, combine them with utility estimates, and must also have a way of learning these general computations. Over recent years an increasing number of studies in neuroscience have asked these basic questions of how the building blocks of optimal decision-making are implemented in the nervous system. Many of these studies are discussed in detail in this book.

The most fundamental question probably is how the brain represents probabilities. To compute probabilistically the nervous system must represent currently available information. It needs to represent its belief about the world, which is the information about the current state of the world obtained up to any given point in time. Toward this aim it needs to constantly combine newly acquired information with prior information obtained over long periods of time. A number of theoretical approaches, as well as experimental recordings, have addressed how a population of neurons can represent probabilities. Various proposals have been made on very different levels of explanation. However, how these sources of information are supplied to the motor system to produce efficient movement remains unclear.

At the level of the brain as a whole it has been proposed [56] that neuromodulators such as acetylcholine (ACh) and norepinephrine (NE) encode the general state of uncertainty of the animal: ACh should represent expected uncertainty (i.e. I expect uncertainty when I throw dice) while NE represents unexpected uncertainty (i.e. I will be very surprised if all of a sudden my car starts to fly). By supplying this information to all of the cortex it should be possible to tune a Bayesian inference algorithm.

At the level of single neurons there is more experimental evidence and it has been shown in recordings from the lateral intraparietal area that some neurons modulate their firing rate relative to the probability of a saccade ending within the receptive field of a neuron [42] and even represent how probabilities change over time [25]. Similarly, it has been shown that even neurons in the early visual system [46] seem to encode the probability of saccades. More importantly, neurons in the dopaminergic system, which is responsible for reward encoding, also show such firing behavior [11]. In summary, the way the brain represents external stimuli does seem to encode probabilities of events. How such probability estimates emerge from a combination of sensory inputs and prior knowledge remains to be elucidated in future research. The motion-processing pathway, including area V5/MT, might be a good candidate to find out how prior and likelihood are combined. In that system it is known that a prior that favors low velocities is combined with likelihood stemming from visual perception. The prior for velocities is well characterized [47] and at the same time the electrophysiology is well advanced to the point where decisions can be analyzed [17] and influenced using current injections [6, 39]. We can hope that such simple well characterized systems will allow a first look at the way the brain combines prior with new evidence.

A second fundamental question is how the nervous system represents rewards and expected rewards. Some recent findings show that neurons in the brain of monkeys do represent the values of expected rewards [44]. Some recent fMRI results show that the nervous system of humans also represents expected reward [30]. The brain thus clearly has ways of representing the expected rewards. Newer research even shows how high-level rewards are represented. For example, a recent study showed how having punished a person who has not collaborated with us leads to brain activation similar to having received a monetary reward [8]. To learn to use a strategy that maximizes expected monetary reward, the brain will have to use a learning algorithm. Reinforcement learning is the framework in which such decision learning problems are usually phrased. A recent study showed that the outputs of some dopaminergic neurons actually represent the change of the expected reward [40]. Such a signal is a necessary component of most reinforcement learning algorithms. It is an important question if utility functions for movements that contain loss terms deriving from energy expenditure or weak precision are represented the same way as utility signals in other modalities.

Finally, the nervous system must combine probabilities with utilities to come up with a decision about how to move. Unfortunately, little is known about how the nervous system makes decisions. Some research indicates how information is combined over time to make a decision in the presence of uncertainty [17] and how values in simple situations may be computed [48]. While there are some studies that address this fascinating question, we are still far from understanding how the nervous system solves this problem. Moreover, whether the decision-making process for high-level cognitive questions is the same as the process used for making decisions about movements remains to be seen. Some early evidence suggests that it indeed is a different process [36] and that we behave optimally in the sense of decision theory in the case of the kinds of movement decisions that we do on a regular basis.

However, while there is some evidence that the nervous system possesses the necessary ingredients to make decisions as predicted by decision theory, it remains to be shown how the nervous system solves these tasks. It is still unclear at the moment how probabilities are encoded in the nervous system. Other chapters within this book analyze in detail which kinds of codes could be used to encode for the probability of events and signals. It is also unclear how probability is combined with estimates of utility and how the decision process works. While much research has been ignoring the fact that the only task of the nervous system is to make decisions, there is a surge of studies now moving in the direction of understanding the ingredients of decision-making. We can expect this to shed light on the way people decide how to move.

13.5   Discussion

The inference problems that are discussed in this chapter are all of a simple nature: we essentially want to find out about a one-dimensional variable and the choice made is itself described by a one-dimensional variable. In the case of movements we, however, make decisions about a sequence of motor commands, the trajectory, that can be very complicated. Nevertheless, optimal control approaches allow in many cases accurate prediction of human movement from a decision-theoretic perspective [20, 50]. However, many of our movements are in the context of complicated tasks such as social interaction. In such cases, coming up with a good Bayesian model can be arbitrarily complicated as it involves a Bayesian inference about the state of the world, including the mental state of other people. From the movements of other people we can start inferring their internal state. While this is theoretically possible [54] it will ultimately involve inferring the utility functions of others, which is a computationally hard problem [38]. While it is not very hard to formulate a generative model it has not been possible to get anywhere close to the abilities of people to solve such problems. However, novel Bayesian approaches are beginning to be able to describe how people make causal inference, how they find out that something causes something else, a skill that people are particularly good at [49, 5, 43, 18, 53]. In general, Bayesian inference from complicated generative models that are good at describing the world is proving prohibitively hard from a computational perspective. Quite possibly, the brain is using efficient approximations to the general problem that allow it to perform that well.

Beyond those algorithmic problems it is also important to consider possible constraints and biases in making inferences that are imposed by the brain. The brain is the substrate that is being used to support us doing Bayesian inference. The way the brain is built, acquired through the course of evolution, will already supply us with some knowledge about what kind of a world to expect; it will thus already define what class of generative models can be implemented and moreover what kind of inference algorithms the brain will have to use.

While there are an increasing number of studies that analyze how human behavior can be understood in terms of Bayesian decision theory, it is important to look for studies that report deviations from the Bayesian solution. The finding that the brain gives us the statistically best solution to a problem does not very much constrain the kind of algorithm the brain uses. Any algorithm that does decent learning should in some way converge to the optimal solution. If, however, we find tasks in which people perform very differently from the way they should, then we may get additional insight into the way the nervous system computes. There are already some known problems that seem hard to explain in Bayesian terms and therefore might actually explain us something about the function of the brain. An example is the size-weight illusion in motor control. People perceive objects that have less volume to be heavier than objects with more volume even if the weight is exactly identical. In a Bayesian framework, the opposite should be expected. If an object has more volume it is a priori more likely that it will be heavy. People should thus, if anything, estimate objects with a large volume as being heavier. While some such findings point toward deviations from the brain being perfectly Bayesian we can look forward to understanding more about the brain by looking at its deviations from being optimal in a decision-theoretic framework.

In conclusion, Bayesian decision theory predicts many of the properties of the movement system and is a coherent framework in which to think about movement decisions. How the brain solves the underlying inference problems and how it represents its information is an important question for further research.

References

[1] Alais D, Burr D (2004) The ventriloquist effect results from near-optimal bimodal integration. *Current Biology*, 14:257-62.

[2] Bentham J (1780) *An Introduction to the Principles of Morals and Legislation*. Oxford: Clarendon Press.

[3] Bernanke BS, Woodford M. (1997) Dynamic effects of monetary policy. *Journal of Money, Credit and Banking*, 29: 653-84.

[4] Bernoulli D (1738) Specimen theoriae novae de mensura sortis. *Comentarii academiae scientarium imperialis Petropolitanae (for 1730 and 1731)*, 5: 175-92.

[5] Buehner MJ, Cheng PW, Clifford D (2003) From covariation to causation: a test of the assumption of causal power. *Journal of Experimental Psychology: Learning, Memory, and Cognition*, 29:1119-40.

[6] Celebrini S, Newsome WT (1995) Microstimulation of extrastriate area MST influences performance on a direction discrimination task. *Journal of Neurophysiology*, 73: 437-48.

[7] Cox RT (1946) Probability, frequency and reasonable expectation,. *American Journal of Physics*, 17: 1-13.

[8] de Quervain DJ, Fischbacher U, Treyer V, Schellhammer M, Schnyder U, et al. (2004) The neural basis of altruistic punishment. *Science*, 305: 1254-8.

[9] Ernst MO, Banks MS (2002) Humans integrate visual and haptic information in a statistically optimal fashion. *Nature*, 415: 429-33.

[10] Fehr E, Rockenbach B (2004) Human altruism: economic, neural, and evolutionary perspectives. *Current Opinion in Neurobiology*, 14: 784-90.

[11] Fiorillo CD, Tobler PN, Schultz W (2003) Discrete coding of reward probability and uncertainty by dopamine neurons. *Science*, 299: 1898-902.

[12] Flash T, Hogan N (1985) The coordination of arm movements: an experimentally confirmed mathematical model. *Journal of Neuroscience*, 5: 1688-703.

[13] Freedman DA (1995) Some issues in the foundation of statistics. *Foundations of Science*, 1: 19–83.

[14] Ghahramani Z (1995) Computational and psychophysics of sensorimotor integration. Ph.D. thesis, Massachusetts Institute of Technology.

[15] Geisler WS, Kersten D (2002) Illusions, perception and Bayes. *Nature Neuroscience*, 5(6):508-10.

[16] Gibbons R, Katz LF, Lemieux T, Parent D (2005) Comparative advantage, learning, and sectoral wage determination. *Journal of Labor Economics*, 23.

[17] Gold JI, Shadlen MN (2002) Banburismus and the brain: decoding the relationship between sensory stimuli, decisions, and reward. *Neuron*, 36: 299-308.

[18] Griffiths TL, Tenenbaum JB (2005) Structure and strength in causal induction. *Cognitive Psychology*, 51:334?84.

[19] Guiso L, Jappelli T, Terlizzese D (1996) Income risk, borrowing constraints, and portfolio choice. *American Economic Review*, 86: 158-72.

[20] Harris CM, Wolpert DM (1998) Signal-dependent noise determines motor planning. *Nature*, 394: 780-4.

[21] Hartung B, Schrater PR, Bulthoff HH, Kersten D, Franz VH (2005) Is prior knowledge of object geometry used in visually guided reaching? *Journal of Vision*, 5(6):504-14.

[22] Holt CA, Laury SK (2002) Risk aversion and incentive effects. *American Economic Review*, 92: 1644-55.

[23] Huber PJ (1981) *Robust Statistics*. New York: Wiley.

[24] Jacobs RA (1999) Optimal integration of texture and motion cues to depth. *Vision Research*, 39:3621-9.

[25] Janssen P, Shadlen MN (2005) A representation of the hazard rate of elapsed time in macaque area LIP. *Nature Neuroscience*, 8: 234-41.

[26] Kagel JH, Roth AE (1995) *The Handbook of Experimental Economics*. Princeton, NJ: Princeton University Press.

[27] Kahneman D, Tversky A (1979) Prospect Theory: An Analysis of Decision Under Risk, *Econometrica*, 47: 263-291.

[28] Kalman RE (1960) A new approach to linear filtering and prediction problems. *Journal of Basic Engineering (ASME)*, 82D: 35-45.

[29] Knill DC, Richards W (1996) *Perception as Bayesian Inference*. Cambridge, UK: Cambridge University Press.

[30] Knutson B, Westdorp A, Kaiser E, Hommer D (2000) fMRI visualization of brain activity during a monetary incentive delay task. *Neuroimage*, 12: 20-7.

[31] Körding KP, Fukunaga I, Howard IS, Ingram JN, Wolpert DM (2004) A neuroeconomics approach to inferring utility functions in sensorimotor control. *PLoS Biology*, 2:e330.

[32] Körding KP, Ku SP, Wolpert DM (2004) Bayesian Integration in force estimation. *Journal of Neurophysiology*, 92(5):3161-5.

[33] Körding KP, Wolpert DM (2004) Bayesian integration in sensorimotor learning. *Nature*, 427: 244-7.

[34] Körding KP, Wolpert DM (2004) The loss function of sensorimotor learning. *Proceedings of the National Academy of Sciences*, 101:9839-42.

[35] Körding KP, Wolpert DM (2006) Bayesian decision theory in sensorimotor control. *Trends in Cognitive Science*, 10(7), 319-26.

[36] Maloney LT, Trommershauser J, Landy MS (2006) Questions without words: a comparison between decision making under risk and movement planning under risk. In W Gray, eds., *Integrated Models of Cognitive Systems*. New York: Oxford University Press.

[37] Miyazaki M, Nozaki D, Nakajima Y (2005) Testing Bayesian models of human coincidence timing. *Journal of Neurophysiology*, 94: 395-9.

[38] Ng AY, Russell S (2000) Algorithms for inverse reinforcement learning. Presented at 17th International Conference on Machine Learning.

[39] Nichols MJ, Newsome WT (2002) Middle temporal visual area microstimulation influences veridical judgments of motion direction. *Journal of Neuroscience*, 22: 9530-40.

[40] O'Doherty J, Dayan P, Schultz J, Deichmann R, Friston K, Dolan RJ (2004) Dissociable roles of ventral and dorsal striatum in instrumental conditioning. *Science*, 304: 452-4.

[41] Pan P, Peshkin MA, Colgate JE, Lynch KM (2005) Static single-arm force generation with kinematic constraints. *Journal of Neurophysiology*, 93(5):2752-65.

[42] Platt ML, Glimcher PW (1999) Neural correlates of decision variables in parietal cortex. *Nature*, 400: 233-8.

[43] Saxe R, Tenenbaum JB, Carey S (2005) Secret agents: inferences about hidden causes by 10- and 12-month-old infants. *Psychological Science*, 16:995-1001.

[44] Schultz W, Tremblay L, Hollerman JR (2000) Reward processing in primate orbitofrontal cortex and basal ganglia. *Cerebral Cortex*, 10: 272-84.

[45] Shams L, Ma WJ, Beierholm U (2005) Sound-induced flash illusion as an optimal percept. *Neuroreport*, 16:1923-7.

[46] Sharma J, Dragoi V, Tenenbaum JB, Miller EK, Sur M (2003) V1 neurons signal acquisition of an internal representation of stimulus location. *Science*, 300: 1758-63.

[47] Stocker A, Simoncelli EP (2005) Constraining a Bayesian model of human visual speed perception. In Saul LK, Weiss Y, Bottou L, eds., *Advances in Neural Information Processing Systems. 17*, pages 1361-1368, Cambridge, MA: MIT Press.

[48] Sugrue LP, Corrado GS, Newsome WT (2004) Matching behavior and the representation of value in the parietal cortex. *Science*, 304: 1782-7.

[49] Tenenbaum JB, Niyogi S (2003) Learning causal laws. Presented at 25th Annual Conference of the Cognitive Science Society.

[50] Todorov E, Jordan MI (2002) Optimal feedback control as a theory of motor coordination. *Nature Neuroscience*, 5: 1226-35.

[51] Trommershauser J, Maloney LT, Landy MS (2003) Statistical decision theory and the selection of rapid, goal-directed movements. *Journal of the Optical Society of America A*, 20: 1419-33.

[52] Van Beers RJ, Sittig AC, Gon JJ (1999) Integration of proprioceptive and visual positioninformation: An experimentally supported model. *Journal of Neurophysiology*, 81:1355?64.

[53] Waldmann MR (2000) Competition among causes but not effects in predictive and diagnostic learning. *Journal of Experimental Psychology: Learning, Memory, and Cognition*, 26:53?76.

[54] Wolpert DM, Doya K, Kawato M (2003) A unifying computational framework for motor control and social interaction. *Philosophical Transactions of the Royal Society London. Series B. Biological Sciences*, 358: 593-602.

[55] Wolpert DM, Ghahramani Z, Jordan MI (1995) An internal model for sensorimotor integration. *Science*, 269: 1880-2.

[56] Yu AJ, Dayan P (2005) Uncertainty, neuromodulation, and attention. *Neuron*, 46: 681-92.

Contributors

Anne K. Churchland   achurchl@cshl.edu
Cold Spring Harbor Laboratory
Cold Spring Harbor, NY, USA

Kenji Doya   doya@oist.jp
Okinawa Institute of Science and Techonlogy
Onna, Okinawa, Japan

Adrienne Fairhall   fairhall@u.washington.edu
University of Washington
Seattle, WA, USA

Karl Friston   k.friston@fil.ion.ucl.ac.uk
Wellcome Department of Imaging Neuroscience
University College London
London, UK

Timothy D. Hanks   tdhanks@u.washington.edu
University of Washington
Seattle, WA, USA

Shin Ishii   ishii@i.kyoto-u.ac.jp
Kyoto University
Koyto, Japan

Roozbeh Kiani   roozbeh@u.washington.edu
University of Washington
Seattle, WA, USA

David C. Knill   knill@cvs.rochester.edu
University of Rochester
Rochester, NY, USA

Konrad P. Körding   konrad@koerding.com
Northwestern University
Chicago, IL, USA

Peter Latham   pel@gatsby.ucl.ac.uk
Gatsby Computational Neuroscience Unit
University College London
London, UK

Tai Sing Lee   tai@cnbc.cmu.edu
Carnegie Mellon University
Pittsburgh, PA, USA

William D. Penny   wpenny@fil.ion.ucl.ac.uk
Wellcome Department of Imaging Neuroscience
University College London
London, UK

Jonathan Pillow   pillow@mail.utexas.edu
University of Texas at Austin
Austin, TX, USA

Alexandre Pouget   alex@bcs.rochester.edu
University of Rochester
Rochester, NY, USA

Rajesh P. N. Rao   rao@cs.washington.edu
University of Washington
Seattle, WA, USA

Barry J. Richmond   bjr@ln.nimh.nih.gov
National Institutes of Health
Bethesda, MD, USA

Michael N. Shadlen   shadlen@u.washington.edu
University of Washington
Seattle, WA, USA

Emanuel Todorov   todorov@cs.washington.edu
University of Washington
Seattle, WA, USA

Matthew C. Wiener   matthew_wiener@merck.com
Merck Research Laboratories
Rahway, NJ, USA

Daniel M. Wolpert   wolpert@eng.cam.ac.uk
University of Cambridge
Cambridge, UK

Tianming Yang   tyang@shadlen.org
University of Washington
Seattle, WA, USA

Alan L. Yuille   yuille@stat.ucla.edu
University of California, Los Angeles
Los Angeles, CA, USA

Richard S. Zemel   zemel@cs.toronto.edu
University of Toronto
Toronto, ON, Canada

Index